BASIC STATISTICS AND PHARMACEUTICAL STATISTICAL APPLICATIONS

Biostatistics: A Series of References Books and Textbooks

Series Editor

Shein-Chung Chow

StatPlus, Inc., Yardley, and
Temple University, Philadelphia, Pennsylvania

1. *Design and Analysis of Animal Studies in Pharmaceutical Development*, edited by Shein-Chung Chow and Jen-pei Liu
2. *Basic Statistics and Pharmaceutical Statistical Applications*, James E. De Muth

ADDITIONAL VOLUMES IN PREPARATION

Basic Statistics and Pharmaceutical Statistical Applications

James E. De Muth

University of Wisconsin–Madison
Madison, Wisconsin

MARCEL DEKKER, INC.   NEW YORK · BASEL

DEKKER

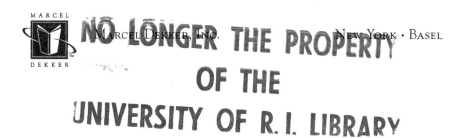

Library of Congress Cataloging-in-Publication Data

De Muth, James E.
   Basic statistics and pharmaceutical statistical applications / James E. De Muth.
      p. cm.-(Biostatistics; 2)
   Includes bibliographical references and index.
   ISBN 0-8247-1967-0 (alk. paper)
     1. Pharmacy-Statistical methods.   2. Statistics.   I. Title   II. Series:
Biostatistics (New York, N. Y.); 2.
   RS57.D46   1999
   615.1'072-dc21   99-30733
                                                             CIP

This book is printed on acid-free paper.

Headquarters
Marcel Dekker, Inc.
270 Madison Avenue, New York, NY 10016
tel: 212-696-9000; fax: 212-685-4540

Eastern Hemisphere Distribution
Marcel Dekker AG
Hutgasse 4, Postfach 812, CH-4001 Basel, Switzerland
tel: 41-61-261-8482; fax: 41-61-261-8896

World Wide Web
http://www.dekker.com

The publisher offers discounts on this book when ordered in bulk quantities. For more information, write to Special Sales/Professional Marketing at the headquarters address above.

Current printing (last digit):
10 9 8 7 6 5 4

PRINTED IN THE UNITED STATES OF AMERICA

To Judy,
Jenny, and Betsy

Series Introduction

The primary objectives of the Biostatistics series are to provide useful reference books for researchers and scientists in academia, industry, and government, and also to offer textbooks for undergraduate and/or graduate courses in the area of biostatistics. This series gives comprehensive and unified presentations of statistical designs and analyses of important applications in biostatistics, such as those in biopharmaceuticals. A well-balanced summary will be given of current and recently developed statistical methods and interpretations for both statisticians and researchers/scientists with minimal statistical knowledge who are engaged in applied biostatistics. The series is committed to providing easy-to-understand, state-of-the-art references and textbooks. In each volume, statistical concepts and methodologies will be illustrated by real examples.

As indicated in the preface to this book, statistics provide useful methods for analyzing the world around us, to help us make beneficial and useful decisions. Statistics, that support scientific evaluation for addressing research questions are especially helpful for researchers/scientists in the pharmaceutical industry. However, statistics have been ignored, misused, and abused in the past several decades in pharmaceutical research and development. As a result, *good statistics practice* (GSP) is needed to provide a fair and valid statistical/scientific evaluation with certain assurance regarding the uncertainty of the pharmaceutical product under investigation. As indicated by Chow (1), in essence, GSP is the foundation of good pharmaceutical practices including *good laboratory practice* (GLP), *good clinical practice* (GCP) and *current good manufacturing practice* (cGMP). The implementation of GSP is a team project that involves statisticians,

v

pharmaceutical scientists, and regulatory agents as well. The success of GSP depends on mutual communication, confidence, respect, and cooperation among statisticians, pharmaceutical scientists, and regulatory agents. This volume serves as a bridge among statisticians, pharmaceutical scientists, and regulatory agents by providing a good understanding of key statistical concepts.

Shein-Chung Chow

Reference

1. Chow, S.C. (1997). Good statistics practice in the drug development and regulatory approval process. Drug Information Journal, 31, 1157–1166.

Preface

Statistics provides useful methods for analyzing the world, evaluating the findings, and hopefully making beneficial and useful decisions. These various tests provide a methodology for answering questions faced by pharmacists and members of the pharmaceutical industry. Currently, a popular phrase in the profession is "outcome measurements." Statistics provides the only method for summarizing data and making constructive decisions about the observed outcomes and their potential impact. This organized approach to evaluating observed data helps us avoid jumping to conclusions and making choices that may be unwise or even dangerous to individuals served by our profession.

Unfortunately, many individuals fear, or even hate, statistics. Why? There appear to be two major reasons for this disposition. The first is the belief that statistics is associated with higher mathematics and therefore difficult to learn. On the contrary, as seen in the following pages, most basic statistical tests involve four-function math ($+$, $-$, $\times$, $\div$), with a few square roots thrown in for good measure. By avoiding "heavy duty" mathematics in this book, even one who struggles with mathematics will benefit and gain confidence using these procedures. The second strike against this area of mathematics is the association of unpleasant past experiences with statistics. In many cases, undergraduate and graduate courses are taught by individuals who are deeply concerned and interested in how statistical formulae work and the rationale behind the manipulation of the data. Unfortunately, they may spend too much time on the derivation of the statistical tests, rather than focusing on practical day-to-day uses for these tools and the successful interpretation of their results.

An example of this perceived fear of statistics appears in the opening sentence of an October 1992 *PC World* announcement of SPSS for Windows software, "Until now, statistics was a course most of us took in college and happily forgot." This also illustrates a related problem, namely that researchers have become increasingly dependent on computers to answer their statistical problems. Computers offer the advantage of speed and accuracy. Unfortunately, without a good understanding of how the tests work and, more importantly, how to interpret their results, the computer outputs (those mysterious p, t, F, Z or χ^2 values) may be useless or misleading if interpreted incorrectly.

The primary goal of this book is to dispel some of the fear and anxiety associated with the basic statistical tests used in the pharmacy profession and to assist individuals using statistical computer software to help them interpret their results correctly.

A greater knowledge of statistics can assist pharmacy students, pharmacists, and individuals working in the pharmaceutical industry in at least three ways:

1. When reading articles in a refereed journal we assume that the material has been thoroughly checked and the information presented is accurate. Unfortunately, reviews of the medical literature have found numerous errors. Studies of various medical journals, discussed in Chapter 20, have found at least one statistical error in 40-75% of all articles reviewed. It is important to be cognizant of possible statistical mistakes when reading the literature.

2. Pharmacists and pharmacy decision-makers are constantly gathering data to improve or justify their professional services. Appropriate manipulation of data can assist in supporting new programs or expanded services. However, we must be careful to use appropriate statistical tests and avoid errors that could eventually come back to haunt us.

3. For pharmacists, the Board of Pharmaceutical Specialties has developed Board Certification for pharmacotherapy with the designation "Board Certified Pharmacotherapy Specialist." Certification requires the candidate to pass a rigorous examination that includes therapeutics, research design, basic data analysis and biostatistics, clinical pharmacokinetics and a knowledge of physical examination findings. In addition, some schools are proposing Board Certification for entry into nontraditional Pharm.D. programs. An increased comfort level with statistical tests can assist with either endeavor.

Purposes

The primary purpose of this book is to serve as an introduction to statistics for undergraduate and graduate students in pharmacy, as well as a reference guide for individuals in various pharmacy settings, including the pharmaceutical industry. It is designed for individuals desiring a brief introduction to the field of statistics, as well as those in need of a quick reference for statistical problem solving. It does not deal with the theoretical basis or derivation of most of the formulae presented; rather, it serves as a quick and practical tool for the application of the most commonly employed statistical tests.

This book represents the tenth revision of an instructional manual originally developed in 1973 to serve as a tutorial aid and reference for graduate students in the pharmacy continuing education program at the University of Wisconsin-Madison. Over the years sections have been added and older ones modified. The manual was primarily intended as a supplement to statistical short courses for individuals in various areas of pharmaceutical development and manufacturing.

Contents

Let us imagine for a moment a heavy object suspended in midair, held in place by a rope. By definition a rope is a flexible line composed of fibers twisted together to give tensile strength to the line. The strength of a rope is based on the interwoven nature of this series of fibers. The individual fibers by themselves can support very little weight, but combined and wrapped with other fibers can form a product capable of supporting a great deal of weight. Statistics can be thought of in similar terms. A very useful and powerful device, a statistical test is based on a number of unique interwoven areas, such as types of variables, random sampling, probability, measures of central tendency, and hypothesis testing. In order to understand how statistical tests work, it's necessary to have a general understanding of how these individual areas (fibers) work together to make the test (rope) a strong and effective procedure. By the same token a poorly knotted rope will eventually weaken and untie. Similarly, poorly designed experiments and/or inappropriate statistical tests will eventually fail, producing erroneous results.

Therefore, the first section of this book, Chapters 1 through 7, will briefly explore some of the basic fibers involved in strengthening this rope we call statistics. The later chapters will focus on: 1) the most commonly used tests; 2) when these tests should be used; 3) conditions that are required for their correct use; and 4) how to properly interpret the results. The incorrect use of statistics (through their inappropriate application) or misinterpretation of the results of the statistical test can be as dangerous as using faulty or biased data to reach the decision. Our statistical rope could quickly fray and the object come crashing to the ground.

The second section, Chapters 8 through 19, presents the various statistical tests commonly found in pharmacy and the pharmaceutical literature. Table 1 presents information identifying the most commonly used statistical tests appearing in the pharmacy literature of the 1970s. This was the result of a survey of 140 issues of the *American Journal of Hospital Pharmacy, Drug Intelligence and Clinical Pharmacy, Hospital Formulary, American Pharmacy*, and *Hospital Pharmacy*. The same authors of this 1978 article presented an unpublished report in 1991 indicating approximately the same frequencies of occurrence. A cursory view of today's literature indicates that these same tests are still commonly used. With the exception of two procedures, all of the tests presented in Table 1 will be discussed in this book as well as many other statistical procedures that may also be useful to the reader. Each chapter includes example problems and their answers. The problems are derived from the areas of pharmacy, analytical chemistry, and clinical drug trials.

The last section includes tables of critical values needed to make appropriate decisions from the statistical tests.

Structure

Designed to serve as both a teaching aid and reference manual, each chapter is divided into two major sections. The first is a description of each statistical test or subject matter. Most statistical tests are discussed briefly with respect to their appropriate use, applications, limitations, and specific mathematical formulae. With each procedure, decision-making models are specified (hypotheses, decision rules, abbreviated tables of critical values, and interpretation of the findings). The second section consists of a series of example problems. The best approach to learning statistics is through examples; thus most statistical tests will have at least one example problem to aid the learner in observing the practical applications of each test and the evaluating the results. The problems in this book try to illustrate practical examples found in a variety of pharmacy settings and contain the full mathematical computations and interpretation of the test results.

Acknowledgements

Many people have contributed directly and indirectly to the completion of this book. A thank you to the participants in short courses for their challenging questions regarding the practical application of statistics to their

Table 1. Most Frequently Used Statistics in the Pharmacy Literature

Statistical term or analytical procedure	Freq.	Statistical term or analytical procedure	Freq.
t-test	81	Yates correction for Chi Square	3
Mean	77	Two-way ANOVA	3
One-way ANOVA	57	Duncan's multiple-range test	3
Chi Square	43	Tukey test	3
Standards Deviation	29	Spearman rank correlation	3
Wilcoxon test	24	Ridit analysis	2
Covariant analysis	18	Sign test	2
Regression	17	Kruskal-Wallis ANOVA	2
Correlation coefficient	15	Median	1
Standard error of the mean	14	Mode	1
Range	13	Path analysis	1
Factor analysis	6	Neuman-Keuls procedure	1
Sequential analysis	5	Method of Cox	1
Fisher exact test	5	Binomial test	1
Ratio	4	Kolmogorov-Smirnov	1
Z score	4	McNemar Test	1
Mann-Whitney U	4	Median Test	1
Kendall's Tau	4	Cochran Q	1

From: Moore, R., et al. (1978). "Statistical background needed to read professional pharmacy journals," American Journal of Pharmaceutical Education 42:251-254.

professional responsibilities. Appreciation is expressed to the undergraduate students, now pharmacists, who reviewed the chapters for readability and understanding and for rechecking the mathematical calculations to insure their accuracy: Megan Margenau, Gina Rottino, and Garret Newkirk. Additional thanks to numerous colleagues in the pharmaceutical industry who provided me with "real life" data to include in example problems, especially Peter Billiaert of Novopharm and Jerry Flesland, formerly with S.C. Johnson.

My gratitude to my academic mentors: Drs. C. Boyd Granberg of Drake University and Melvin H. Weinswig of the University of Wisconsin-Madison. Boyd provided the role model for my professional values and skills, and Mel encouraged my interest in statistics and provided me with the freedom to teach on- and off-campus short courses. Additional thanks to Professor Emeritus Jens Carstensen for allowing me the opportunity to team-teach the industrial short course "Statistics and Stability Prediction," which lead to the development of many other solo short courses for pharmaceutical manufacturers and professional audiences. Special thanks to Dr. Joel R. Levin at the University of Wisconsin-Madison. Joel was the first and finest statistics professor I have had the opportunity to study under. His teaching style made statistics interesting and exciting, and forged my fascination with this mathematical discipline.

Finally, special and loving thanks to my wife Judy and daughters, Jenny and Betsy, for their support, encouragement, and patience with my frequent nocturnal trips to the basement to work on this book.

James E. De Muth

Contents

Symbols

α (alpha)	Type I error, probability used in statistical tables
α_{ew}	experimentwise error rate = $1 - (1-\alpha)^C$
β (beta)	Type II error
$1-\beta$	power
η (eta)	correlation ratio
θ (theta)	equivalence interval
μ (mu)	population mean
μ_0	target mean in control charts
μ_d	mean population difference (matched-pair t test)
$\mu_{\bar{X}}$	mean of the sampling distribution of $\bar{X}$
ν (nu)	degrees of freedom
ρ (rho)	Spearman rank correlation coefficient; population correlation coefficient
σ (sigma)	population standard deviation
σ^2	population variance
$\sigma_{\bar{X}}$	standard deviation of the sampling distribution of $\bar{X}$
ϕ (phi)	phi coefficient (phi)
χ^2	chi square coefficient (chi)
$\chi^2_{corrected}$	Yate's correction for continuity
$\chi^2_{McNemar}$	McNemar test
χ^2_{MH}	Mantel-Haenszel Chi Square test
ψ_i	estimator for Scheffé's procedure (psi)
a	y-intercept, intercept of a sample regression line
b	slope, slope of a sample regression line

c or C	number of columns in a contingency table
cf	cumulative frequency
CI	confidence interval
CV	coefficient of variation
d	difference between pairs of values or ranks
df	degrees of freedom
$\bar{d}$	mean difference
e	2.7183, the base of natural logarithms
E	event or expected frequency with chi square
f	frequency
F	analysis of variance coefficient
FN	false-negative results
FP	false-positive results
H	Kruskal-Wallis test statistic
H_0	null hypothesis
H_1	alternate hypothesis
Log	logarithm to the base 10
M	median
MS_B	mean square between
MS_W	mean square within
n	number of values in a sample
N	number of values in a population, total number of observations
n!	factorial
O	observed frequency with chi square
p	probability, level of significance
$p(E)$	probability of event E
$p(E_1 \text{ and } E_2)$	probability that both events E_1 and E_2 will occur
$p(E_1 \cap E_2)$	probability that both events E_1 and E_2 will occur
$p(E_1 \text{ or } E_2)$	probability that either events E_1 and E_2 will occur
$p(E_1 \cup E_2)$	probability that either events E_1 and E_2 will occur
$p(E_1 \mid E_2)$	probability that event E_1 will occur, given E_2 has occurred
$_nP_x$	permutation notation
Q_1	25th percentile
Q_3	75th percentile
r	correlation coefficient, Pearson's correlation
r or R	number of rows in a contingency table
rf	relative frequency
r^2	coefficient of determination
r_{xy}	reliability coefficient

Symbols

R_1, R_2	sum of ranks for samples of n_1, n_2 in Mann-Whitney U test
R^2	coefficient of multiple determination
RSD	relative standard deviation
S or SD	sample standard deviation
S^2	sample variance or Scheffé's value
S_p^2	pooled variance
S_r	residual standard deviation
SD	sample standard deviation
SEM	standard error of the mean
SIQR	semi-interquartile range
t	t-test statistic
T	Wilcoxon signed rank test statistic
TN	true-negative results
TP	true-positive results
U	Mann-Whitney U test statistic
x	any variable, variable used to predict y in regression model
$\overline{X}$	sample mean
$\overline{X}_G$	grand mean
y	variable used to predict x in regression model
z	z-test statistic

1

Introduction

Statistics can be simply defined as the acquisition of knowledge through the process of observation. We observe information or data about a particular phenomena and from these observations we attempt to increase our understanding of the event which that data represents. Physical reality provides the data for this knowledge and statistical tests provide the tools by which decisions can be made.

Types of Statistics

As noted by Daniel (1978) "...statistics is a field of study concerned with (1) the organization and summarization of data, and (2) the drawing of inferences about a body of data when only a part of the data are observed." All statistical procedures can be divided into two general categories - descriptive or inferential. **Descriptive statistics**, as the name implies, describe data that we collect or observe (**empirical data**). They represent all of the procedures that can be used to organize, summarize, display, and categorize data collected for a certain experiment or event. Examples include: the frequencies and associated percentages; the average or range of outcomes; and pie charts, bar graphs or other visual representations for data. These types of statistics communicate information, they provide organization and summary for data or afford a visual display. Such statistics must be: 1) an accurate representation of the observed outcomes; 2) presented as clear and understandable as possible; and 3) be as efficient and effective as possible.

1

Inferential statistics represent a wide range of procedures that are traditionally thought of as statistical tests (i.e., t-test, analysis of variance or chi square test). These statistics infer or make predictions about a large body of information based on a sample (a small subunit) from that body. It's important to realize that the performance of an inferential statistical test involves more than simple mathematical manipulation. The reason for using these statistical tests is to solve a problem or answer a question. Therefore, inferential statistics actually involves a series of steps: 1) establishing a research question; 2) formulating a hypothesis that will be tested; 3) selecting the most appropriate test based on the type of data collected; 4) selecting the data correctly; 5) collecting the required data or observations; 6) performing the statistical test; and 7) making a decision based on the result of the test. This last step, the decision making, will result in either the rejection of or failure to reject the hypothesis and will ultimately answer the research question posed in the first step of the process. These seven steps will be discussed in more detail at the end of this chapter.

The first sections of this book will deal mainly with descriptive statistics, including presentation modes (Chapter 4) and with data distribution and measures of central tendency (Chapters 5 and 6). These measured characteristics of the observed data have implications for the inferential tests that follow. Chapter 7 on hypothesis testing will give guidance toward the development of statements that will be selected by the decisions reached through the inferential statistics. The information beginning with Chapter 8 covers specific inferential statistical tests that can be used to make decisions about an entire set of data based on the small subset of information selected.

In fact, statistics deal with both the known and unknown. As researchers, we collect data from experiments and then we present these initial findings in concise and accurate compilations (known as descriptive statistics). However, in most cases the data that we collect is only a small portion (a **sample**) of a larger set of information (a **population**) for that we desire information. Through a series of mathematical manipulations the researcher will make certain guesses (unknown, inferential statistics) about this larger population.

Parameters and Statistics

As mentioned, statistical data usually involve a relatively small portion of an entire population, and through numerical manipulation, decisions and interpretations (inferences) are made about that population. To illustrate the use of statistics and some of the terms presented later in this chapter, consider the following example:

A pharmaceutical manufacturing company produces a specific dosage form of a drug in batches (lots) of 50,000 tablets. In other words, one complete production cycle is represented by 50,000 tablets.

Parameters are characteristics of populations. In this particular case the population would be composed of one lot of 50,000 units. To define one of the populations parameters, we could weigh each of the 50,000 tablets and then be able to: 1) calculate the average weight for the entire lot; and 2) determine the range of weights within this one particular batch, by looking at the extreme weights (lightest and heaviest tablets). This would give us the exact weight parameters for the total batch; however, it would be a very time consuming process. An even more extreme situation would be to use a Stokes or Strong-Cobb Hardness Tester to measure the hardness of each tablet. We could then determine the average hardness of the total batch, but in the process we would destroy all 50,000 tables. This is obviously not a good manufacturing procedure.

In most cases, calculating an exact population parameter may be either impractical or impossible (due to required destructive testing as shown in the second example). Therefore, we sample from a given population, perform a statistical analysis of this information, and make a statement (inference) regarding the population. **Statistics** are characteristics of samples, they represent summary measures computed on observed sample values. For the above example, it would be more practical to periodically withdraw 20 tablets during the manufacturing process, then perform weight and hardness tests, and assume these sample statistics are representative of the entire population of 50,000 units.

Continuing with our manufacturing example, assume that we are interested in the average weight for each tablet (the research question). We assume there is some variability, however small, in the weights of the tablets. Using a process described in Chapter 3, we will sample 20 tablets which are representative of the 50,000 tablets in the lot and these will become our best "guess" of the true average weight. These 20 tablets are weighed and their weights are averaged to produce an average sample weight. With some statistical manipulation (discussed in Chapter 6) we can make an educated guess about the actual average weight for the entire population of 50,000 tablets. As explained in Chapter 6, we would create a confidence interval and make a statement such as "with 95% certainty, the true average weight for the tablets in this lot is somewhere between 156.3 and 158.4 milligrams." Statistical inference is the degree of confidence we can place on the accuracy of the measurements to represent the population parameter.

It is important to note (and will be further discussed in Chapter 7) that if we are careful and accurate about our sample collection and summary, then our descriptive statistic should be 100% accurate. However, when we make inferences or statements about a larger population from which we have sampled, because it is an educated guess, we must accept a percentage of chance that this inference may be wrong. Therefore, descriptive statistics can be considered accurate, but inferential statistics are always associated with a certain (hopefully small) chance of error (Figure 1.1).

For consistency in this book, parameters or population values are usually represented by Greek symbols (for example μ, σ, ψ) and sample descriptive statistics are denoted by letters (for example $\overline{X}$, S^2, r).

Samples, which we have noted are only a small subset of a much larger population, are used for nearly all statistical tests. Through the use of formulas these descriptive sample results are manipulated to make predictions (inferences) about the population from which they were sampled.

Sampling and Independent Observations

One of the underlying assumptions for any inferential test is that the data obtained from a population is collected through some random **sampling** process. As discussed in Chapter 3, in a completely random sample, each individual member or observation in the population has an equal chance of being selected for the sample. In the above example, sampling was conducted in such a matter that each of the 50,000 tablets theoretically has an equal chance of being selected.

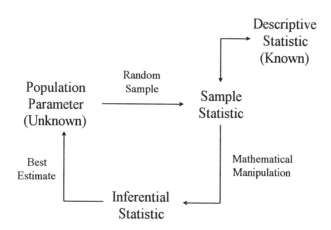

Figure 1.1 Descriptive and inferential statistics.

The second required assumption for any inferential statistical test is that the observations be measured independent of each other. Therefore, no member of the sample should affect the outcome of any other member of the sample. The simplest example of this type of **independence** would be the proctoring of an examination to insure that students do not cheat, thereby assuring independent performance by each person being tested. In the case of laboratory analysis, equipment should be properly cleaned and calibrated, so that the seventh sample assayed is not influenced by the sixth sample and the seventh sample does not affect any remaining assays. In other words, an independent observation or result must represent an outcome not dependent on the result of any other observation, either past or future.

Types of Variables

A variable is any attribute, characteristic or measurable property that can vary from one observation to another. Any observation could have an infinite number of variables, such as height, weight, color or density. For example, consider pharmacy students in a specific graduating class (at the moment each receives their degree) and just a few of the numerous variables that could be associated with each student:

> sex
> height
> weight
> marital status
> class rank
> previous undergraduate degree (yes/no)
> systolic blood pressure
> blood type (A,B,AB,O)
> blood glucose level
> employed/unemployed
> accepted into graduate school (yes/no)
> final examination score in Physical Pharmacy

The number of possible variables is limited only by our imagination. Also, the fact that we can measure a certain characteristic implies that students will differ with respect to that characteristic, and thus becomes a variable. Variables may be either discrete or continuous. The determination of whether a variable is discrete or continuous is critical in selecting the appropriate test required for statistical analysis.

A **discrete variable** is characterized by gaps or interruptions. Variables are also referred to as "qualitative," "category," or "nominal" (from the Latin word nominalis meaning "of a name"). These variables involve placing observations into a specific, finite number of categories or classifications. Examples include distinct colors, dosage form (tablets vs. capsules), and passage or failure of a specific assay criteria. Discrete variables can represent predetermined blocks of data, such as above and below a midpoint in a distribution. With relationship to the population, discrete variables for a sample must be both exhaustive and mutually exclusive. Levels of a discrete variable are **exhaustive** when the categories of that variable account for all possible outcomes. For example, males and females are exhaustive for the population of human beings based on sex; whereas age groups 0-20, 21-40, 41-60, and 61-80 are not exhaustive because there are humans over 80 years old. Similarly, levels of a discrete variable must be set to be **mutually exclusive** where categories do not have members in common with each other. Age groupings 0-20, 20-40, 40-60, and 60-80 are not mutually exclusive because ages 20, 40, and 60 are included in two of the discrete groups. To represent a mutually exclusive and exhaustive set of categories, the age groupings should be as follows: 20 years or less, 21-40 years, 41-60 years, or 61 and older. A second example might be a predetermined dissolution criteria for tablets. In this case the outcomes represented by two mutually exclusive and exhaustive results – either the tablet passes or fails the specified criteria. From the above list of possible variables for pharmacy graduates, discrete variables include:

>sex
>marital status
>previous undergraduate degree (yes/no)
>blood type (A,B,AB,O)
>employed/unemployed
>accepted into graduate school (yes/no)

In contrast, a **continuous variable** has no gaps or interruptions. Also referred to as a "quantitative" variable, they are probably the most commonly encountered variables in pharmacy research. Where discrete variables usually imply some form of counting, continuous variables involve measurements. Examples include age, weight, viscosity, or blood glucose levels. In the case of our pharmacy graduates, continuous variables would include:

>height
>weight
>class rank

systolic blood pressure
blood glucose level
final examination score in Physical Pharmacy

With a discrete variable, outcomes or measures are clearly separated from one another (i.e., males and females). With continuous variables it's possible to imagine more possible values between them. Theoretically, no matter how close two measures are together, a difference could be found if a more accurate instrument were used. Consider age, which is a continuous variable; it can be measured by years, months, days, hours, minutes, seconds or even fractions of a second. Therefore, any measurement result for a continuous variable actually represents a range of possible outcomes and in theory, any value for a continuous variable is considered to occupy a distance or interval from half a unit below to half a unit above the value. These numbers ("real limits") are useful in providing an accurate interpretation of statistical tests using interval or ratio scales, which are discussed below. To illustrate this, assume the most precise analytical balance in a laboratory measures the weight of a sample to be 247 mg. If we could use a more exact balance we might find that the sample actually weighs 247.2 mg. An even more precise instrument could identify the weight in micrograms. Therefore, our original weight of 247 mg. actually represents an infinite range of weights from the real limits 246.5 to 247.5 mg. The major limitation in measuring a continuous variable is the sensitivity of the instrumentation used with that value.

Occasionally, a continuous variable is presented on a **rating scale** or modified into a discrete variable. For example, study results may be: 1) dichotomized into either above or below the midpoint, 2) arbitrarily classified as high, medium or low results, or 3) measured on a continuum which either "passes" or "fails" a predefined level. Even though each of these examples represent the results of a continuous measurement, by placing them *a priori* (before the test) on a rating scale they can be handled as discrete variables.

Parallel nomenclature for measurements of a variable could be in terms of types of scales, with a **scale** implying a set of numbers. As mentioned, discrete variables would involve the simplest type, a **nominal scale**, where observations are qualitatively classified based on a characteristic that was being measured. They differ only in kind and cannot be arranged in any meaningful order (i.e., largest to smallest). Examples of nominal scale measurements would be male vs. female, a tablet vs. a capsule vs. a solution, or survival vs. death.

The second type of measure scale is the **ordinal scale**, in which quantitative observations are related to each other or some predetermined criteria. There is a hierarchy to the levels of the scale with some type of rank order. We are not concerned here with the amount of difference between two observations, but their relative position (for example, if the second observation is less than, equal to or greater than the first observation). Ordinal scales may be used when it is not possible to make more precise measurements. For example, asking patients to rank their pain on a ten-point scale. The numbers are attached simply to show the arranged order, not the magnitude of difference between the various measures. In fact the distance between each consecutive observation becomes equal. Ordinal scales are extremely important in nonparametric statistical procedures (Chapter 17). Both nominal and ordinal scales are sometimes referred to as **non-metric scales**.

The third type of measurement scale is the **interval scale**, where the difference between each level of the scale is equal. The scales represent a quantitative variable with equal difference between scale values, however, ratios between the scale values have no meaning because of an arbitrary zero. For example the ratio between 40°C and 20°C, doesn't imply that the former measure is twice as hot as the second. Other examples include calendar years and interval scales such as Likert scales commonly used in questionnaires and evaluations.

If a genuine zero is within an interval scale it becomes a **ratio scale**; for example, measures of weight or height. If an object weights 500 mg and a second object weights 250 mg, the first object is twice the weight of the second. Other examples of ratio scales would include percentage scales and frequency counts. With interval and ratio scales most arithmetic operations (i.e., addition and subtraction) are permissible with these numbers. Ratio and interval scales are sometimes referred to as **metric scales**.

Independent and Dependent Variables

In addition to a variable being defined as continuous or discrete, it may also be considered independent or dependent. Most statistical tests require at least one **independent variable** that is established in advanced and controlled by the researcher. Also called a **predictor variable**, the independent variable allows us to control some of the research environment. At least one or more **dependent variables** are then measured against their independent counterparts. These **response** or **criterion variables** are beyond our control and dependent on the levels of the independent variable used in the study. Independent variables are usually qualitative (nominal) variables and may be either continuous or discrete. For example, subjects in a clinical trial are assigned to a new drug therapy or control group, their selection is made before the study and this becomes the independent variable (treatment vs. control). The therapeutic outcomes (i.e., decreased blood pressure, pharmacokinetic data, length of hospitalization) are variables dependent on the group to which they were assigned. A second example is a measure of hardness for the core tablet portion of an enteric coated tablet for the same medication, using the same process, at three different manufacturing facilities (New Jersey, England and Puerto Rico). The independent variable is the facility location (a discrete variable with two levels) and the dependent variable would be the average content (amount of active ingredient) of the drug at each facility. Note in the second example that only three facilities are used in the study and samples must come from one of these sites and cannot come from two different locations at the same time; thus representing mutually exclusive and exhaustive observations that fulfill the requirements for a discrete variable. It is assumed that samples were selected appropriately (through some random process, discussed in Chapter 3) and hardness is measured using the same apparatus and the same procedures and conducted in such a manner that each result is independent of any other sample.

In designing any research study, the investigator must control or remove as many variables as possible, measure the outcome of only the dependent variable, and compare these results based on the different levels or categories of the independent variable(s). The extraneous factors that might influence the dependent variable's results are known as **confounding** or **nuisance variables**. In the previous example, using different hardness testers at different sites may produce different results even though the tablets are the same at all three sites.

Selection of the Appropriate Statistical Test

In order to select the correct inferential test procedure, it is essential that as researchers, we understand the variables involved with our data. Which variables are involved for a specific statistical test? Which variable or variables are under the researcher's control (independent) and are not (dependent)? Is the independent variable discrete or continuous? Is the dependent variable continuous or discrete? As seen in Appendix A, answering these questions automatically gives direction toward the correct statistical procedure. All the statistical procedures listed in the flow chart in Appendix A will be discussed in Chapters 8 through 17. To illustrate the use of this Appendix, consider the previous example on clinical trials (measure of therapeutic outcomes based on assignment to the treatment or control group). Starting in the box in the upper left corner of Panel A in Appendix A, the first question would be - is there an independent, researcher-controlled variable? The answer is yes, we assign volunteers to either the experimental or control groups. Therefore, we would proceed down the panel to the next box: is the independent variable continuous or discrete? It is discrete, because we have two nominal levels which are mutually exclusive and exhaustive. Continuing down Panel A, are the results reported as a percentage or proportion? Assuming that our results are length of hospital stay in days, the answer would be no and we again continue down the page to the next decision box. Is the dependent variable continuous or discrete? Obviously number of days is a continuous measure; therefore we proceed to Panel B. The first question in Panel B asks the number of discrete independent variables. In this example there is only one, whether the volunteer received the study drug or control. Moving down Panel B, what is the number of levels (categories) within the independent variable? There are only two, therefore we continue down this panel. The next decision will be explained in Chapter 8, but for the moment we will accept the fact that the data is not paired and moved down once again to the last box on the left side of Panel B. Similarly, for the point of our current discussion we will assume that the population variance is unknown and that our sample is from a population in which the dependent variable is normally distributed and that both levels produce a similar distribution of values (these will be explained in Chapter 6). Thus, we continue to the right and then down to the last point on the right side of the panel and find that the most appropriate inferential statistical test for our clinical trial would be a two-sample t-test.

Procedures for Inferential Statistical Tests

Most individuals envision statistics as a labyrinth of numerical machinations. Thus, they are fearful of exploring the subject. As mentioned in the Preface, the statistics in this book rely primarily on the four basic arithmetic functions and an occasional square root. The effective use of statistics requires more than knowledge of the mathematical required formulas. This is especially true today, when personal computers can quickly analyze sample data. There are several important parts to completing an appropriate statistical test.

1. **Establish a research question.** It is impossible to acquire new knowledge and to conduct research without a clear idea of what you wish to explore. For example, we would like to know if three batches of a specific drug are the same regarding their content uniformity. Simply stated: are these three batches equal?

2. **Formulate a hypothesis.** Although covered in a later chapter, we should formulate a hypothesis that will be either rejected or not rejected based on the results of the statistical test. In this case, the hypothesis which is being tested is that Batch A equals Batch B equals Batch C. The only alternative

to this hypothesis is that the batches are not equal to each other.

3. **Select an appropriate test**. Using information about the data, the dependent and independent variables and the correct test is selected based on whether these variables are discrete or continuous. For example, batches A, B, and C represent an independent variable with three discrete levels and the assay results for the drug's contents is a continuous variable dependent upon the batch from which it was selected. Therefore, the most appropriate statistical test would be one that can handle a continuous dependent variable to a discrete independent variable with three categories. If we once again proceeded through Appendix A we would conclude that the "analysis of variance" test would be most appropriate (assuming normality and homogeneity of variance, terms discussed later in this book). A common mistake is to collect the data first, without consideration of the requirements of the statistical tests, only to realize a that statistical judgement cannot be made because of the arbitrary format of the data.

4. **Sample correctly**. The sample should be randomly selected from each batch (Chapter 3). An appropriate sample size should be selected to provide the most accurate results (Chapter 7).

5. **Collect data**. The collection should insure that each observed result is independent of any other assay.

6. **Perform test**. Only this portion of the statistical process actually involves the number crunching associated with mathematical analysis. Many statistical computer packages are available to save us the tedium of detailed mathematical manipulations.

7. **Make a decision**. Based on the data collected and statistically manipulated from the samples, a statement (inference) is made regarding the entire population from which the sample was drawn. In our example, based on the results of the test statistics, the hypothesis that all three batches are equal (based on content uniformity), is either

rejected or the sample does not provide enough information to reject the hypothesis. As discussed in Chapter 7, the initial hypothesis can be rejected, but never proven true.

To comprehend the principles underlying many of the inferential statistical tests it is necessary that we have a general understanding of probability theory and the role that probability plays in statistical decision making. The next chapter focuses on this particular area.

Reference

Daniel, W.W. (1978). Biostatistics: A Foundation for Analysis in the Health Sciences, John Wiley and Sons, New York, p.1.

Suggested Supplemental Readings

Bolton, S. (1997). Pharmaceutical Statistics: Practical and Clinical Applications, Marcel Dekker, Inc., New York, p.538-541.

Zar, J.H. (1984). Biostatistical Analysis, Prentice Hall, Englewood Cliffs, NJ, pp. 1-4, 14-17.

Example Problems

1. Which of the following selected variables associated with clinical trials of a drug are discrete variables and which are continuous?

    Experimental vs. controls (placebo)
    Dosage form - table/capsule/other
    Bioavailability measurements (C_{max}, T_{max}, AUC)
    Test drug vs. reference standard
    Fed vs. fasted state (before/after meals)
    Prolactin levels (ng/l)
    Manufacturer (generic vs. brand)
    Male vs. female subjects
    Age (in years)
    Smoking history (cigarettes per day)
    "Normal" vs. geriatric population

2. Which of the following selected variables associated with a random sample of 50,000 tablets, mentioned earlier in this chapter, are discrete variables and which are continuous?

    Amount of active ingredient (content uniformity)
    Dissolution test - pass or fail criteria
    Disintegration rate
    Change in manufacturing process - old process vs. new
    Friability - pass or fail criteria
    Hardness
    Impurities - present or absent
    Size - thickness/diameter
    Tablet weight
    Immediate release or sustained release
    Formulation A, B or C

3. The ability to select or identify independent and dependent variables, and determine if these variables are discrete or continuous is critical to statistical testing. In the examples listed below, identify the following:

    Is there an independent variable? Is this variable continuous or discrete? What is the dependent variable? Is this variable continuous or discrete?

    a. During a clinical trial, volunteers were randomly divided into two groups and administered either: 1) the Innovators antipsychotic medication or 2) Acme Chemical generic equivalent of the same drug. Listed below are the results of the trial (C_{max}). Is there any difference between the two manufacturer's drugs based on this one pharmacokinetic property?

        Result of Clinical Trial for C_{max} (ng/ml)

	Innovator	Acme Chemical
Mean	289.7	281.6
S.D.	18.1	20.8
n	24	23

    b. During a cholera outbreak in a war devastated country, records for one hospital were examined for the survival of children contracting the disease. These records also reported the children's nutritional status. Was there a significant relationship between their nutrition and survival rate?

Nutritional Status

	Poor (N$_1$)	Good (N$_2$)
Survived (S$_1$)	72	79
Died (S$_2$)	87	32

c. Samples were taken from a specific batch of drug and randomly divided into two groups of tablets. One group was assayed by the manufacturer's own quality control laboratories. The second group of tablets was sent to a contract laboratory for identical analysis.

Percentage of Labeled Amount of Drug

Manufacturer		Contract Lab	
101.1	98.8	97.5	99.1
100.6	99.0	101.1	98.7
100.8	98.7	97.8	99.5

d. An instrument manufacturer ran of series of tests to compare the pass/fail rate of a new piece of disintegration equipment. Samples were taken from a single batch of uncoated tablets. Two different temperatures were used and tested for compendia recommended times. Success was defined as all six tablets disintegrating in the disintegration equipment.

	Success	Failure	
39°C	96	4	100
35°C	88	12	100
	184	16	200

e. Three physicians were selected for a study to evaluate the length of stay for patients undergoing a major surgical procedure. All these procedures occurred in the same hospital and were without complications. Eight records were randomly selected from patients treated over the past twelve months. Was there a significant difference, by physician, in the length of stay for these surgical patients?

Days in the Hospital

Physician A	Physician B	Physician C
9	10	8
12	6	9
10	7	12
7	10	10
11	11	14
13	9	10
8	9	8
13	11	15

f. Acme Chemical and Dye received from the same raw material supplier three batches of oil from three different production sites. Samples were drawn from drums at each location and compared to determine if the viscosity was the same for each batch.

Batch A	Batch B	Batch C
10.23	10.24	10.25
10.33	10.28	10.20
10.28	10.20	10.21
10.27	10.21	10.18
10.30	10.26	10.22

g. Two different scales were used to measure patient anxiety levels upon admission to a hospital. Method A was an established test instrument, while Method B (which had been developed by the researchers) was quicker and an easier instrument to administer. Was there a correlation between the two measures?

Method A	Method B	Method A	Method B
55	90	52	97
66	117	36	78
46	94	44	84
77	124	55	112
57	105	53	102
59	115	67	112
70	125	72	130
57	97		

Answers to Problems

1. Discrete variables:
Experimental vs. controls (placebo)
Dosage form - table/capsule/other
Test drug vs. reference standard
Fed vs. fasted state (before/after meals)
Manufacturer (generic vs. brand)
Male vs. female subjects
"Normal" vs. geriatric population

Continuous variables:
Bioavailability measurements (C_{max}, T_{max}, AUC)
Prolactin levels (ng/l)
Age (in years)
Smoking history (cigarettes per day)

2. Discrete variables:
Dissolution - pass or fail criteria
Friability - pass or fail criteria
Impurities - present or absent
Change in manufacturing process –
    old process vs. new
Immediate release or sustained release
Formulation A, B or C

Continuous variables:
Amount of active ingredient (content uniformity)
Disintegration rate
Hardness
Size - thickness/diameter
Tablet weight

3. a. Independent variable: Two manufacturers (Innovator vs. Acme)
             Discrete

    Dependent variable: Pharmacokinetic measure (C_{max})
             Continuous

  b. Independent variable: Nutritional status (poor vs. good)
             Discrete

    Dependent variable: Survival (lived vs. died)
             Discrete

  c. Independent variable: Laboratory (manufacturer vs. contract lab)
             Discrete

    Dependent variable: Assay results (% labeled amount of drug)
             Continuous

  d. Independent variable: Temperature (39°C vs. 35°C)
             Discrete

    Dependent variable: Disintegration results (pass vs. fail)
             Discrete

  e. Independent variable: Physician (A vs. B vs. C)
             Discrete

    Dependent variable: Length of stay in hospital (days)
             Continuous

  f. Independent variable: Batch of raw material (batch A vs. B vs. C)
             Discrete

    Dependent variable: Viscosity
             Continuous

   g. Independent variable: Method A (gold standard)
                                           Continuous

       Dependent variable: Method B
                                           Continuous

2

Probability

As mentioned in the previous chapter, statistics involve more than simply the gathering and tabulating of data. Inferential statistics are concerned with the interpretation and evaluation of data and making statements about larger populations. The development of the theories of probability have resulted in an increased scope of statistical applications. Probability can be considered the "essential thread" which runs throughout all statistical inference (Kachigan, 1991).

Classic Probability

Statistical concepts covered in this book are essentially derived from probability theory. Thus, it would be only logical to begin our discussion of statistics by reviewing some of the fundamentals of probability. The **probability** of an event [p(E)] is the likelihood of that occurrence. It is associated with discrete variables. The probability of any event is the number of times or ways an event can occur (m) divided by the total number of possible associated events (N):

$$p(E) = \frac{m}{N} \qquad \text{Eq. 2.1}$$

In other words, probability is the fraction of time that the event will occur, given many opportunities for its occurrence. For example, if we toss a fair coin, there are only two possible outcomes (a head or a tail). The likelihood that one event, for example a tail, is 1/2 or p(T) = 0.5.

$$p(T_{ail}) = \frac{1}{2} = 0.50$$

A synonym for probability is **proportion**. If the decimal point is moved two numbers to the right, the probability can be expressed as a percentage. In the previous example, the proportion of tails is 0.5 or there is a 50% chance of tossing a tail or 50% of the time we would expect a tail to result from a toss of a fair coin.

The **universe** (N), which represents all possible outcomes is also referred to as the **outcome space** or **sample space**. Note that the outcomes forming this sample space are mutually exclusive and exhaustive. The outcomes that fulfill these two requirements are called **simple outcomes**. Other common examples of probabilities can be associated with a normal deck of playing cards. What is the probability of drawing a red card from a deck of playing cards? There are 52 cards in a deck, of which 26 are red; therefore, the probability of drawing a red card is

$$p(R_{ed}) = \frac{26}{52} = \frac{1}{2} = 0.50$$

Note that cards must be red or black, and cannot be both; thus representing mutually exclusive and exhaustive simple outcomes. What is the probability of drawing a queen from the deck? With four queens per deck the probability is

$$p(Q_{ueen}) = \frac{4}{52} = \frac{1}{13} = 0.077$$

Lastly, what is the probability of drawing a diamond from the deck? There are 13 diamonds per deck with an associated probability of

$$p(D_{iamond}) = \frac{13}{52} = \frac{1}{4} = 0.25$$

Does this guarantee that if we draw four cards one will be a diamond? No. Probability is the likelihood of the occurrence of an outcome over the "long run." However, if we draw a card, note its suit, replace the card, and continue to do this 100, 1,000 or 10,000 times we will see the results close to if not equal to 25% diamonds.

There are three general rules regarding all probabilities. The first is that a probability cannot be negative. Even an impossible outcome would have $p(E)$ = 0. Second, the sum of probabilities of all mutually exclusive outcomes for a discrete variable is equal to one. For example, with the tossing of a coin, the probability of a head equals 0.50, the probability of a tail also equals 0.50 and the sum of both outcomes equals 1.0. Thus the probability of an outcome cannot be less than 0 or more than 1.

$$0 \leq p(E) \leq 1$$

A probability equal to zero indicates that it is impossible for that event to occur. In contrast, a probability of 1.0 means that particular event will occur with utter certainty.

At times our primary interest may not be in a single outcome, but with a group of simple outcomes. Such a collection is referred to as a **composite outcome**. Because of the **addition theorem**, the likelihood of two or more mutually exclusive outcomes equals the sum of their individual probabilities.

$$p(E_i \text{ or } E_j) = p(E_i) + p(E_j) \qquad \text{Eq. 2.2}$$

For example, the probability of a composite outcome of drawing a face card (jack, queen or king) would equal the sum of their probabilities.

$$p(Face\ card) = p(King) + p(Queen) + p(Jack) = \frac{1}{13} + \frac{1}{13} + \frac{1}{13} = \frac{3}{13} = 0.231$$

For any outcome E, there is a complementary event ($\overline{E}$), which can be considered "not E." Since either E or $\overline{E}$ must occur, but cannot occur at the same time then $P(E) + P(\overline{E}) = 1$ or written for the complement

$$p(\overline{E}) = 1 - p(E) \qquad \text{Eq. 2.3}$$

The complement is equal to all possible outcomes minus the event under consideration. For example, in one of the previous examples, it was determined that the probability of drawing a queen from a deck of cards is 0.077. The complimentary probability, or the probability of "not a queen" is

$$p(\overline{Q}_{ueen}) = 1 - p(Q_{ueen}) = 1 - 0.077 = 0.923$$

Our deck of cards could be considered a universe or a population of well defined objects. Probabilities can then be visualized using simple schematics as illustrated in Figure 2.1. Figure 2.1-A illustrates the previous example of the likelihood of selecting a queen or a card that is not a queen. Note that the two outcomes are visually mutually exclusive and exhaustive. This type of figure can be helpful when more than one variable is involved.

Probabilities can be either theoretical or empirical. The previous examples with a deck of cards can be considered **theoretical probabilities** because we can base our decision on formal or logical grounds. In contrast, **empirical probabilities** are based on prior experience or observation of prior behavior. For example the likelihood of a 25 year-old female dying of lung cancer can not be based on any formal or logical considerations. Instead, probabilities associated with risk factors and previous mortalities would contribute to such an empirical probability.

A visual method for identifying all of the possible outcomes in a probability exercise is the **tree diagram**. Branches from the tree correspond to the possible results. Figure 2.2 displays the possible outcome from tossing

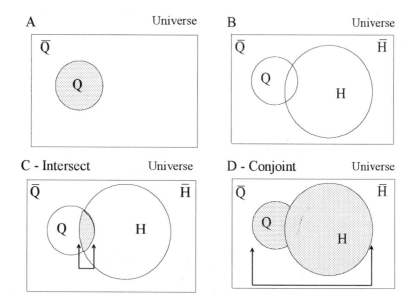

Figure 2.1 Schematics of various probability distributions.

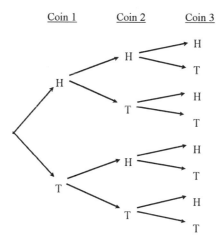

Figure 2.2 Tree diagram of the result of tossing three fair coins.

three fair coins.

Probability Involving Two Variables

In the case of two different variables (i.e., playing card suit and card value), it is necessary to consider the likelihood of both variables occurring, p(A) and p(B), which are not mutually exclusive. A **conjoint** or **union** (A∪B) is used when calculating the probability of either A or B occurring. An **intersect** (A∩B) or **joint probability** is employed when calculating the probability of both A and B occurring at the same time. The probability of an intersect is either given, or in the case of theoretical probabilities, easily determined using the **multiplication theorem**, in which p(A∩B) = p(A) x p(B) if A and B are independent of each other.

$$p(A\ and\ B) = p(A)\ x\ p(B)$$ Eq. 2.4

For example what is the probability of drawing a card which is both a queen and a heart (Figure 2.1-C)?

$$p(\ queen\ and\ heart\ ) = p(\ Q \cap H\ ) = 1\ /\ 52$$

$$p(\ queen\ and\ heart\ ) = p(\ queen\ )xp(\ heart\ ) = 1\ /\ 13\ x\ 1\ /\ 4 = 1\ /\ 52$$

In this case there is obviously only one queen of hearts in a deck of cards. What is the probability of drawing either a queen or a red card. Looking at Figure 2.1-D it is possible to see that using the addition theorem the probability of queen and the probability of a heart could be added together. However, the intersect represents an overlapping of the two probabilities or the p(A or B) equals the sum of the two probabilities minus the probability associated with the intersect.

$$p(A \cup B) = p(A) + p(B) - p(A \cap B) \qquad\qquad \text{Eq. 2.5}$$

Therefore, if we subtract one of the two intercept areas seen in Figure 2.1.C we can compute the conjoint:

$$p(\text{queen or heart}) = p(Q \cup H) = p(Q) + p(H) - p(Q \cap H)$$

$$p(\text{queen or heart}) = 4/52 + 13/52 - 1/52 = 16/52$$

Here there are 13 heart cards and four queens for a total of 17, but one of the queens is also a heart, thus the 16 possible outcomes.

To illustrate these points further, consider the following example using empirical probability data. In a recent randomized national survey on the availability of various types of hardware required to utilize different methods of programming for continuing pharmaceutical education, it was found that out of the 807 respondents: 419 had access to a personal computer capable of downloading external software; 572 had cable television in their homes; and 292 had both personal computers and cable television. Assuming that this sample is representative of pharmacists nationally, what is the probability of selecting a pharmacist at random and finding that this individual has access to a personal computer?

$$p(PC) = \frac{m(PC)}{N} = \frac{419}{807} = 0.519$$

What is the probability of selecting a pharmacist at random and finding that this individual has cable television?

$$p(TV) = \frac{m(TV)}{N} = \frac{572}{807} = 0.709$$

What is the probability of selecting a pharmacist at random and finding that this individual <u>does not</u> have cable television?

$$p(noTV) = \frac{m(noTV)}{N} = \frac{(807 - 572)}{807} = 0.291$$

or considering p(noTV) as a compliment

$$p(noTV) = 1 - p(TV) = 1 - 0.709 = 0.291$$

Note that the sum of all possible outcomes for cable television equals 1.

$$Total \; p(cable \, TV) = p(TV) + p(noTV) = 0.709 + 0.291 = 1.000$$

What is the probability of selecting a pharmacist at random who has both access to a personal computer and cable television?

$$p(PC \cap TV) = \frac{m(PC \cap TV)}{N} = \frac{292}{807} = 0.362$$

Conditional Probability

Many times it is necessary to calculate the probability of an outcome, given that a certain value is already known for a second variable. For example, what is the probability of event A occurring given the fact that only a certain level (or outcome) of a second variable (B) is considered.

$$p(A) \; given \; B = p(A \mid B) = \frac{p(A \cap B)}{p(B)} \qquad \text{Eq. 2.6}$$

For example, what is the probability of drawing a queen from a stack of cards containing all the red cards from a single deck?

$$p(queen \mid heart) = \frac{p(Q \cap H)}{p(H)} = \frac{1/52}{13/52} = 1/13$$

In this example, if all the hearts are removed from a deck of cards, 1/13 is the probability of selecting a queen from the extracted hearts.

Another way to consider the multiplication rule in probability is based on conditional probabilities. The probability of the joint occurrence (A∩B) is equal to the product of the conditional probability of A given B times the probability of B:

$$p(A \cap B) = p(A \mid B)\, p(B) \qquad\qquad \text{Eq. 2.7}$$

From the previous example, if a selected pharmacist has a personal computer, what is the probability that this same individual also has cable television?

$$p(TV \mid PC) = \frac{p(PC \cap TV)}{p(PC)} = \frac{(0.362)}{(0.519)} = 0.697$$

If the selected pharmacist has cable television, what was is the probability that this same individual also has access to a personal computer?

$$p(PC \mid TV) = \frac{p(PC \cap TV)}{p(TV)} = \frac{(0.362)}{(0.709)} = 0.511$$

Conditional probability can be extremely useful in determining if two variables are independent of each other or if some type of interaction occurs. For example, consider the above example of pharmacists with cable television and/or personal computers. The data could be arranged as follows, with those pharmacists having both cable television and personal computers counted in the upper left box.

	Cable TV	No Cable TV
Computer		
No Computer		

Assume for the moment that only 300 pharmacists were involved in the sample and by chance 50% of these pharmacists had personal computers:

	Cable TV	No Cable TV	
Computer			150
No Computer			150
	200	100	300

If there is no relationship between cable TV and personal computer ownership (independence) then we would expect the same proportion of computer owners and those not owning computers to have cable TV service (100 and 100 in each of the left boxes) and the same proportion of individuals not receiving cable:

	Cable TV (A)	No Cable TV ($\overline{A}$)	
Computer (B)	100	50	150
No Computer ($\overline{B}$)	100	50	150
	200	100	300

In this example:

$$p(Cable\,TV \mid Computer) = p(Cable\,TV \mid No\,Computer) = p(Cable\,TV)$$

Thus, p(A∩B) will equal p(A) if the outcomes for A and B are independent of each other. This aspect of conditional probability is extremely important when discussing the Chi Square Test of Independence in Chapter 15.

Probability Distribution

A **discrete random variable** is any discrete variable with levels that have associated probabilities and these associated probabilities can be displayed as a distribution. Many times a graph or table can be used to illustrate the outcomes for these discrete random variables. For example, consider the rolling of two fair dice. There is only one possible way to roll a two: a one (on die 1) and a one (on die 2). Two outcomes could produce a three: a one (on die 1) and a two (on die 2); or a two (on die 1) and a one (on die 2). Table 2.1 represents all the possible outcomes from rolling two dice.

Knowing the frequency of each possible outcome and the total number of possible events (N), it is possible to calculate the probability of any given outcome (Eq. 2.1). If fair dice are used the probability of rolling a two is:

$$p(2) = \frac{1}{36} = 0.0278$$

Whereas the probability of a three is:

$$p(3) = \frac{2}{36} = 0.0556$$

Therefore it is possible to construct a table of probabilities for all outcomes for this given event (rolling two dice). As seen in Table 2.2, the first column represents the outcome, and the second and third columns indicate the associated frequency and probability for each outcome, respectively. The fourth column is the accumulation of probabilities from smallest to largest outcome. For example, the cumulative probability for four or less is the sum of the

Table 2.1 Outcomes Expected from Rolling Two Dice

Outcome	Die 1	Die 2	Freq.	Outcome	Die 1	Die 2	Freq.
2	1	1	1	8	2	6	5
					3	5	
3	1	2	2		4	4	
	2	1			5	3	
					6	2	
4	1	3	3				
	2	2		9	3	6	4
	3	1			4	5	
					5	4	
5	1	4	4		6	3	
	2	3					
	3	2		10	4	6	3
	4	1			5	5	
					6	4	
6	1	5	5				
	2	4		11	5	6	2
	3	3			6	5	
	4	2					
	5	1		12	6	6	1
7	1	6	6				
	2	5					
	3	4			Total possible ways = 36		
	4	3					
	5	2					
	6	1					

Table 2.2 Probability of Outcomes Expected from Rolling Two Dice

Outcome	Frequency	Probability	Cumulative Probability
2	1	0.0278	0.0278
3	2	0.0556	0.0834
4	3	0.0833	0.1667
5	4	0.1111	0.2778
6	5	0.1389	0.4167
7	6	0.1666	0.5833
8	5	0.1389	0.7222
9	4	0.1111	0.8333
10	3	0.0833	0.9166
11	2	0.0556	0.9722
12	1	0.0278	1.0000
$\sum$ =	36	1.0000	

probabilities of one, two, three and four (Eq. 2.2). Obviously the probabilities for any discrete probability distribution when added together should add up to 1.0 (except for rounding errors) since it represents all possible outcomes and serves as a quick check to determine that all possible outcomes have been considered. In order to prepare a probability table, two criteria are necessary: 1) each outcome probability must be equal to or greater than zero and less than or equal to one; and 2) the sum of all the individual probabilities must equal 1.00. Note once again that these are mutually exclusive and exhaustive outcomes. If two dice are rolled on a hard flat surface there are only 11 possible outcomes (3.5, 6.7 or 11.1 are impossible outcomes). Also, two different results cannot occur at the same time.

Many of the founders of probability were extremely interested in games of chance and in some cases were compulsive gamblers (Bernstein, 1996). Therefore, for those readers interested in vacationing or attending conventions in Las Vegas or Atlantic City, Table 2.3 presents a summary of the possible hands one could be dealt during a poker game. Notice these also represent mutually exclusive and exhaustive events. Half the time you will get a hand with nothing, only 7.6% of the time will you receive two pairs or better (1- 0.9238). Note also that we are dealt only one hand at a time. Each hand that is dealt should be independent of the previous hand, assuming we have an

Table 2.3 Probabilities of Various Poker Hands

Possible Hands	Ways to Make	p
Royal flush (Ace through ten, same suit)	4	.000002
Straight flush (five cards in sequence, same suit)	40	.000015
Four of a kind	624	.00024
Full house (three of a kind and a pair)	3,744	.0014
Flush (five cards the same suit)	5,108	.0020
Straight (five cards in sequence)	10,200	.0039
Three of a kind	54,912	.0211
Two pairs	123,552	.0475
One pair	1,098,240	.4226
Nothing	1,302,540	.5012
Totals	2,598,964	.99996

Modified from: Kimble, G.A. (1978). How to Use (and Misuse) Statistics. Prentice-Hall, Englewood Cliffs, NJ, p. 91.

honest dealer and that numerous individual decks are combined to produce the dealer's deck. Therefore, the cards received on the tenth deal should not be influenced by the ninth hand. This fact dispels the **gambler's fallacy** that eventually the cards will improve if one plays long enough. As a parallel, assume that a fair coin is tossed ten times and the results are all heads. The likelihood of this occurring is 0.1%, which we'll prove later. Wouldn't it be wise to call tails on the sixth toss? Not really, if the coin is fair you still have a 50/50 chance of seeing a head on the sixth throw.

Counting Techniques

   With the previous example, it is relatively easy to calculate the number of possible outcomes of rolling two dice. However, larger sets of information become more difficult and time consuming. The use of various counting techniques can assist with these calculations.

   Factorials are used in counting techniques. Written as *n*!, a factorial is the product of all whole numbers from 1 to n.

$$n! = n(n-1)(n-2)(n-3)...(1)$$
Eq. 2.8

For example:

$$8! = 8 \cdot 7 \cdot 6 \cdot 5 \cdot 4 \cdot 3 \cdot 2 \cdot 1 = 40,320$$

Because it is beyond the scope of this book, we will accept by definition that:

$$0! = 1.0$$
Eq. 2.9

Permutations represent the number of possible ways objects can be arranged where *order is important*. For example, how many different orders (arrangements) can be assigned to five sample tablets in a row (tablets A,B,C,D, and E)? First let's consider the possible arrangements if tablet A is selected first (Figure 2.3). Thus, if A is first, there are 24 possible ways to arrange the remaining tablets. Similar results would occur if Tablets B, C, D or E are taken first. The resultant number of permutations being:

$$24 \cdot 5 = 120 \ possible \ arrangements$$

This is identical to a five factorial arrangement:

$$5! = 5 \cdot 4 \cdot 3 \cdot 2 \cdot 1 = 120$$

Thus, when order is important, a permutation for n objects is $n!$.
If the permutation involves less than the total n, a factorial adjustment is easily calculated. In the above example how many possible ways could three of the five tablets be arranged? Once again, let us look at the possibilities if tablet A is selected first (Figure 2.4). In this case, there are 12 possible ways to arrange the tablets when A is assayed first. Thus, the total possible ways to assay 3 out of 5 tablets is:

$$12 \cdot 5 = 60 \ ways$$

An easier way to calculate these permutations is to use the formula:

$$_nP_x = \frac{n!}{(n-x)!}$$
Eq. 2.10

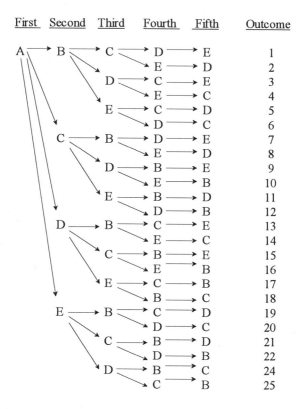

First	Second	Third	Fourth	Fifth	Outcome

Figure 2.3 Possible ways to arrange five tablets with tablet "A" first.

where n is the total number of possible objects and x is the number in the arrangement. In the example cited above, the possible number of arrangements for selecting five tablets, three at a time, is:

$$_5P_3 = \frac{n!}{(n-x)!} = \frac{5!}{2!} = \frac{5x4x3x2x1}{2x1} = 60$$

Combinations are used when the order of the observations is <u>not</u> important. For example, assume we want to assay three of the five tablets described above instead of arranging them in a row. The important feature is which three are selected not the order in which they are chosen. As discussed in the previous chapter, independence is critical to any statistical analysis. Therefore, the order in which they are selected is irrelevant.

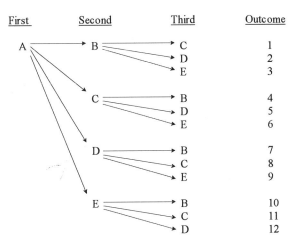

First	Second	Third	Outcome
A	B	C	1
		D	2
		E	3
	C	B	4
		D	5
		E	6
	D	B	7
		C	8
		E	9
	E	B	10
		C	11
		D	12

Figure 2.4 Possible ways to arrange three out of five tablets with tablet "A" first.

In the above example of five sample tablets, the results of the assay of three out of five tablets is the important aspect, not the order in which the tablets were assayed. Orders A-B-C (*1* in Figure 2.4), B-C-A, C-A-B, B-A-C, A-C-B (*4* in Figure 2.4), and C-B-A would yield the same results. Thus the total possible combinations regardless of order is reduced from 60 to only ten possibilities. Using factorials for calculating larger combinations, the formula would be as follows:

$$\binom{n}{x} = \frac{n!}{x!(n-x)!}$$

Eq. 2.11

Once again, n is the total number of possible objects and x is the number of objects selected for the combination. In the example previously cited:

$$\binom{n}{x} = \frac{n!}{x!(n-x)!} = \frac{5!}{3!2!} = \frac{5x4x3x2x1}{(3x2x1)(2x1)} = 10$$

Consider the following example. During the production of a parenteral agent, the manufacturer samples 25 vials per hour for use in various quality control tests. Five of the vials sampled each hour are used for tests of contamination. How many possible ways could these vials be selected for contamination testing for one specific hour?

$$\binom{25}{5} = \frac{25!}{20!\,5!} = \frac{25x24x23x22x21x20!}{5x4x3x2x1x20!} = 53,130$$

In this particular case, the order with which the samples are evaluated is unimportant and therefore produces 53,130 possible sample combinations.

In a second example involving a dose proportionality study, 60 volunteers are randomly assigned to ten groups of six subjects each for the various segments (or legs) of a study. The first group receives the lowest dose, the second group receives the second lowest dose, up to the last group which receives the largest dose. At the last minute the sponsor of the study decides to reduce the maximum dose and will require only the first six segments of the study. How many ways can the assigned groups be selected for this abbreviated study?

$$_6 P_{10} = \frac{10!}{10-6!} = \frac{10x9x8x7x6x5x4!}{4!} = 151,200$$

With the groupings of subjects, order is important since each group will receive progressively larger dosages of the drug. With the order being important, there are 151,200 different way of selecting six of the ten groups of volunteers.

Binomial Distribution

The binomial distribution is one of the most commonly encountered probability distributions. It consists of two mutually exclusive outcomes, sometimes referred to as **Bernoulli Trials**. The simplest example would be a coin toss, where the probability of tossing a head is .50 and a tail is .50. If we toss two fair coins the possible results are displayed in the upper half of Figure 2.5. Note that these probabilities are excellent examples of the multiplication theorem. The first example is an example of two mutually exclusive outcomes (heads on the first coin and heads on the second coin).

$$p(H_1 \cap H_2) = p(H_1)p(H_2) = (0.50)(0.50) = 0.25$$

This is identical to the third possible outcome of zero heads, as seen in Figure 2.5. In the case of one head, we see a conditional probability.

Two Coins

Coin 1	Coin 2		Outcome	Probability
H	H		1/4	0.25 of 2 heads
H	T		1/2	0.50 of 1 head
T	H			
T	T		1/4	0.25 of 0 heads

Three Coins

Coin 1	Coin 2	Coin 3	Outcome	Probability
H	H	H	1/8	0.125 of 3 heads
H	H	T	3/8	0.375 of 2 heads
H	T	H		
T	H	H		
H	T	T	3/8	0.375 of 1 head
T	H	T		
T	T	H		
T	T	T	1/8	0.125 of 0 heads

Figure 2.5   Probability of outcomes from tossing two or three coins.

$$p(H_2 \mid H_1) = \frac{p(H_2 \cap H_1)}{p(H_1)} = \frac{0.25}{0.50} = 0.50$$

The total outcomes for two coins are three combinations and four permutations. If we increase the number of fair coins to three we see the results in the bottom of Figure 2.5, where there are four combinations and eight permutations.

Obviously, the possible combinations and permutations become more difficult to define as the number of coins or observations increase. In 1303 Chu Shih-chieh, a Chinese mathematician created what he called the "precious mirror of the four elements" (Bernstein, 1996, p.64). This later became know as **Pascal's Triangle** and provides a method for calculating outcomes associated with events where the likelihood of success is 50% and failure is 50%. Figure 2.6 illustrates this triangle, the numbers in the upper portion represent frequency counts and the lower half are proportions or probability. With respect to the frequencies, the two numbers in the top line of the bolded triangles are summed to create the third lower point of the triangle. The total of all the frequencies for each row is summed in the far right column. To create the lower triangle in Figure 2.6, each frequency is divided by the sum of frequencies for that row. The result is a matrix that gives the probability of various outcomes (given a 50% chance of success). Notice the second and third rows in the probability matrix are identical to the results reported in Figure 2.5 for two and three coin tosses.

For example, assume we toss a coin six times, what is the probability

Frequency Matrix

$\underline{n}$				1					$\underline{f}$
1				1	1				2
2			**1**	**2**	1				4
3			1	**3**	3	1			8
4		1	4	6	4	1			16
5		1	5	10	10	5	1		32
6	1	6	15	20	**15**	**6**	1		64
7	1	7	21	35	35	**21**	7	1	128

Probability Matrix

$\underline{n}$									$\underline{p}$
1				.5000	.5000				1.00
2			.2500	.5000	.2500				1.00
3			.1250	.3750	.3750	.1250			1.00
4		.0625	.2500	.3750	.2500	.0625			1.00
5		.0313	.1562	.3125	.3125	.1562	.0313		1.00
6	.0156	.0938	.2344	.3125	.2344	.0938	.0156		1.00
7	.0078	.0547	.1641	.2734	.2734	.1641	.0547	.0078	1.00

Figure 2.6 Pascal's triangle.

that we will get two heads? Referring to Figure 2.6, we would go down the sixth row of the probability matrix. The first probability (.0156) is associated with no heads, the second (.0938) is the probability of one head, the third (.2344) for two heads, and so on to last probability (.0156) associated with all six tosses being heads. Thus, if we toss a fair coin six times, we would expect two heads approximately 23% of the time.

Unfortunately Pascal's Triangle works only for dichotomous outcomes which represent a 50/50 chance of occurring (each outcome has a probability of .50). The binomial equation, which follows Pascal's Triangle, is based on the experiments of Jacob Bernoulli in the late 1600s (Bernstein, 1996, p.123). This can be used to calculate the likelihood associated with any number of successful outcomes regardless of the probability associated with that success, providing the probabilities of the independent events are known. The probability for each individual outcome can be calculated using the following formula:

$$p(x) = \binom{n}{x} p^x q^{n-x} \qquad \text{Eq. 2.12}$$

where n is the number of possible outcomes, x is number of successful outcomes, p is probability of success and q is the probability of failure (or not success $1-p$). For example, what is the probability of having 2 heads out of 6 coin tosses?

$$p(x) = \binom{n}{x} p^x q^{n-x} = p(2) = \binom{6}{2} (.5)^2 (.5)^{6-2}$$

$$p(2) = \frac{6!}{2!4!} (.5)^2 (.5)^4 = 15(0.25)(0.0625) = 0.2344$$

Here we produce the exact same results as seen with Pascal's Triangle.

Four conditions must be met in order to calculate a binomial equation: 1) there must be a fixed number of trials (n); 2) each trial can result in only one of two possible outcomes that are defined as a success or failure; 3) the probability of success (p) is constant; and 4) each of the trials produce independent results, unaffected by any previous trial.

Using the binomial equation we can create a probability table to represent the associated probabilities. Again, let us use the example of coin tossing. The possible outcomes for heads based on ten tosses of a fair coin (or tossing ten separate fair coins at one time) would result in the distribution presented in Table 2.4. Using a binomial table it is possible to answer all types

Table 2.4 Possible Results from Tossing a Fair Coin Ten Times

Outcome - f(x) (number of heads)	p(f(x))	Cumulative p(f(x))
0	0.001	0.001
1	0.010	0.011
2	0.044	0.055
3	0.117	0.172
4	0.205	0.377
5	0.246	0.623
6	0.205	0.828
7	0.117	0.945
8	0.044	0.989
9	0.010	0.999
10	0.001	1.000

of probability questions by referring to the individual probabilities or the cumulative probabilities. For example, what is the probability of 1 head in 10 tosses of a fair coin?

$$p(1) = 0.010$$

What is the probability of less than 3 heads in 10 tosses?

$$p(0,1,2) = p(0) + p(1) + p(2) = 0.001 + 0.010 + 0.044 = 0.055$$

or, to read off the cumulative table, $p(<3) = 0.055$. What is the probability of 7 or more heads in 10 tosses?

$$p(7,8,9,10) = 0.117 + 0.044 + 0.010 + 0.001 = 0.172$$

or, to read off the cumulative table for $1 - p(<7) = 1 - 0.828 = 0.172$. What is the probability of 4 to 6 heads in 10 tosses?

$$p(6 \text{ or less}) - p(< 4) = 0.828 - 0.172 = 0.656$$

$$p(4,5,6) = 0.205 + 0.246 + 0.205 = 0.656$$

The binomial distribution can be applied to much of the data that is encountered in pharmacy research. For example:

- LD50 determination (animals live or die after dosing; used to determine the dose which kills 50% of the animals).
- ED50 determination (drug is effective or not effective; used to determine the dose which is effective in 50% of the animals).
- Sampling for defects (in quality control; product is sampled for defects and tablets are acceptable or unacceptable).
- Clinical trials (treatment is successful or not successful).
- Formulation modification (palpability preference for old and new formulation) (Bolton, 1984).

Poisson Distribution

Another discrete probability distribution is the Poisson distribution. As will be discussed in Chapter 6, the binomial distribution tends to be bell-shaped as n increases for any fixed value of p. However, dichotomous outcomes in which one of the two results has a small probability of occurrence, the binomial distribution will more than likely not produce a desired bell-shaped distribution. The Poisson process can be used to calculate probabilities associated with various events when p is relatively small:

$$p(x) = \frac{\mu^x}{x!} e^{(-\mu)} \qquad \text{Eq. 2.13}$$

where e is the constant 2.7183, the base of natural logarithms. In this case the best estimate of μ is np. Therefore the formula can be rewritten:

$$p(x) = \frac{(np)^x}{x!} e^{(-np)} \qquad \text{Eq. 2.14}$$

It can be shown, for every x, that p(x) is equal to or greater than zero and that the sum of all the p(x) equals 1, thus satisfying the requirements for a probability distribution. This produces a slightly more conservative distribution, with larger p-values associated with 0 and smaller numbers of outcomes. Because the two events of the Poisson distribution are mutually exclusive they can be summed similar to our discussion of a probability distribution.

For example, during production of a dosage form, the pharmaceutical company normally expects to have 2% of the tablets in a batch to have less than 95% of the labeled amount of a drug. These are defined as defective. If 20 tablets are randomly sampled from a batch, what is the probability of finding three defective tablets? In this example: p = .02, the probability of a defect; n is 20 for the total sample size and x is 3 for the outcome of interest:

$$p(3) = \frac{[(20)(.02)]^3}{3!} e^{(-0.4)} = (.01)(.6703) = .006758$$

There is less than a 1% likelihood of randomly sampling and finding three defective tablets out of 20. What is the probability of finding one defect:

$$p(1) = \frac{[(20)(.02)]^1}{1!} e^{(-0.4)} = (.4)(.6703) = .2681$$

Listed below is a comparison of the difference between results using the binomial and Poisson processes:

Number of defective tablets	Poisson p(f(x))	Binomial p(f(x))
0	0.6703	0.6676
1	0.2681	0.2725
2	0.0536	0.0528
3	0.0067	0.0065
4	0.0007	0.0005

It is possible to take this one step further and create a binomial distribution table for the probability of defective tablets and criteria for batch acceptance or rejection. Based on a sample of 20 tablets:

Defective tablets	Poisson p(f(x))	Cumulative p(f(x))
0	0.6703	0.6703
1	0.2681	0.9384
2	0.0536	0.9920
3	0.0067	0.9987
4	0.0005	0.9992

Thus, there is a 94% chance of finding one or no defective tablets in 20 samples if there is an expected 2% defect rate. Finding more than one defect is a rare occurrence and can serve as a basis for rejecting a production batch, depending upon the manufacturer's specifications.

References

Bernstein, P.L. (1996). Against the Gods: The Remarkable Story of Risk, John Wiley and Sons, New York.

Bolton, S. (1984). Pharmaceutical Statistics: Practical and Clinical Applications, Marcel Dekker, Inc., New York, p.82.

Kachigan, S.A. (1991). Multivariate Statistical Analysis, 2nd Ed., Radius Press, New York, p. 59.

Suggested Supplemental Readings

Daniel, W.W. (1991). Biostatistics: A Foundation for Analysis in the Health Sciences, John Wiley and Sons, New York, pp. 44-63.

Forthofer, R.N. and Lee, E.S. (1995). Introduction to Biostatistics: A Guide to Design, Analysis and Discovery, Academic Press, San Diego, pp. 93-102, 125-141.

Example Problems

1. A total of 150 healthy females volunteered to take part in a multi-center study of a new urine testing kit to determine pregnancy. One-half of the volunteers were pregnant, in their first trimester. Urinary pHs were recorded and 62 of the volunteers were found to have a urine pH less than 7.0 (acidic) at the time of the study. Thirty-six of these women with acidic urine were also pregnant.

    If one volunteer is selected at random:

    a. What is the probability that the person is pregnant?

    b. What is the probability that the person has urine that is acidic, or less than a pH 7?

c. What is the probability that the person has a urine which is basic or a pH equal to or greater than 7?

d. What is the probability that the person is both pregnant <u>and</u> has urine which is acidic or less than pH 7?

e. What is the probability that the person is either pregnant <u>or</u> has urine which is acidic or less than pH 7?

f. If one volunteer is selected at random from only those women with acidic urinary pHs, what is the probability that the person is also pregnant?

g. If one volunteer is selected at random from only the pregnant women, what is the probability that the person has a urine pH of 7.0 or greater?

2. Three laboratory technicians work in a quality control laboratory with five different pieces of analytical equipment. Each technician is qualified to operate each piece of equipment. How many different ways can the equipment be assigned to each technician?

3. Ten tablets are available for analysis, but because of time restrictions you are only able to sample five tablets. How many possible ways can the tablets be sampled?

4. With early detection, the probability of surviving a certain type of cancer is 0.60. During a mass screening effort eight individuals were diagnosed to have early manifestations of this cancer.

a. What is the probability that all eight patients will survive their cancer?

b. What is the probability that half will die of the cancer?

5. A newly designed shipping containers for ampules was compared to the existing one to determine if the number of broken units could be reduced. One hundred shipping containers of each design (old and new) were subjected to identical rigorous abuse. The containers were evaluated and failures were defined as containers with more than 1% of the ampules broken. A total of 15 failures were observed and 12 of those failures were with the old container. If one container was selected at random:

a. What is the probability that the container will be of the new design?

b.   What is the probability that the container will be a "failure"?

c.   What is the probability that the container will be a "success"?

d.   What is the probability that the container will be both an old container design and a "failure"?

e.   What is the probability that the container will be either of the old design or a "failure"?

f.   If one container is selected at random from only the new containers, what is the probability that the container will be a "failure"?

g.   If one container is selected at random from only the old container design, what is the probability that the container will be a "success"?

6.   An in-service director for Galaxy Drugs is preparing a program for new employees. She has eight topics to cover and they may be covered in any order.

a.   How many different programs is it possible for her to prepare?

b.   At the last minute she finds that she has time for only six topics. How many different programs is it possible for her to present if all are equally important?

If order is important?

If order is not important?

7.   Calculate the following:

a. $\binom{6}{2}$ b. $\binom{9}{5}$ c. $\binom{30}{3}$

Answers to Problems

1. 150 healthy female volunteers in a multi-center study for a new pregnancy test. The probability of randomly selecting one volunteer:

    a. Who is pregnant

    $$p(PG) = \frac{m(PG)}{N} = \frac{75}{150} = 0.500$$

    b. Who has acidic urine

    $$p(pH \downarrow) = \frac{m(pH \downarrow)}{N} = \frac{62}{150} = 0.413$$

    c. Who has non-acidic urine

    $$p(pH \uparrow) = 1 - p(pH \downarrow) = 1 - 0.413 = 0.587$$

    d. Who is both pregnant <u>and</u> has acidic urine

    $$p(PG \cap pH \downarrow) = \frac{m(PG \cap pH \downarrow)}{N} = \frac{36}{150} = 0.240$$

    e. Who is either pregnant <u>or</u> has acidic urine

    $$p(PG \cup pH \downarrow) = p(PG) + p(pH \downarrow) - p(PG \cap pH \downarrow)$$

    $$p(PG \cup pH \downarrow) = 0.500 + 0.413 - 0.240 = 0.673$$

    f. Who is pregnant from those women with acidic urine

    $$p(PG \mid pH \downarrow) = \frac{p(PG \cap pH \downarrow)}{p(pH \downarrow)} = \frac{0.24}{0.413} = 0.581$$

    g. Who has non-acidic urine from those women who are pregnant

$$p(pH \uparrow | PG) = \frac{p(PG \cap pH \uparrow)}{p(PG)} = \frac{0.260}{0.500} = 0.520$$

2. The ways of assigning three laboratory technicians to five pieces of equipment:

$$\binom{n}{x} = \frac{n!}{x!(n-x)!} = \binom{5}{3} = \frac{5!}{3!2!} = \frac{5 \cdot 4 \cdot 3 \cdot 2 \cdot 1}{(3 \cdot 2 \cdot 1)(2 \cdot 1)} = 10$$

3. The possible ways to sample five out of ten tablets:

$$\binom{n}{x} = \frac{n!}{x!(n-x)!} = \binom{10}{5} = \frac{10!}{5!5!} = \frac{10 \cdot 9 \cdot 8 \cdot 7 \cdot 6 \cdot 5!}{(5 \cdot 4 \cdot 3 \cdot 2 \cdot 1)(5!)} = 252$$

4. The outcomes for eight patients where the survival rate is 0.60:

   a. That all eight patients will survive:

$$p(8) = \binom{8}{0}(0.60)^8(0.40)^0 = (1)(0.0168)(1) = 0.017$$

   b. That half will die:

$$p(4) = \binom{8}{4}(0.60)^4(0.40)^4 = (70)(0.1296)(0.0256) = 0.232$$

5. 200 containers of an old and new design were subjected to identical rigorous abuse. The probability of randomly selecting a container:

   a. Of the new design:

$$p(New) = \frac{m(New)}{N} = \frac{100}{200} = 0.500$$

   b. That is a "failure":

$$p(F) = \frac{m(F)}{N} = \frac{15}{200} = 0.075$$

c. That is a "success":

$$p(S) = 1 - p(F) = 1 - 0.075 = 0.925$$

d. That is both an old container design and a "failure":

$$p(Old \cap F) = \frac{m(Old \cap F)}{N} = \frac{12}{200} = 0.060$$

e. That is either an old design or a "failure":

$$p(Old \cup F) = p(Old) + p(F) - p(Old \cap F)$$

$$p(Old \cup F) = 0.500 + 0.075 - 0.060 = 0.515$$

f. That the container is a "failure" if selected from only the new containers:

$$p(F \mid New) = \frac{p(F \cap New)}{p(New)} = \frac{0.015}{0.500} = 0.030$$

g. That the container is a "success" if selected from only the old containers:

$$p(S \mid Old) = \frac{p(S \cap Old)}{p(Old)} = \frac{0.440}{0.500} = 0.880$$

6. An in-service director for Galaxy Drugs prepared a program for new employees. She had eight topics to cover, and they could be covered in any order.

a. How many different programs is it possible for her to prepare?

$$8! = 40,320$$

b. At the last minute she finds that she has time for only six topics. How many different programs is it possible for her to present if all are equally important?

If order is important - a permutation:

$$\frac{8!}{(8-6)!} = \frac{8!}{2!} = 20,160$$

If order is not important – combination:

$$\binom{8}{6} = \frac{8!}{6! \, 2!} = 28$$

7. Calculate the following:

a.

$$\binom{6}{2} = \frac{6!}{2! \, 4!} = \frac{6 \times 5 \times 4!}{2 \times 1 \times 4!} = \frac{30}{2} = 15$$

b.

$$\binom{9}{5} = \frac{9!}{5! \, 4!} = \frac{9 \times 8 \times 7 \times 6 \times 5!}{4 \times 3 \times 2 \times 1 \times 5!} = 126$$

c.

$$\binom{30}{3} = \frac{30!}{3! \, 27!} = \frac{30 \times 29 \times 28 \times 27!}{3 \times 2 \times 1 \times 27!} = 4060$$

3

Sampling

Samples from a population represent the best estimate we have of the true parameters of that population. Two underlining assumptions for all statistical tests are: 1) that the samples are randomly selected and 2) that observations are measured independently of each other. Therefore, insuring that samples are randomly selected from the study population is critical for all statistical procedures. Rees (1989) has defined a random sample as "one for which each measurement in the population has the same chance (probability) of being selected."

Random Sampling

As mentioned in Chapter 1, as researchers we will be interested in identifying characteristics of a population (parameters). In most cases it will not be possible to obtain all the information about that particular characteristic. Instead, a sample will be obtained which will hopefully represent a suitably selected subset of the population. The probability theories presented in Chapter 2, and upon which statistics is based, require randomness.

In order to be a random sample, all elements of the population must have an equal chance (probability) of being included in the sample. In other words, each of the 50,000 tablets coming off a scale-up production line should have an equal likelihood of being selected for analysis. If the manufacturer in the above example sampled tablets only at the beginning or the end of the production run, the results may not be representative of all the tablets. A procedure should be developed to ensure periodic sampling; for example, every 30 minutes during the production run. Randomization may be accomplished for a smaller number of units by using a random numbers table or by numbers generated at random using a calculator or computer. For example, assume that we are in a quality control department and want to analyze a batch of ointments. Samples have been collected during the production run and 250 tubes are available in the quality control department (these tubes are numbered in order from the first sample to the 250th tube). Because of time and expense, we are only able to analyze 10 tubes. The ten samples would be our best guess of the population consisting of 250 ointment tubes.

The best way to select the ten ointment tubes is through the use of a **random numbers table** (Table B1, Appendix B). Random numbers tables, usually generated by computers, are such that each digit (1, 2, 3, etc.) has the probability of occurring (.10) and theoretically each pair of numbers (21, 22, 23, etc.) or triplicate (111, 112, 113, etc.) would have the same probability of occurrence, .01 and .001 respectively. We would begin using a random numbers table by dropping a pencil or pen point on the table to find an arbitrary starting point. To illustrate the use of this table, assume the pencil lands at the beginning of the sixth column, eighth row in our Table B1:

$$23616$$

We have decided **a priori** (before the fact; before the dropping of the pencil point) to select numbers moving to the right of the point. We could have also decided to move to the left, up or down the table. Because we are sampling tubes between 001 and 250, the number would be selected in groupings of three digits.

$$\underline{236}16$$

Thus, the first number would be 236 or the 236th ointment sample would be selected. The next grouping of three digits to the right would include the last two digits of this column and the first digit of the next column to the right.

$$236\underline{16} \quad \underline{4}5170$$

The 164th ointment tube would be the second sample. The third set of three digits (517) exceeds the largest number (250) and would be ignored. Continuing to the right in, groups of three digits, the third sample would be the 78th tube.

$$23616 \quad 4517\underline{0} \quad \underline{78}646$$

To this point the first three samples would be ointment tubes 236, 164 and 078. The next three groupings all exceed 250 and would be ignored.

23616 45170 78<u>646</u> 77552 01582
23616 45170 78646 <u>775</u>52 01582
23616 45170 78646 775<u>52</u> <u>0</u>1582

The next sample that can be selected from this row is 158. The fourth sample is the 158th ointment tube.

23616 45170 78646 77552 0<u>158</u>2

The researcher has decided to continue down the page (the individual could have used the same procedure moving up the page). Therefore, the last digit in the eighth row is combined with the first two digits in the ninth row to create the next sampling possibility.

23616 45170 78646 77552 0158<u>2</u>
<u>11</u>004

With the 211th tube as the fifth sample, the remaining samples are selected moving across the row and ignoring numbers in excess of 250.

11<u>004</u> 06949 40228 95804 06583 10471 83884 27164 50516 89635
11004 0<u>694</u>9 40228 95804 06583 10471 83884 27164 50516 89635
11004 06949 4<u>022</u>8 95804 06583 10471 83884 27164 50516 89635
11004 06949 40228 95804 0<u>658</u>3 10471 83884 27164 50516 89635
11004 06949 40228 95804 06583 1<u>047</u>1 83884 27164 50516 89635

If any of the three digit number combinations had already been selected, it would also be ignored and the researcher would continue to the right until ten numbers were randomly selected. In this particular random sampling example, the ten tubes selected to be analyzed were:

Tubes	
004	078
022	158
047	164
065	211
069	236

Dropping the pencil at another location would have created an entirely different set of numbers. Thus, using this procedure, all of the ointment tubes have an equal likelihood of being selected.

Many calculators have the capability of generating random numbers. A simple BASIC computer program to print a list of random numbers would be as follows:

```
10      CLS:CLEAR
20      RANDOMIZE
30      INPUT "NUMBER OF RANDOM NUMBERS"; E
40      R=RND(1)
50      N = N+1
60      LPRINT R
70      IF N<E GOTO 40
80      END
```

One program produced the following numbers:

.3503473
.0234021
.5161394
.6897221
.6510906
.0081350
.1510521

Assume that fifty volunteers are enrolled for a clinical trial to evaluate the difference in response between an active drug and a placebo. These volunteers are to be randomly divided into two groups of 25 subjects. Based on the above computer generated random numbers, the first subjects assigned to the treatment group would be numbers 35, 02 and 15 (using the first two places to the right of the decimal point). In a similar manner, most calculators will also provide a random number's key (i.e., Casio[Inv][Ran#]; HP48G [Mth][Nxt][Prob][Rand] or TI-85 [2nd][Math] [Prob][Rand]). In this case the output may look as follows:

.560
.369
.783
.437
.853
.222

Using the same clinical trials example, the hand-held calculator generated numbers would select subjects 36, 43 and 22 as the first three selected for the treatment group.

Other Sampling Procedures

Selective sampling, in contrast to random sampling can be considered a "nonprobability" sampling method. It is often used because it is convenient, relatively easy to accomplish, and is often more realistic than pure random sampling. Selective sampling offers a practical means for producing a sample that is representative of all the units in the population. A sample is biased when it is not representative and every attempt should be made to avoid this situation. There are three alternative techniques: systematic, selective, and cluster sampling.

Systematic sampling is a process by which every *nth* object is selected. Consider a mailing list for a survey. The list is too large for us to mail to everyone in this population. Therefore, we select every 6th or 10th name from the list to reduce the size of the mailing while still sampling across the entire list (A-Z). The limitation is that certain combinations may be eliminated as possible samples (i.e., spouses or identical twins with the same last names); therefore, producing a situation where everyone on the mailing does not have an equal chance of being selected. In the pharmaceutical industry this might be done during a production run of a certain tablet where at selected time periods (every 30 or 60 minutes) tablets are randomly selected as they come off the tablet press and weighed to ensure the process is within control specifications. In this production example, the time selected during the hour can be randomly chosen in an attempt to detect any periodicity (regular pattern) in the production run.

In **stratified sampling** the population is divided into groups (strata) with similar characteristics and then individuals or objects can be randomly selected from each group. For example, in another study we may wish to insure a certain percentage of smokers (25%) are represented in both the control and experimental groups in a clinical trial (n=100 per group). First the volunteers are stratified into smokers and non-smokers. Then, 25 smokers are randomly selected for the experimental group and an additional 25 smokers are randomly selected as controls. Similarly two groups of 75 non-smoking volunteers are randomly selected to complete the study design. Stratified sampling is recommended when the strata are very different from each other and all of the objects or individuals within each stratum are similar.

Also known as "multistage" sampling, **cluster sampling** is employed when there are many individual "primary" units that are clustered together in "secondary", larger units that can be subsampled. For example, individual tablets (primary) are contained in bottles (secondary) sampled at the end of a production run. For example, assume that 150 containers of a bulk powder chemical arrive at a pharmaceutical manufacturer and the quality control laboratory needs to sample these for the accuracy of the chemical or lack of contaminants. Rather than sampling each container we randomly select ten containers. Then within each of the ten containers we further extract random samples (from the top, middle and bottom) to be assayed.

In the final analysis, the selective sampling procedure that is chosen by the investigator depends on the experimental situation. There are several factors to be considered when choosing a sampling technique. They include: 1) cost of sampling, both associated expense and labor; 2) practicality, using a random number table for one million tablets during a production run would be unrealistic if not impossible to accomplish; 3) the nature of the population the sample is taken from - periodicity, unique strata or clustering of smaller units within larger ones; and 4) the desired accuracy and precision of the sample.

Precision, Accuracy and Bias

As mentioned, it is desirable that sample data be representative of the true population from which it is sampled and every effort should be made to ensure this is accomplished.

Precision refers to how closely data are grouped together or the compactness of the sample data. Illustrated in Figure 3.1 are data where there is less scatter, or closely clustered data, which have greater precision (Samples A and C). Also included is Sample B with a great deal of scatter and which does not have great precision. Precision measures the variability of a group of measurements. A precise set of measurements is compact and, as discussed in Chapter 5, is reflected by a small relative standard deviation.

However, assume that the smaller box within Samples A, B and C represent the true value for the population from which the samples were taken. In this example, even though Samples A and C have good precision, only Sample C is accurate as a predictor of the population. **Accuracy** is concerned with "correctness" of the results and refers to how closely the sample data represents the true value of the population. It is desirable to have data that is both accurate and precise.

An analogy for precision and accuracy is to consider Figure 3.1 as an example of target shooting with the smaller box representing the bulls eye. Sample C is desired because all of the shots are compacted near or within the bulls eye of the target. Sample B is less precise, yet some shots reach the center of the target. Sample A is probably the most precise, but it lacks accuracy. This lack of accuracy is bias. **Bias** can be thought of as **systematic error** which causes some type of constant error in the measurement or idiosyncrasy with the measurement system. In the example of target shooting, the system error might be improper adjustment of the aiming apparatus or failure to account for wind velocity, either of which would cause a constant error. Ideally, investigators should use random sampling to avoid "selection bias." **Selection bias** occurs when certain characteristics make potential

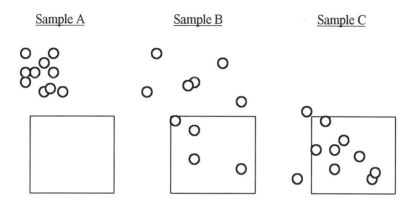

Figure 3.1 Samples comparing precision and accuracy.

observations more (or less) likely to be included in the study. For example, always sampling from the top of storage drums may bias the results based on particle size, assuming smaller particles settle to the lower regions of the drums. Bias can result from an incorrect sampling, inappropriate experimental design, inadequate blinding, or mistakes (blunders) in observing or recording the data.

Even random samples of the same pool of objects (i.e., tablets of a particular batch) are very unlikely to be exactly the same. For example, the average weight of ten tablets will vary from sample to sample. Multiple samples from the same pool or population will result in a distribution of possible outcomes, which is called the sampling distribution (Chapter 6). All data points in a set of data are subject to two different types of error: systematic and random errors. **Random errors**, or chance errors, are unpredictable and will vary in sign (+ or -) and magnitude; but systematic errors always have the same sign and magnitude, and produce biases.

Reliability and Validity

Closely related to the accuracy of the sample data is its reliability and validity. **Reliability** is a collection of factors and judgments that, when taken together, are a measure of reproducibility. Reliability is the consistency of measures and deals with the amount of error associated with the measured values. In order for data to be reliable, all sources of error and their magnitude should be known, including both constant errors (bias) and random or chance errors. With respect to this measure of reproducibility, if subjects are tested twice and there is a strong relationship between successive measurements (correlation, Chapter 12) this is referred to as **test-retest reliability**. It is a method of pairing the scores on the first test and the retest to determine the reliability. A second type of reliability measure, in the case of a knowledge test, is to divide the test into two portions: one score on the odd items and one score on the even items (or first half and second half of the test). If there is a strong relationship between the scores on the two halves it is called **split-half reliability**. Reliability is basic to every measurement situation and interpretation that we place on our sample data.

Validity refers to the fact that the data represents a true measurement. A valid piece of data describes or measures what it is suppose to represent. In other words, to be a valid measurement it must reflect what it is intended to measure. It is possible for a sample to be reliable without being valid, but it cannot be valid without being reliable. Therefore, the degree of validity for a set of measurements is limited by its degree of reliability. Also, if randomness is removed from the sampling technique used to collect data, it potentially removes the validity of our estimation of a population parameter.

Table 3.1   Results of Weights for Fifteen Tabets (mg)

Sample	Weight	Sample	Weight	Sample	Weight	Sample	Weight
1	649	14	653	27	645	40	650
2	654	15	646	28	650	41	651
3	644	16	644	29	656	42	639
4	648	17	649	30	649	43	648
5	650	18	647	31	649	44	652
6	636	19	650	32	657	45	648
7	652	20	652	33	643	46	669
8	662	21	646	34	653	47	647
9	646	22	648	35	645	48	664
10	650	23	655	36	650	49	649
11	648	24	651	37	647	50	653
12	651	25	642	38	651		
13	660	26	647	39	654		

Reference

Rees, D.G. (1989). <u>Essential Statistics</u>, Chapman and Hall, New York, p.78

Suggested Supplemental Readings

Bolton, S. (1997). <u>Pharmaceutical Statistics: Practical and Clinical Applications</u>, Marcel Dekker, New York, pp. 102-109.

Forthofer, R.N. and Lee, E.S. (1995). <u>Introduction to Biostatistics: A Guide to Design, Analysis and Discovery</u>, Academic Press, San Diego, pp. 23-35.

Example Problems

1. Using the random numbers table presented as Table B1 in Appendix B, randomly sample three tablets from Table 3.1. Calculate the average for the three values obtained by the sample (add the three numbers and divide by three).

2. Repeat the above sampling exercise five times and record the average for each sample. Are these averages identical?

3. From the discussion in Chapter 2, how many possible samples (n=3) could be randomly selected from the data in Table 3.1?

Answers to Problems

1. Answers will vary based on the sample.

2. Chances are the five samples will all be different and the averages could vary from 639 to 665 mg depending on which three samples are selected. The most common results will be near the center (650 mg) for all 50 measurements. The reason for this will be explained in Chapter 6 where sample distributions are discussed.

3. There are 19,600 possible samples:

$$\binom{n}{x} = \frac{n!}{x!\,(n-x)!} = \frac{50!}{3!\,(50-3)!} = \frac{50 \cdot 49 \cdot 48 \cdot 47!}{(3 \cdot 2 \cdot 1)(47!\,)} = 19,600$$

4

Presentation Modes

Data can be communicated in one of four different methods: 1) verbal; 2) written descriptions; 3) tables; or 4) graphic presentations. This chapter will focus on the latter two methods for presenting descriptive statistics. Often the graphic representation of data may be beneficial for describing and/or explaining research data. The main purpose in using a graph is to present a visual representation of the data and the distribution of observations.

The old adage "a picture is worth a thousand words" can be especially appropriate with respect to graphic representation of statistical data. Visualizing data can be useful when reviewing preliminary data, for interpreting the results of inferential statistics, and for detecting possible extreme or erroneous data (outliers). A variety of graphic displays exist and a few of the most common are presented in this chapter. The only limitation to their use is the amount of research creativity.

Tabulation of Data

The simplest and least informative way to present experimental results is to list the observations (raw scores). For example, working in a quality control laboratory we are requested to sample 30 tetracycline capsules during a production run and to report to the supervisor the results of this sample. Assume the information in Table 4.1 represents the assay results for the random sample of 30 capsules. Data presented in this format is relatively useless other then to simply report the individual results.

We could arrange the results of the 30 samples in order from the smallest

Table 4.1 Results from the Assay of 30 Tetracycline Capsules

Capsule #	mg	Capsule #	mg	Capsule #	mg
1	251	11	250	21	250
2	250	12	253	22	254
3	253	13	251	23	248
4	249	14	250	24	252
5	250	15	249	25	251
6	252	16	252	26	248
7	247	17	251	27	250
8	248	18	249	28	247
9	254	19	246	29	251
10	245	20	250	30	249

Table 4.2 Rank Ordering from Smallest to Largest

Rank	mg	Rank	mg	Rank	mg
1	245	11	249	21	251
2	246	12	250	22	251
3	247	13	250	23	251
4	247	14	250	24	252
5	248	15	250	25	252
6	248	16	250	26	252
7	248	17	250	27	253
8	249	18	250	28	253
9	249	19	251	29	254
10	249	20	251	30	254

assay result to the largest (Table 4.2). With this ordinal ranking of the data we begin to see certain characteristics about our data: 1) most of the observations cluster near the middle of the distribution (i.e., 250 mg) and 2) the spread of outcomes varies from as small as 245 mg to as large as 254.

The purpose of descriptive statistics is to organize and summarize information, therefore, tables and graphics can be used to present this data in a more useful format. What we are doing is called the process of **data reduction**, trying to take data and reduce it down to more manageable information. The assay results seen in Tables 4.1 and 4.2 represent a continuous variable (mg of drug present). As mentioned in Chapter 1, continuous data can be grouped together to form categories and then handled as a discrete variable. Assume that the desired amount (labeled amount) of tetracycline is 250 mg per capsule. The data can be summarized to report results: 1) focusing on those which meet or exceed the labeled amount:

Outcome	n	%
< 250 mg	11	36.7
≥ 250 mg	19	63.3
Total	30	100.0

(n representing the number of occurrences in a given level); 2) showing those which do not exceed the labeled amount:

Outcome	f	%
≤ 250 mg	18	60.0
> 250 mg	12	40.0
Total	30	100.0

(the number of occurrences can also be listed as frequency of outcomes); or 3) listing those observations which exactly meet the label claim and those which fall above or below the desired amount:

Outcome	f	cf	%	cum. %
< 250 mg	11	11	36.7	36.7
= 250 mg	7	18	23.3	60.0
> 250 mg	12	30	40.0	100.0

Notice in this last table that the cumulative frequencies and cumulative percentages are reported, in addition to the frequency and percentage. The **frequency** (f) or number of observations for each discrete level appears in the second column. The third column represents the **cumulative frequency** (cf) which is obtained by adding the frequency of observations at each discrete level point to those frequencies of the preceding level(s). The last two columns report the percentages associated with each level of the discrete variable. The fourth column is the **relative frequency** (rf) which is the frequency converted into the percentage of the total number of observations. The last column shows the cumulative outcomes expressed as **cumulative percent** or proportion of the observations. One of the problems associated with converting a continuous, quantitative variable into a categorical discrete variable is a loss of information. Notice in the last table that 10 different values (ranging from 245 to 254 mg) have been collapsed into only three intervals.

Visual Displays for Discrete Variables

Often simple data, such as the previous example, can be presented in graphic form. **Bar graphs** are appropriate for visualizing the frequencies associated with different levels of a discrete variable. Also referred to as **block diagrams**, they are drawn with spaces between the bars symbolizing the discontinuity among the levels of the variable (this is in contrast to histograms for continuous data that will be discussed later). In Figure 4.1, information is presented using the three mutually exclusive and exhaustive levels created for the data in Table 4.2. In preparing bar graphs, the horizontal plane (x-axis or **abscissa**) usually represents observed values or the discrete levels of the variable (in this case <250, =250 or >250 mg.). The vertical axis (y-axis or **ordinate**) represents the frequency or proportion of observations (in this case the frequency).

A **line chart** is similar to a bar chart except that thin lines, instead of thicker bars, are used to represent the frequency associated with each level of the discrete variable. **Point plots** are identical to line charts; however, instead of a line a number of points or dots equivalent to the frequency are stacked vertically for each value of the horizontal axis. Also referred to as **dot diagram**, point plots are useful for small data sets. Using the data presented in

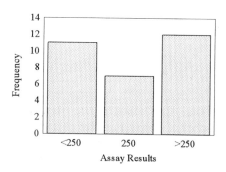

Figure 4.1 Example of a bar graph.

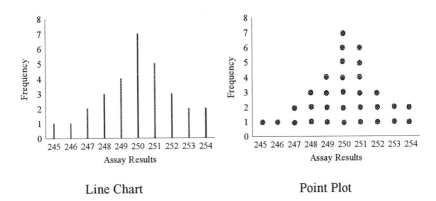

Line Chart   Point Plot

Figure 4.2 Examples of a line chart and point plot.

Table 4.2, a corresponding line chart and dot diagram are presented in Figure 4.2.

Pictograms are similar to bar charts. They present the same type of information, but the bars are replaced with a proportional number of icons. This type of presentation for descriptive statistics dates back to the beginning of civilization when pictorial images were used to record numbers of people, animals or objects (Figure 4.3).

Pie charts provide a method for viewing and comparing levels of a discrete variable in relationship to that variable as a whole. Whenever a data set can be divided into parts, a pie chart may provide the most convenient and effective method for presenting the data (Figure 4.4).

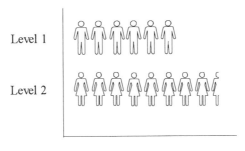

Frequency

Figure 4.3 Example of a pictogram.

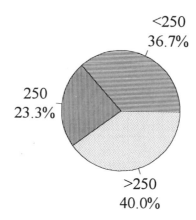

Figure 4.4 Example of a pie chart.

Visual Displays for Continuous Variables

Stem-and-leaf plot. Also called a **stemplot**, the stem-and-leaf plot is a visual representation for continuous data. It was developed by John Tukey in the 1960s. It contains features common to both the frequency distribution and dot diagrams. Digits, instead of bars are used to illustrate the spread and shape of the distribution. Each piece of data is divided into "leading" and "trailing" digits. For example, based on the range of data points, the observation *125* could be divided into the either *12* and *5*, or *1* and *25*, as the leading and trailing digits. All the leading digits are sorted from lowest to highest and listed to the left of a vertical line. These digits become the stem. The trailing digits are then written in the appropriate location to the right of the vertical line. These become the leaves. The frequency or "depth" of the number of leaves at each value in the lead digit of the stem are listed on the left side and can be used to calculate the median, quartiles, or percentiles. An M and Q are placed on the vertical line to identify the **median** and **quartiles**. These measures of central tendency will be discussed in the next chapter. For the present, the median represents that value below which 50% of the observations fall. The quartiles are the values below which 25% and 75% of the data would be located, respectively. For example, the data presented for *125* patients in Table 4.3 can be graphically represented by the following stemplot (Figure 4.5).

Frequency	Stem		Leaves
1	70		6
2	71		48
8	72		00455889
18	73		001122244456788999
19	74	Q	0011113333355556699
31	75	M	00111112222234445555555556668999
28	76	Q	000111222334445555666666677789
12	77		000124455588
4	78		0058
2	79		03
125			

Figure 4.5 Example of a stem-and-leaf plot.

Table 4.3 C_{max} Calculations for Bigomycin in Micrograms (mcg)

739	775	765	751	761	738	759	761	764	765	749	767
764	743	739	759	752	762	730	734	759	745	743	745
751	760	768	766	756	741	741	774	756	749	760	765
743	752	729	735	725	750	745	745	738	763	752	737
706	769	760	755	767	750	728	778	740	741	771	752
756	746	788	743	725	765	754	766	755	772	758	763
734	728	755	778	785	718	730	731	714	752	770	732
770	755	720	754	764	731	790	793	753	780	732	751
766	751	762	734	755	761	740	767	775	755	766	736
755	755	770	741	751	774	780	724	720	746	754	766
743	743	775	732	762							

Formulation A		Formulation B
97	11	
98766655321100	12	27899
6553310	13	0002236688
0	14	0112589
	15	01

Figure 4.6 Example of a back-to-back stem-and-leaf plot.

The appearance of the stemplot is similar to a horizontal bar graph (rotated 90 degrees from the previous example of a bar graph), however, individual data values are retained. Also shown are the maximum and minimum scores, and also the range (distance from the largest to smallest observation) can be easily calculated. The stem-and-leaf plot could also be expanded to provide more information about the distribution. In the above example, if each stem unit was divided into halves (upper and lower), then the leaves would be established for 70.0-70.4, 70.5-70.9, 80.0-80.4, etc.

A **back-to-back stemplot** could be used to visually compare two sets of data. For example the information in Table 4.4 is plotted in Figure 4.6. Visually the data obtained for the two formulations appear to be different. In Chapter 8, we will reevaluate this data to determine if there is a statistically significant difference or if the difference could be due to some type of random difference.

Similar to the back-to-back stemplot, the **cross diagram** is a simple graphic representation for two or more levels of a discrete independent variable

Table 4.4 C_{max} Values for Two Formulations of the Same Drug

Formulation A						Formulation B					
125	130	135	126	140	135	130	128	127	149	151	130
128	121	123	126	121	133	141	145	132	132	141	129
131	129	120	117	126	127	133	136	138	142	130	122
119	133	125	120	136	122	129	150	148	136	138	140

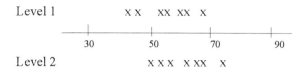

Level 1   x x   xx xx   x

      30   50   70   90

Level 2   x x x   x xx   x

Figure 4.7 Example of a cross diagram.

and a dependent continuous variable. The values for the dependent variable are represented on a horizontal or vertical line. Data are plotted on each side of the line based on which level of the independent variable they represent.

One simple plot that displays a great deal of information about a continuous variable is the **box-and-whisker plot.** The box plot illustrates the bulk of the data as a rectangular box in which the upper and lower lines represent the third quartile (75% of observations below Q_3) and first quartile (25% of observations below Q_1), respectively. The second quartile (50% of the observations below this point) is depicted as a horizontal line through the box. The arithmetic average may or may not be shown as an x. Vertical lines (whiskers) extend from the top and bottom lines of the box to an upper and lower **adjacent value.** The adjacent values equal three **semi-interquartile ranges** (SIQR) above and below the median. The SIQR is the distance between the upper or lower quartile and the median, or:

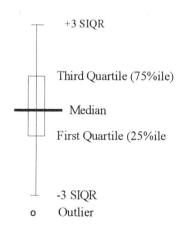

Figure 4.8 Example of a box and whisker plot.

$$SIQR = \frac{(Q_3 - Q_1)}{2}$$ Eq. 4.1

Observations that fall above or below the adjacent values can be identified as potential outliers (Chapter 19).

Similar to bar charts and point plots, **histograms** are useful for displaying the distribution for a continuous variable, especially as sample sizes become larger or if it becomes impractical to plot each of the different values observed in the data. The vertical bars are connected and reflect the continuous nature of the observed values. Each bar represents a single value or a range of values within the width of that bar. For example, a histogram representing the 30 tetracycline capsules listed in Table 4.1 is presented in Figure 4.9. Each value represents a continuous variable and the equipment used had precision to measure to only the whole mg (i.e., 248 or 251 mg.). If more exact instruments were available, the measurements might be in tenths or hundredths of a milligram. Therefore, the value of 248 really represents an infinite number of possible outcomes between 0.5 below and 0.5 mg above that particular measure (247.5 to 248.5 mg). Similarly, the value 250 represents all possible results between 249.5 and 250.5 mg. The histogram representing this continuum is presented in Figure 4.10.

The data in Figure 4.10 represents an **ungrouped frequency distribution**, which is a visual representation of each possible outcome and its

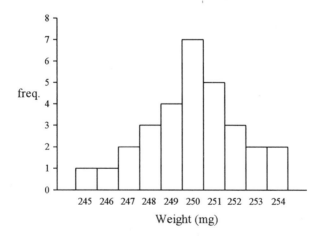

Figure 4.9 Example of a histogram.

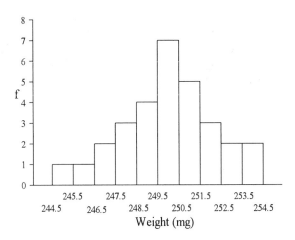

Figure 4.10 Example of a histogram with correction for continuity.

associated frequency. Such a distribution shows the extremes of the outcomes, as well as how they are distributed and if they tend to concentrate in the center or to one end of the scale. Unfortunately, with large data sets, ungrouped frequency distributions may become cumbersome and produce a histogram with many points on the abscissa with frequency counts of only one or two per level. A more practical approach would be to group observed values or outcomes into **class intervals**. In a **grouped frequency distribution**: 1) all class intervals must be the same width, or size; 2) the intervals are mutually exclusive and exhaustive; and 3) the interval widths should be assigned so the lowest interval includes the smallest observed outcome and the top interval includes the largest observed outcome. The number of class intervals and their size (boundaries) must be specified. Two questions exist regarding these intervals: how many intervals should be used and what should be the width for each interval? To illustrate this process, consider the pharmacokinetic data presented in Table 4.3, representing a sample of patients (n=125) receiving the fictitious drug bigomycin. As mentioned previously, the range is the difference between the largest and smallest value in a set of observations and represents the simplest method for presenting the dispersion of the data. In this example the largest observation is 792 mcg and the smallest is 706 mcg. This represents the **range** of the observations:

$$792 \, mcg - 706 \, mcg = 86 \, mcg$$

But into how many class intervals should this data be divided? Some authors provide approximations such as ten to 20 (Snedecor and Cochran, 1989), eight to 12 (Bolton, 1984), or five to 15 intervals (Forthofer and Lee, 1995). However, **Sturges' rule** (Sturges, 1926) provides a less arbitrary guide to determine the number of intervals based on the sample size (n):

$$K_{intervals} = 1 + 3.32 \log_{10}(n) \qquad \text{Eq. 4.2}$$

A quick reference on the number of intervals for various sample sizes based on Sturges' rule is presented in Table 4.5. The interval width is found by dividing the range by the prescribed number of intervals:

$$width \ (w) \ = \ \frac{range}{K} \qquad \text{Eq. 4.3}$$

In our current example, for a sample size of 125 and a range of 86, the number of intervals and width of those intervals would be:

$$K = 1 + 3.32 \log_{10}(125) = 1 + 3.32(2.10) = 7.97 \approx 8 \ intervals$$

$$w = \frac{range}{K} = \frac{86}{8} = 10.75 \approx 11 \ mcg$$

Table 4.5 Number of Intervals for Various
Sample Sizes Using Sturges' Rule

Sample Size	K Intervals
23-45	6
46-90	7
91-181	8
182-363	9
364-726	10
727-1454	11
1455-2909	12

Table 4.6 Example of Intervals Created Using Sturges' Rule

Interval	Interval Boundary values	Frequency
706-716	705.5-716.5	2
717-727	716.5-727.5	6
728-738	727.5-738.5	18
739-749	738.5-749.5	22
750-760	759.5-760.5	35
761-771	760.5-771.5	28
772-782	771.5-782.5	10
783-793	782.5-793.5	4

Thus, the most representative histogram would consist of 8 intervals, each with a width of 11. In order to include the smallest and largest values the sections of the histogram would be divided as seen in the first column of Table 4.6. However, the values represent a continuous variable; therefore, correcting for continuity, the true boundaries (**interval boundary values**) of each interval of the histogram and their associated frequencies would be the second column of Table 4.6.

Note that the distribution represents eight intervals that are mutually exclusive and exhaust all possible outcomes. The histogram would appear as presented in Figure 4.11. The center of this distribution can be calculated, as well as a measure of dispersion and these will be discussed in the following chapter.

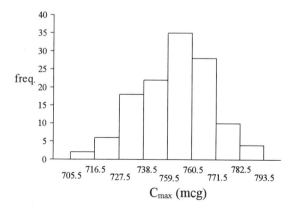

C_{max} (mcg)

Figure 4.11 Histogram for data presented in Table 4.3.

A **frequency polygon** can be constructed by placing a dot at the midpoint for each class interval in the histogram and then these dots are connected by straight lines. This frequency polygon gives a better conception of the shape of the distribution. The **class interval midpoint** for a section in a histogram is calculated as follows:

$$Midpoint = \frac{highest + lowest\ point}{2}$$ Eq. 4.4

For class interval 705.5 to 716.6 the midpoint would be:

$$Midpoint = \frac{highest + lowest\ point}{2} = \frac{705.5 + 716.5}{2} = 711$$

The midpoints for the above histogram are:

Class Interval	Midpoint (m_i)	Frequency (f_i)
705.5-716.5	711	2
716.5-727.5	722	6
727.5-738.5	733	18
738.5-749.5	744	22
749.5-760.5	755	35
760.5-771.5	766	28
771.5-782.5	777	10
782.5-793.5	788	4
	Total =	125

The frequency polygon is then created by listing the midpoints on the x-axis, frequencies on the y-axis, and drawing lines to connect the midpoints for each interval as presented in Figure 4.12 for the previous data. The midpoint of the class interval represents all the values within that interval and will be used in drawing frequency polygons and in the calculation of measures of central tendency (Chapter 5). Unfortunately there is some loss of precision with grouped frequency distribution because only one value (the midpoint) represents all the various data points within the class interval.

At times it may be desirable to prepare graphs which show how the values accumulate from lowest class intervals to highest. These **cumulative frequency polygons** display the frequency or percentage of the observed values

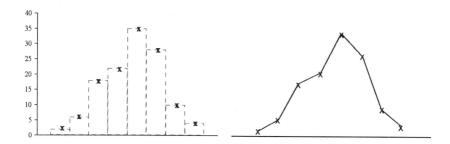

Figure 4.12 Example of a frequency polygon.

falling below each interval. By using such a drawing it is possible to establish certain percentiles. Figure 4.13 shows a cumulative frequency polygon for the same data presented in the above frequency polygon (data from Table 4.3). Note that lines are drawn from the 25th (Q1), 50th (Q2), and 75th (Q3) percentile on the y-axis (point at which 25, 50, and 75% of the results fall below) and where they cross the polygon is the approximation of each percentile. If the population from which the sample approximates a normal or bell-shaped distribution, the cumulative distribution is usually S-shaped or **ogive**.

If there were an infinite number of midpoints (the interval width approaches zero), it would be represented by a smooth curve. The skewness of a distribution describes the direction of the stringing out of the tail of the curve

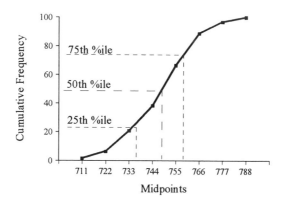

Figure 4.13 Example of a cumulative frequency polygon.

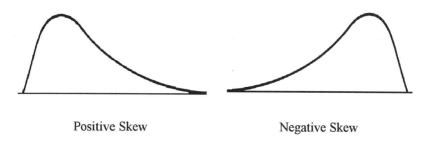

Positive Skew   Negative Skew

Figure 4.14 Examples of skewed dirstributions.

(Figure 4.14). In a **positively skewed distribution** most of the values in the frequency distribution are at the left end of the distribution with a few high values causing a tapering of the curve to the right side of the distribution. In contrast, a **negatively skewed distribution** has most of the values at the right side of the distribution with a few low values causing a tapering of the curve to the left side of the distribution.

If a sample were normally distributed it would not be skewed to the left or right and would be symmetrical in shape. The normal distribution and its characteristics will be discussed in great length in Chapter 6.

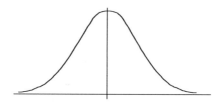

Kurtosis is a property associated with a frequency distribution and refers to the shape of the distribution of values regarding its relative flatness and peakedness. **Mesokurtic** is a frequency distribution that has the characterists of a normal bell-shaped distribution. If the normal distribution is more peaked than a traditional bell shaped curve is it termed **leptokurtic** and **platykurtic** refers to a shape that is less peaked or flatter than the normal bell-shaped curve.

Visual Displays for Two or More Continuous Variables

Scatter diagram or scatter plot. A scatter diagram is an extremely useful presentation for showing the relationship between two continuous variables.

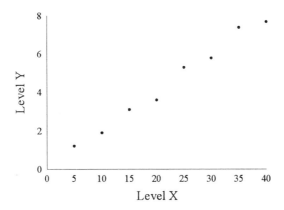

Figure 4.15 Example of a scatter diagram.

The two dimensional plot has both horizontal and vertical axes which cover the ranges of the two variables. Plotted data points represent paired observations for both the x and y variable (Figure 4.15). These types of plots are valuable for correlation and regression inferential tests (Chapters 12 and 13).

A **sequence plot** is a plot where the horizontal axis represents a logical or physical sequencing of data. An example might be a measurement of successive lots of a particular product, where the vertical axis is a continuous variable and the horizontal axis represents the first lot, followed by the second, then the third, etc. If time is considered, then data is arranged chronologically

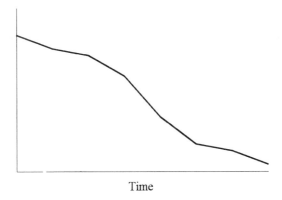

Figure 4.16 Example of a sequence plot.

on the horizontal axis. This **time series graph** is a visual representation of changes in data over time, in which the dependent variable is placed on the y-axis (Figure 4.16).

Further data reduction techniques for continuous data will be presented in the next chapter where we will explore methods to define the center of distributions and how data disperses from that center. However, visual/graphic techniques should be considered as a possible alternative to obtain a "feel" for the shape of the statistical descriptive data.

References

Snedecor, G.W. and Cochran, W.G. (1989). Statistical Methods. Iowa State University Press, Ames, p. 18.

Bolton, S. (1997). Pharmaceutical Statistics: Practical and Clinical Applications. Marcel Dekker, Inc., New York, p.43.

Forthofer, R.N. and Lee, E.S. (1995). Introduction to Biostatistics. Academic Press, San Diego, p.52.

Sturges, H.A. (1926). "The choice of a class interval." Journal of the American Statistical Association, 21:65-66.

Suggested Supplemental readings

Daniel, W.W. (1991). Biostatistics: A Foundation for Analysis in the Health Sciences, John Wiley and Sons, New York, pp. 6-16.

Mason, R.L., Gunst, R.F. and Hess, J.L. (1989). Statistical Design and Analysis of Experiments, John Wiley and Sons, New York, pp. 44-62.

Fisher, L.D. and van Belle, G. (1993). Biostatistics: A Methodology for the Health Sciences, John Wiley and Sons, New York, pp. 35-52.

Example Problems

1. During clinical trials, observed adverse effects are often classified by the following scale:

> Mild: Experience was trivial and did not cause any real problem.
>
> Moderate: Experience was a problem but did not interfere significantly with patient's daily activities or clinical status.
>
> Severe: Experience interfered significantly with the normal daily activities or clinical status.

Based on 1109 patients involved in the Phase I and II clinical trials for bigomycin, it was observed that 810 experienced no adverse effects, while 215, 72, and 12 subjects suffered from mild, moderate, and severe adverse effects, respectively. Prepare visual and tabular presentations for this data.

2. The following assay results (percentage of label claim) were observed in 50 random samples during a production run.

102	100	96	99	101	102	100	105	97	100
92	103	101	100	99	102	96	100	101	98
107	95	98	100	100	99	97	104	101	103
98	101	100	105	99	101	102	100	87	98
101	103	93	99	101	97	100	102	99	104

Report these results as a box-and-whisker plot, stemplot and histogram.

3. During a study of particle sizes for a blended powder mixture, the results of percent of powder retained on the various sites were 50.1%, 27.2%, 10.4%, 6.0%, and 5.1% in sieve mesh sizes of 425, 180, 150, 90, and 75 μM, respectively. Only 1.2% was captured on the pan (<75 μM). Prepare a visual and tabular presentation for this data.

4. Comparison of two methods for measuring anxiety in patients is listed below:

Method A	Method B		Method A	Method B
55	90		52	97
66	117		61	110
46	94		44	84
63	124		55	112
57	105		53	102
59	115		67	112
70	125		72	130
57	97			

Prepare a scatter plot to display the relationship between these two variables.

Answers to Problems

1. Incidence of reported adverse drug effects:

   a. Tabular results

Severity of Adverse Effects

Severity	n	%	Cum. %
none	810	73.0	73.0
mild	215	19.4	92.4
moderate	72	6.5	98.9
severe	12	1.1	100.0
	1109	100.0	

   b. Bar graph

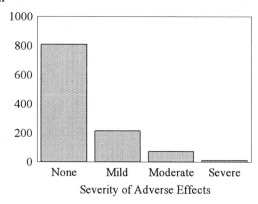

Severity of Adverse Effects

c. Pie chart

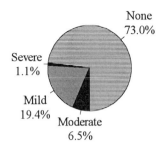

None
73.0%

Severe
1.1%

Mild
19.4%

Moderate
6.5%

2. Distribution of assay results:

a. Box-and-whisker plot

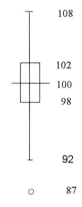

108

102
100
98

92

○   87

b. Stemplot

Frequency	Stem		Leaves
0	8		
1			7
2	9		23
16		Q	5667778888999999
28	10	MQ	00000000001111111112222233344
3			557
50			

c.   Histogram

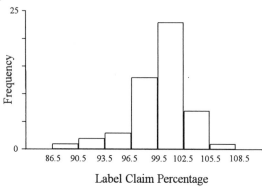

Label Claim Percentage

3.   Particle size determination:

a.   Tabular results

Percent of Particles Retained on Various Sieve Screens

Mesh Size (μM)	% Retained	Cum. % Retained
425	50.1	50.1
180	27.2	77.3
150	10.4	87.7
90	6.0	93.7
75	5.1	98.8
pan (<75)	1.2	100.0
	100.0	

b.   Pie chart

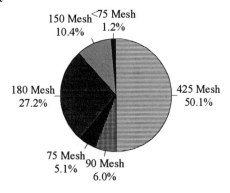

c. Bar chart

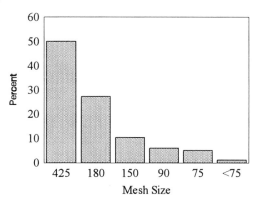

4. Scatter plot

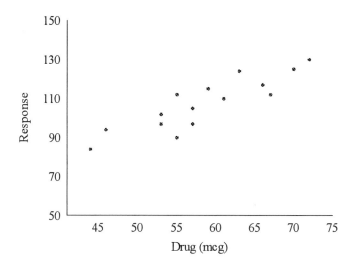

5

Measures of Central Tendency

Central tendency involves description statistics for the observed results of a continuous variable and takes into consideration two important aspects: 1) the center of that distribution and 2) how the observations are dispersed within the distribution. Three points are associated with the center (mode, median and mean) and three other measures are concerned with the dispersion (range, variance and standard deviation).

Measures of central tendency can be used when dealing with ordinal, interval or ratio scales. It would seem logical with any of these continuous scales to be interested in where the center of the distribution is located and how observations tend to cluster around or disperse from this center. Many inferential statistical tests involve continuous variables (see Appendix A) and all require information about the central tendency of associated sample data.

Centers of a Continuous Distribution

The **sample mode** is simply that value with the greatest frequency of occurrence. In other words, that value which is most "popular" in a continuous distribution of scores. For example, what is the mode for the following group of observations?

2,6,7,5,3,8,7,6,5,3,2,5,4,6,8,3,4,4,7,6,5,1,5

Graphically the distribution would look as presented in Figure 5.1. In this distribution of observations, the **modal value** is 5 because it has the greatest

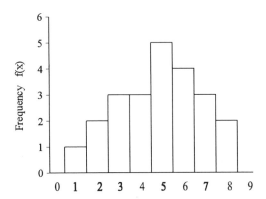

Figure 5.1 Histogram of sample data.

frequency. The mode is the simplest, but least useful measure of the center of a distribution. The mode is most useful when continuous data has been divided into categories (i.e., a histogram) or where it represents the category with the greatest frequency.

A distribution may be multi-modal and have several different values that have the same greatest relative frequency. Such a distribution may have several peaks. An example of a **bimodal distribution** appears below with slow and fast metabolizers of isoniazid (Figure 5.2). The first peak (to the left) represents a central point for the rapid metabolizers (a lower concentration of drug at six hours) and the second peak depicts the slow metabolizers where higher concentrations are seen at the same point in time.

The **sample median** is the center point for any distribution of scores. It represents that value below which 50% of all scores are located. The median (from the Latin word *medianus* or "middle") divides the distribution into two equal parts (the 50th **percentile**). For example, using the same data as the previous example for the mode, a rank ordering of the scores from lowest to highest would produce the following:

Example 5A: 1,2,2,3,3,3,4,4,4,5,5, 5, 5,5,6,6,6,6,7,7,7,8,8

In this case 5 is the median, which is the value that falls in the exact center of the distribution. If there is an even number of observations, the 50th percentile is between the two most central values and the median would be the average of those two central scores. For example, in the following set of numbers the median (represented by a underlined area) in located between the two center

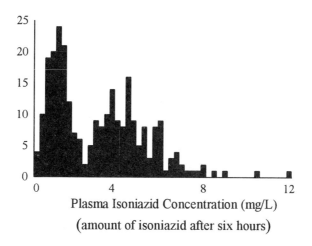

Plasma Isoniazid Concentration (mg/L)

(amount of isoniazid after six hours)

Figure 5.2 Bimodal distribution (Evans, 1960).

values:

Example 5B: 20,22,23,24,24,24,25,25,25,25, __
                26,26,26,27,27,28,28,28,29,30

The calculation of the median would be:

$$\frac{25+26}{2} = 25.5$$

The **median value** is a better estimate of the center of a distribution than the mode. However, it is neither effected by, nor representative, of extreme values in the sample distribution. For example, consider the following two samples:

Example 5C -   Sample 1   36,45,48,50, 50, 51,51,53,54
Table weights in mg: Sample 2   47,48,49,50, 50, 51,52,57,68

Even though both samples have the same median (50 mg), Sample 1 appears to have more observations which are relatively small and Sample 2 has more samples which are high. The two samples appear to be different, yet both produce the same median. If possible, a measure of the center for a given distribution should consider all extreme data points (i.e., 36 and 68). However, at the same time, it's inability to be affected by extreme values also represents one of the advantages of using the median as a measure of the center. As will be seen in Chapter 19, an outlier or atypical data point, can strongly effect the arithmetic center of the distribution, especially in small sample sizes. The median is insensitive to these extreme values.

The median is a relative measure, in that it is defined by its position in relation to the other ordered values for a set of data points. In certain cases it may be desirable to describe a particular value with respect to its position related to other values. The most effective way to do this is in terms of its **percentile location** (the percent of observations that the data point exceeds):

$$percentile = \frac{number\ of\ values\ less\ than\ the\ given\ value}{total\ number\ of\ values} \times 100 \qquad \text{Eq. 5.1}$$

For example consider Table 4.2 where 30 tetracycline capsules were placed in ranked order from smallest to largest. If one were interested in the percentile for 252 mg (the 24th largest value) the calculation would be

$$percentile = \frac{23}{30} \times 100 = 77\ percentile$$

Thus, 252 mg represents the 77 percentile for the data presented in Table 4.2. At the same time, when using percentiles, it is possible to calculate variability in a distribution, especially a skewed distribution. In this case, the measure would be the **interquartile range** or inter-range (the distance between the 25th and the 75th percentiles).

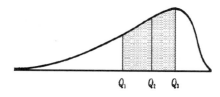

$$Q_1 \qquad Q_2 \qquad Q_3$$

The **sample mean** is what is commonly referred to as the **average**. It is the weighted center point of a distribution, and is computed by summing up all the observations or scores and dividing by the total number of observations.

$$\overline{X} = \frac{x_1 + x_2 + x_3 + \ldots + x_n}{n}$$

The character $\overline{X}$ (x-bar) will be used to symbolize the sample mean. The observed values of a given variable are designated with the same letter (usually x) and each individual value is distinguished with a subscript number or letter. For example x_i indicates the ith observation in a set of data. The symbol sigma (Σ) indicates the addition (summation) of all variable observations. Also referred to as the **arithmetic mean**, the formula for this equation is written as follows:

$$\overline{X} = \frac{\sum_{i=1}^{n} x_i}{n} \qquad \text{Eq. 5.2}$$

In this equation, all observations (x_i) for variable x are added together from the first ($i=1$) to the last (n) and divided by the total number of sample observations (n). Equation 5.2 can be simplified as follows:

$$\overline{X} = \frac{\sum x}{n}$$

The advantage in using the mean over the other measures of central tendency is that it takes into consideration how far the scores or values spread apart and allows for extreme scores. Other measures do not account for this consideration. The mean can be thought of as a balancing point or center of gravity for our distribution. For the above Example 5A the mean would be:

$$\overline{X} = \frac{2 + 6 + 7 + \ldots 5}{23} = 4.9$$

We typically calculate a mean (and other measures of central tendency) to one decimal point beyond the accuracy of the observed data.

The relative positioning of the three measures of a continuous variable's center can give a quick, rough estimate of the shape of the distribution. As will be discussed in the next chapter, in a normal (bell-shaped) distribution the mode = median = mean; in the case of a positively skewed distribution the mode < median < mean and for a negatively skewed distribution the mode > median > mean.

If data is normally distributed, or assumed to be sampled from a normally distributed population, the mean and standard deviation are the best measures of central tendency. The median is the preferred measure of central tendency in skewed distributions where there are a few extreme values (either small or large). In such cases the inter-quartile range is the appropriate measure of dispersion.

In the third example (Example 5C - tablet weights), the two medians were identical, and the means for the two samples differ because the extreme measures (i.e., 36 and 68 mg) were considered in this weighted measure of central tendency:

$$Sample\ 1: \qquad \overline{X}_1 = 48.7\ mg$$
$$Sample\ 2: \qquad \overline{X}_2 = 52.4\ mg$$

Dispersion Within a Continuous Distribution

The mean is only one dimension in the measure of central tendency, namely the weighted middle of the sampling distribution. Of equal importance is the distribution of all data points around the central point. For example, the two distributions in Figure 5.3 have the exact same median (5) and the same mean (4.9). However, the dispersions of data around the center of these two distributions are considerably different. Thus, measures of central tendency should also be concerned with the spread or concentration of data points around the center of the distribution.

The **sample range** is the simplest method for presenting a distribution of observations and represents the difference between the largest and smallest value in a set of outcomes. In Example 5A the largest observation is 8 and the smallest is 1. The range for these observations is 7. Similarly, the ranges for the two sample batches of tablet weights in Example 5C are:

$$Sample\ 1: \qquad 54\text{-}36 = 18$$
$$Sample\ 2: \qquad 68\text{-}47 = 21$$

Some texts and statisticians prefer to correct for continuity (due to the fact that the continuous variable actually extends to one decimal smaller than the measure). In Sample 1 listed above, 54 to 36, would be 54 to 36 inclusive or 54.5 to 35.5. In this case the range would be:

$$R = (largest\ observation - smallest\ observation) + 1$$

$$R = 54 - 36 + 1 = 19$$

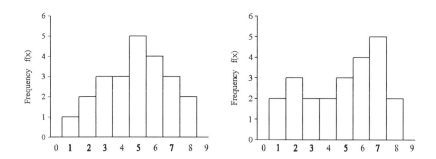

Figure 5.3 Example of distributions with the same mean and median.

If the range were measured in tenths, then 0.1 would be added; if the range is in hundredths, then add an additional 0.01, and so on.

A second measure of dispersion already discussed is the interquartile range. Even though the range and interquartile range are quick and easy measures of dispersion, they possess a limitation similar to the median; specifically they do not account for the actual numerical value of each observation. Much like the mean, a measure is needed to account for how *each* observation varies from the center of the distribution.

One possible measure would be to determine the distance between each value and the center (Figure 5.4). Unfortunately, because the distances to the left and to the right of the mean are equal (since the mean is the weighted center), the sum of all the individual differences ($\sum x_i - \overline{X}$) equals zero and

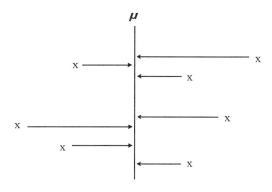

Figure 5.4 Distribution of observations around the mean.

provides no useful information. Therefore, the sum of all the squared differences between the individual observations and the mean is computed, and divided by the number of degrees of freedom (n-1). This produces an intermediate measure known as the **sample variance**:

$$S^2 = \frac{(x_1 - \overline{X})^2 + (x_2 - \overline{X})^2 + (x_3 - \overline{X})^2 + ... + (x_n - \overline{X})^2}{n - 1}$$

Degrees of freedom (*df*) is used to correct for bias in the results that would occur if just the number of observations (*n*) was used. If the **average squared deviation** (the numerator in the variance equation) were divided by *n* observations, it tends to underestimate the variance. The term "degrees of freedom" is best examined by considering the example where the sum of all the deviations $(x_i - \overline{X})$ equals zero. All but one number has the "freedom" to vary. Once we know all but the last data point (*n-1*), we can predict the last value because the sum of all the deviations must equal zero. Therefore, to prevent bias, most statistical analyses involve degrees of freedom (*n-1*) rather than the total sample size (*n*). The sample variance formula can be written:

$$S^2 = \frac{\Sigma(x_i - \overline{X})^2}{n - 1}$$
Eq. 5.3

Obviously as the size of our sample of data increases, the effect of dividing by *n* or *n*-1 becomes negligible. However, for theoretical purposes, degrees of freedom will continually appear in inferential statistical equations.

The variance, using the data from Example 5A (with a mean of 4.9), is calculated as follows:

$$S^2 = \frac{(2 - 4.9)^2 + (6 - 4.9)^2 + (7 - 4.9)^2 + ... (5 - 4.9)^2}{23 - 1} = 3.8$$

An easier method for calculating the variance would be as follows:

$$S^2 = \frac{n(\Sigma x^2) - (\Sigma x)^2}{n(n - 1)}$$
Eq. 5.4

where each observation is squared and both the sum of the observation and the sum of the observations squared are entered into the formula. Algebraically, this produces the exact same results as the original variance formula (Eq. 5.3).

Once again, using data from Example 5A, this method produces the same variance:

x_I	x_I^2
2	4
6	36
...	...
$\underline{5}$	$\underline{25}$
112	628

$$S^2 = \frac{n(\Sigma x^2) - (\Sigma x)^2}{n(n-1)} = \frac{23(628) - (112)^2}{23(22)}$$

$$S^2 = \frac{14444 - 12544}{506} = \frac{1900}{506} = 3.8$$

Variance is only an intermediate measure of dispersion. Each difference ($x_i - \overline{X}$) was squared to produce the variance term. The square root of this result is needed to return to the same measurement scale used for the mean (for example, if the mean is expressed in mg, then the standard deviation will also be expressed as mg).

The **sample standard deviation** (S or SD) is the square root of the variance. It also measures variability about the mean and is most often used to express the dispersion of the observations.

$$S = \sqrt{S^2} \qquad \text{Eq. 5.5}$$

Using the previous set of data as an example:

$$S = \sqrt{3.8} = 1.9$$

It is important to note that the variance has no relevant term of measurement, but the standard deviation is expressed in the same units as the mean. For the sake of illustration, consider the observations for the two samples of tablet weights in Example 5C:

Table 5.1. Data for a Sample of Bottles of Cough Syrup

Original Samples (volume in ml.)				Samples Ordered Smallest to Largest	
Sample	Volume	Sample	Volume		
1	120.7	16	119.0	118.3	120.1
2	120.2	17	121.1	118.5	120.1
3	119.6	18	121.7	118.9	120.1
4	120.1	19	119.2	119.0	120.2
5	121.3	20	120.0	119.0	120.2
6	120.7	21	120.8	119.2	120.4
7	121.0	22	119.9	119.6	120.5
8	119.7	23	119.8	119.7	120.7
9	118.3	24	119.9	119.7	120.7
10	118.9	25	120.2	119.8	120.8
11	120.5	26	120.0	119.8	121.0
12	121.4	27	120.1	119.9	121.1
13	120.4	28	119.0	119.9	121.3
14	118.5	29	120.1	120.0	121.4
15	119.8	30	119.7	120.0	121.7

	$\overline{X}$	S^2	S	n
Sample 1	48.7	29.5	5.4	9
Sample 2	54.4	42.3	6.5	9

In this case the average weights of the tablets in Sample 1 would be 48.7 mg with a standard deviation of 5.43 mg. The variance is simply 29.5, not 29.5 mg or mg squared.

To illustrate the use of central tendency measures, thirty bottles of a cough syrup are randomly sampled from a production line and the results are reported in Table 5.1. The descriptive statistics reporting the measures of central tendency for the sample would be:

Mode: 120.1 ml   (largest frequency of 3 outcomes)

Median: the average of the center two values (15th and 16th ranks)

$$\frac{120.0 + 120.1}{2} = 120.05\,ml$$

Mean: weighted average of all 30 samples

$$\overline{X} = \frac{120.7 + 120.2 + \ldots 119.7}{30} = 120.05\,ml$$

Range: 121.7 - 118.3 = 3.4 ml

Variance:

$$S^2 = \frac{(120.7 - 120.05\,)^2 + \ldots (119.7 - 120.05\,)^2}{30(29)} = 0.70$$

Standard deviation:

$$S = \sqrt{0.70} = 0.84\,ml$$

Lastly, since the standard deviation can be thought of as the square root of the mean of the squared deviations, some textbooks refer to variance as the **root mean square**, or **RMS** value.

Population versus Sample Measures of Central Tendency

The statistics presented thus far have represented means, variances and standard deviations calculated for sample data and not an entire population. The major reason for conducting a statistical analysis is to use sample data as an estimate of the parameters for the entire population of events. For example; it is impractical, and impossible if destructive methods are used, to sample all the tablets in a particular batch. Therefore, compendia or in-house standards for content uniformity testing might consist of a sample of 30 tablets randomly selected from a batch of many thousands of tablets.

Parameters are to populations, as **statistics** are to samples. As seen in Table 5.2, The observed statistics (mean and standard deviation from the sample) are the best estimates of the true population parameters (the population mean and population standard deviation). Note in Table 5.2 that the Greek

Table 5.2   Symbols Used for Sample and Population
Measures of Central Tendency

	Sample Statistic	Population Parameter
Mean	$\overline{X}$	μ
Variance	S^2	σ^2
Standard Deviation	S	σ
Number of observations	n	N

symbols μ (mu) and σ (sigma) are used to represent the population mean and population standard deviation, respectively. Also, in the formulas that follow, N replaces n for the total observations in a population. These symbols will be used throughout the book with Greek symbols referring to population parameters.

The **population mean** is calculated using a formula identical to the sample mean:

$$\mu = \frac{\sum_{i=1}^{N} X_i}{N} \qquad \text{Eq. 5.6}$$

The formula for the **population variance** is similar to that of the sample estimate, except that the numerator is divided by the number of all observations (N). If all the data is known about the population, it is not necessary to use degrees of freedom to correct for bias.

$$\sigma^2 = \frac{\sum_{i=1}^{N} (x_i - \mu)^2}{N} \qquad \text{Eq. 5.7}$$

Similar to the sample standard deviation, the **population standard deviation** is the square root of the population variance.

$$\sigma = \sqrt{\sigma^2} \qquad \text{Eq. 5.8}$$

Measurements Related to the Sample Standard Deviation

The variability of data may often be better described as a relative variation rather than as an absolute variation (i.e., the standard deviation). This can be accomplished by calculating the **coefficient of variation** (CV) that is the ratio of the standard deviation to the mean.

$$CV = \frac{standard\ deviation}{mean} \qquad\qquad \text{Eq. 5.9}$$

The C.V. is usually expressed as a percentage (**relative standard deviation** or **RSD**) and can be useful in many instances because it places variability in perspective to the distribution center.

$$RSD = CV \ x \ 100 \ (percent) \qquad\qquad \text{Eq. 5.10}$$

In the previous Example 5A (CV = 1.94/4.87 = 0.398 and RSD = 0.398 x 100 = 39.8), the standard deviation is 40% of the mean. In the previous example of the liquid volumes (Table 5.1), the coefficient of variation and RSD would be:

$$CV = \frac{0.835}{120.05} = 0.007$$

$$RSD = 0.007 \ x \ 100 = 0.7\%$$

Thus, relative standard deviations present an additional method of expressing this variability, which takes into account its relative magnitude (expressed as the ratio of the standard deviation to the mean). Table 5.3 illustrates the amount of assayed drug and the second and third columns represent 10 and 100 fold increases in the original values. These increases also result in a 10 and 100 fold increase in both the mean and standard deviation, but the relative standard deviation remains constant. In the pharmaceutical industry, this can be used as a measure of precision between various batches of a drug, if measures are based on percent label claim (column 4 in Table 5.3).

    A second example illustrating the relative standard deviation would be the peak area on an HPLC reading:

Table 5.3 Examples with Relative Standard Deviations

	Assayed Amount of Drug			% Labeled Claim
	9.96	99.6	996	99.6
	10.05	100.5	1005	100.5
	9.92	99.2	992	99.2
	9.92	99.2	992	99.2
	9.86	98.6	986	98.6
	9.85	98.5	985	98.5
	10.01	100.1	1001	100.1
	9.90	99.0	990	99.0
	9.96	99.6	996	99.6
	9.86	98.6	986	98.6
Mean =	9.929	99.29	992.9	99.29
S.D. =	0.067	0.666	6.657	0.666
RSD =	0.67%	0.67%	0.67%	0.67%

	HPLC Peak (x)	x^2
Run 1	59.45	3534.30
Run 2	59.50	3540.25
Run 3	58.70	3445.69
Run 4	59.25	3510.56
	236.90	14030.80

Measures of central tendency are as follows:

Mean:

$$\overline{X} = \frac{236.9}{4} = 59.23\,ml$$

Variance:

$$S^2 = \frac{4(14030.8) - (236.9)^2}{4(3)} = 0.13$$

Standard deviation:

$$S = \sqrt{0.13} = 0.36\,ml$$

Coefficient of variation:

$$C.V. = \frac{0.36}{59.23} = 0.0061$$

Relative standard deviation:

$$RSD = 0.0061 \times 100 = 0.61\%$$

Geometric Mean

The geometric mean represents a logarithmic transformation of data to calculate the mean. It is used when data is positively skewed (i.e. most of the values are to the left of the distribution - near zero - and few values are in the right side of the curve). Because of the few extreme values to the right of the curve, the arithmetic mean ($\overline{X}$) would be "pulled" to the right. Performing a logarithmic transformation would produce a distribution that is approximately a normal distribution and the final mean will be more to the "left" and thus closer to the median of the original distribution.

This process involves converting each number to its logarithmic form. These values are summed and divided by the total number of observations to produce an average logarithmic value. This value is then converted back to real numbers by taking the antilog, which represents the geometric mean. Illustrated below are two sets of identical data, with the left on a normal scale

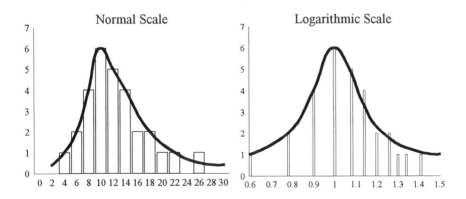

Figure 5.5 Comparisons of data on a normal and logarithmic scale.

Table 5.4 T_{max} Results in Ascending Order

Subject	T_{max}	Log Transformation
3	1.2	0.079
5	1.4	0.146
9	1.5	0.176
10	1.5	0.176
12	1.6	0.204
1	1.6	0.204
6	1.7	0.230
2	1.8	0.255
8	2.1	0.322
4	2.6	0.415
11	3.8	0.580
7	<u>7.2</u>	<u>0.857</u>
$\Sigma =$	28.0	3.644

and the right using a logarithmic scale. Notice the dotted line on the normal scale appears to be skewed while the logarithmic scale appears to be more bell-shaped. A positively skewed distribution, as seen above, is often referred to as a **log-normal distribution** (Figure 5.5).

To illustrate this process, consider the T_{max} data observed in 12 health volunteers, which appears in Table 5.4. The arithmetic mean ($\overline{X}$) is 2.33 and the median is 1.65. The few extreme scores in this skewed distribution have pulled the mean to the right of the median. The conversion to a logarithmic transformation of scores is seen in the last column of Table 5.4. The mean for the logarithmic transformed scores is:

$$Average\ log = \frac{0.079 + 0.146 + ...0.857}{12} = 0.304$$

Converted back to the antilog, the geometric mean is:

$$\overline{X}_G = antilog\ (0.304) = 2.01$$

Notice that the geometric mean is much closer to the median of the original distribution of T_{max} data. An alternate formula for calculating the geometric mean is to take the nth-root of the product of all the observations:

$$\overline{X}_G = \sqrt[n]{product\ of\ all\ data} \qquad \text{Eq. 5.11}$$

This gives the same result as the logarithmic transformation.

$$\overline{X}_G = \sqrt[12]{1.2\ x\ 1.4\ x\ 1.5\ x ...7.2} = 2.01$$

Positively skewed distributions are also referred to as **log-normal distributions**.

Alternative Computational Methods for Calculating Central Tendency

Various other methods can be used to determine sample means and standard deviations. They include calculations from binomial distributions, probability distributions, and frequency distributions.

Binomial Distribution. As mentioned in Chapter 2, the binomial distribution is concerned with two mutually exclusive outcomes. If the probability of one of the outcomes is known, the mean (or **expected value**, $E(x)$) and standard deviation for the distribution can be calculated. In this case the measure of central tendency represents the mean and standard deviation of the values taken by the variable in many repeated binomial experiments. For example, if we flipped a fair coin 1000 times, we would expect on the average to have 500 heads (defined as success with p=0.50). The mean is

$$\overline{X}\ or\ E(x) = n \cdot p \qquad \text{Eq. 5.12}$$

with a variance of

$$S^2\ or\ Var(x) = n \cdot p \cdot q \qquad \text{Eq. 5.13}$$

and standard deviation of

$$S = \sqrt{n \cdot p \cdot q} \qquad \text{Eq. 5.14}$$

where p is the probability of success, q the probability of failure ($1.00 - p$) and n is total number of outcomes or observations. The binomial distribution tends to the normal distribution as n increases, however, in small samples the distribution may be noticeably skewed. For that reason, np should be greater than 5 to use this approximation.

As an example, the probability of rolling a six on one toss of the die is 0.1667. If a single die is tossed 50 times what is the expected number of times a six will appear? What is the variability of this expected outcome? In this case $p(6) = 1/6 = 0.1667$; q(not 6) $= 1 - 0.1667 = 0.8333$; and n is 50 for the sample size.

$$E(x) = np = (50)(0.1667) = 8.3$$

The average number of times six would appear in 50 rolls is 8.3 times. The standard deviation would be:

$$S = \sqrt{npq} = \sqrt{(50)(0.1667)(0.833)} = 2.6$$

Probability Distribution. If the probabilities of all possible outcomes are known, the mean and standard deviation for the distribution can be calculated by first creating a table:

x	p(x)	x·p(x)	x²·p(x)
x_1	$p(x_1)$	$x_1 \cdot p(x_1)$	$x_1 \cdot x_1 \cdot p(x_1)$
x_2	$p(x_2)$	$x_2 \cdot p(x_2)$	$x_2 \cdot x_2 \cdot p(x_2)$
x_3	$p(x_3)$	$x_3 \cdot p(x_3)$	$x_3 \cdot x_3 \cdot p(x_3)$
...	...	...	...
x_n	$p(x_n)$	$x_n \cdot p(x_n)$	$x_n \cdot x_n \cdot p(x_n)$
$\Sigma =$	1.00	$\Sigma(x \cdot p(x))$	$\Sigma(x^2 \cdot p(x))$

where x_i is the occurrence and $p(x_i)$ is the probability of that occurrence. The mean is represented by the third column:

$$\overline{X} = \Sigma(x \cdot p(x)) \qquad \text{Eq. 5.15}$$

The variance and standard deviations involve the sums of the third and fourth columns:

$$S^2 = [\Sigma(x^2 \cdot p(x))] - [\Sigma(x \cdot p(x))]^2 \qquad \text{Eq. 5.16}$$

$$S = \sqrt{[\Sigma(x^2 \cdot p(x))] - [\Sigma(x \cdot p(x))]^2}$$ Eq. 5.17

To illustrate the process, what is the mean and standard deviation for the following values and their respective probabilities of occurrence?

Value	Probability	Value	Probability	Value	Probability
0	0.07776	4	0.11646	8	0.00017
1	0.22680	5	0.04042	9	0.00001
2	0.29700	6	0.00971	10	0.00000
3	0.22995	7	0.00150		

x	$p(x)$	$x \cdot p(x)$	$x^2 \cdot p(x)$
1	0.22680	0.22680	0.22680
2	0.29700	0.59400	1.18800
3	0.22995	0.68985	2.06955
4	0.11646	0.46584	1.86336
5	0.04042	0.20210	1.01050
6	0.00971	0.05826	0.34956
7	0.00150	0.01050	0.07350
8	0.00017	0.00136	0.01088
9	0.00001	0.00009	0.00081
10	0.00000	0.00000	0.00000
$\Sigma =$	1.00000	2.24880	6.79296

$$\overline{X} = \Sigma(x \cdot p(x)) = 2.2488 = 2.25$$

$$S^2 = [\Sigma(x^2 \cdot p(x))] - [\Sigma(x \cdot p(x))]^2$$

$$S^2 = 6.79296 - (2.24880)^2 = 1.74$$

$$S = \sqrt{S^2} = \sqrt{1.74} = 1.32$$

Frequency Distribution. If data is presented that reports the frequency of each occurrence (for example, the frequency of response to a Likert-type scale), the mean and standard deviation can be calculated as follows where x_i is the event and $f(x_i)$ is the frequency associated with that event.

$\underline{x}$	$\underline{f(x)}$	$\underline{x \cdot f(x)}$	$\underline{x^2 \cdot f(x)}$
x_1	$f(x_1)$	$x_1 \cdot f(x_1)$	$x_1 \cdot x_1 \cdot f(x_1)$
x_2	$f(x_2)$	$x_2 \cdot f(x_2)$	$x_2 \cdot x_2 \cdot f(x_2)$
x_3	$f(x_3)$	$x_3 \cdot f(x_3)$	$x_3 \cdot x_3 \cdot f(x_3)$
...	...	...	...
$\underline{x_n}$	$f(x_n)$	$x_n \cdot f(x_n)$	$x_n \cdot x_n \cdot f(x_n)$
$\Sigma =$	$\overline{\Sigma f(x)} = N$	$\overline{\Sigma(x \cdot f(x))}$	$\overline{\Sigma(x^2 \cdot f(x))}$

The mean is:

$$\overline{X} = \frac{\Sigma(x \cdot f(x))}{N}$$

Eq. 5.18

In this case N represents the sum of all the sample frequencies $(n_1 + n_2 ... + n_i)$ and not a population N. The variance is:

$$S^2 = \frac{N[\Sigma(x^2 \cdot f(x))] - [\Sigma(x \cdot f(x))]^2}{N(N-1)}$$

Eq. 5.19

with a standard deviation of:

$$S = \sqrt{\frac{N[\Sigma(x^2 \cdot f(x))] - [\Sigma(x \cdot f(x))]^2}{N(N-1)}}$$

Eq. 5.20

For an example using a frequency distribution, a final examination in which 12 pharmacy students scored 10 points, 28 scored 9, 35 scored 8, 26 scored 7, 15 scored 6, 8 scored 5 and one student scored 4. What is the mean and standard deviation on this final examination?

$\underline{x}$	$\underline{f(x)}$	$\underline{x \cdot f(x)}$	$\underline{x^2 \cdot f(x)}$
10	12	120	1,200
9	28	252	2,268
8	35	280	2,240
7	26	182	1,274
6	15	90	540
5	8	40	200
4	$\underline{1}$	$\underline{4}$	$\underline{16}$
$\Sigma =$	125	968	7,738

$$\overline{X} = \frac{\Sigma(x \cdot f(x))}{N} = \frac{968}{125} = 7.74$$

$$S^2 = \frac{N \left[\Sigma(x^2 \cdot f(x)) \right] - \left[\Sigma(x \cdot f(x)) \right]^2}{N(N-1)} = \frac{125(7738) - (968)^2}{125(124)} = 1.95$$

$$S = \sqrt{S^2} = \sqrt{1.95} = 1.40$$

Central Tendency from a Histogram. An estimate of the mean and standard deviation involves using the frequency distribution and the midpoint of each interval:

$$Midpoint = \frac{highest + lowest\ points}{2} = \frac{705.5 + 716.5}{2} = 711 \qquad \text{Eq. 5.21}$$

A table can be prepared by tabulating the midpoint and their associated frequencies:

Interval Range	Midpoint (m_i)	Frequency (f_i)	$\overline{X}$ $m_i f_i$	S $m_i^2 f_i$
Interval 1	m_1	f_1	$m_1 f_1$	$m_1{}^2 f_1$
Interval 2	m_2	f_2	$m_2 f_2$	$m_2{}^2 f_2$
Interval 3	m_3	f_3	$m_3 f_3$	$m_3{}^2 f_3$
...	...	...	...	...
Interval n	m_n	f_n	$m_n f_n$	$m_n{}^2 f_n$
$\Sigma =$		125	$\Sigma m_i f_i$	$\Sigma m_i^2 f_i$

The midpoint of each class interval, m_i, was weighted by its corresponding frequency of occurrence, f_i. The computation of the mean and standard deviation involves a table similar to that used for frequency distributions discussed under central tendency. With a mean of

$$\overline{X} = \frac{\Sigma m_i f_i}{N} \qquad \text{Eq. 5.22}$$

a variance of

$$S^2 = \frac{n(\sum m_i^2 f_i) - (\sum m_i f_i)^2}{n(n-1)} \qquad \text{Eq. 5.23}$$

and a standard deviation as the square root of the variance or

$$S = \sqrt{\frac{n(\sum m_i^2 f_i) - (\sum m_i f_i)^2}{n(n-1)}} \qquad \text{Eq. 5.24}$$

Using the pharmacokinetic example in Chapter 4 (Table 4.3), the mean and standard deviation are calculated below. How accurate is the measure of the mean and standard deviation using Sturge's Rule to create the histogram? The data is presented in Table 5.5 and the calculation of the mean and standard deviation using the above formulas are presented below. The sample statistics for all the observations presented in the original table of C_{max} is: Mean = 752.4 mcg and S.D. = 16.8 mcg. In this particular case, there is less than 5% difference between the means and standard deviations, which were calculated from the raw data and calculated from the intervals created by Sturge's Rule.

$$\overline{X} = \frac{94,111}{125} = 752.9 \, mcg$$

Table 5.5 Intervals Created Using Sturge's Rule for Table 4.3

Interval Range	Midpoint	Frequency	$m_i f_i$	$m_i^2 f_i$
705.5-716.5	711	2	1,422	1,011,042
716.5-727.5	722	6	4,332	3,127,704
727.5-738.5	733	18	13,194	9,671,202
738.5-749.5	744	22	16,368	12,177,792
759.5-760.5	755	35	26,425	19,950,875
760.5-771.5	766	28	21,448	16,429,168
771.5-782.5	777	10	7,770	6,037,290
782.5-793.5	788	4	3,152	2,483,776
$\sum =$		125	94,111	70,888,849

$$S^2 = \frac{125(70,888,849) - (94,111)^2}{125(124)}$$

$$S^2 = \frac{4,225.804}{15,500} = 272.63$$

$$S = \sqrt{S^2} = \sqrt{272.63} = 16.51 \ mcg$$

Reference

Evans, D.A.P., et al. (1960). "Genetic control of isoniazid metabolism in man." British Medical Journal 2:489.

Suggested Supplemental readings

Daniel, W.W. (1991). Biostatistics: A Foundation for Analysis in the Health Sciences, John Wiley and Sons, New York, pp. 19-38.

Forthofer, R.N. and Lee, E.S. (1995). Introduction to Biostatistics: A Guide to Design, Analysis and Discovery, Academic Press, San Diego, pp. 61-67, 71-77.

Snedecor, G.W. and Cochran W.G. (1989). Statistical Methods, Iowa State University Press, Ames, IA, pp.26-36.

Example Problems

1. Report the various measures for central tendency for the 30 samples of tetracycline capsules presented in Table 4.1.

2. Listed below are the results of a first time in humans clinical trial of a new agent with 90 mg/tablet administered to six healthy male volunteers. Report the measures of central tendency for these C_{max} results.

C_{max} for Initial Pharmacokinetic with New Agent	
Subject Number	C_{max} (ng/ml)
001	60
002	71
003	111
004	46
005	81
006	96

3. Pharmacy students completing the final examination for a pharmacokinetics course received the following scores (Table 5.6). Report the range, median, mean, variance and standard deviation for these results.

Table 5.6   Student Final Examination Results

Student	%	Student	%	Student	%	Student	%
001	85	009	78	017	77	025	97
002	79	010	85	018	83	026	76
003	98	011	77	019	87	027	69
004	84	012	86	020	78	028	86
005	72	013	90	021	60	029	80
006	84	014	84	022	88	030	92
007	70	015	75	023	87	031	85
008	90	016	96	024	82	032	80

4. Listed in Table 5.7 are the times to maximum concentration observed during a clinical trial. It is believed that the data is positively skewed. Calculate the median, mean and geometric mean. Based on the sample, does the population appear to be positively skewed?

Table 5.7   Clinical Trial Results - T_{max} (in hours)

Subject	t_{max}	Subject	t_{max}	Subject	t_{max}
A	1.41	F	1.96	K	1.62
B	1.81	G	0.78	L	1.15
C	3.25	H	1.51	M	2.03
D	1.37	I	1.18	N	2.21
E	1.09	J	2.56	O	0.91

5. Calculate the measures of central tendency for noradrenaline levels (nmol/L) obtained during a clinical trial involving 15 subjects.

2.5	2.6	2.5	2.4	2.4
2.5	2.5	2.6	2.5	2.6
2.3	2.7	2.3	2.8	2.2

6. Calculate the measures of central tendency for prolactin levels (ng/L) obtained during a clinical trial involving 10 subjects.

9.4	7.0	7.6	6.3	6.7
8.6	6.8	10.6	8.9	9.4

7. In a study designed to measure the effectiveness of a new analgesic agent, 8 mg of drug was administered to 15 laboratory animals. The animals were subjected to the Randall-Selitto paw pressure test and the following results (in grams) were observed.

Number	Response	Number	Response	Number	Response
1	240	6	260	11	265
2	295	7	275	12	240
3	225	8	245	13	260
4	250	9	225	14	275
5	245	10	260	15	250

Calculate the mean, median, variance and standard deviation for this data.

Answers to Problems

1. Report the various measures for central tendency for the 30 samples of tetracycline capsules presented in Table 4.1.

   a. Mode = 250

   b. Median = 250

   c. Sample mean

   $$\overline{X} = \frac{\Sigma x}{n} = \frac{251 + 250 + 253 + \ldots 249}{30} = 250 \, mg$$

d. Population mean

$$\mu = \frac{\sum x}{N} = \frac{251 + 250 + 253 + \ldots 249}{30} = 250 \, mg$$

e. Range = 254-245 = 9

f. Sample variance

$$S^2 = \frac{\sum (x_i - \overline{X})^2}{n-1} = \frac{(251 - 250)^2 + \ldots (249 - 250)^2}{29} = 4.90$$

g. Population variance

$$\sigma^2 = \frac{\sum (x_i - \mu)^2}{N} = \frac{(251 - 250)^2 + \ldots (249 - 250)^2}{30} = 4.73$$

h. Sample standard deviation

$$S = \sqrt{S^2} = \sqrt{4.90} = 2.21 \, mg$$

i. Population standard deviation

$$\sigma = \sqrt{\sigma^2} = \sqrt{4.73} = 2.17 \, mg$$

j. Coefficient of variation

$$CV = \frac{S}{\overline{X}} = \frac{2.21}{250} = 0.0088$$

k. Relative standard deviation

$$RSD = CV \times 100 = 0.0088 \times 100 = 0.88\%$$

2. Measures of central tendency for the C_{max} results in the six healthy male volunteers are as follows:

$$
\begin{array}{cc}
\underline{x} & \underline{x^2} \\
60 & 3600 \\
71 & 5041 \\
111 & 12321 \\
46 & 2116 \\
81 & 6561 \\
\underline{96} & \underline{9216} \\
\Sigma = \quad 465 & 38855
\end{array}
$$

a. Mean

$$\overline{X} = \frac{\Sigma x}{n} = \frac{465}{6} = 77.5$$

b. Variance

$$S^2 = \frac{n(\Sigma X^2) - (\Sigma X)^2}{n(n-1)} = \frac{6(38855) - (465)^2}{6(5)} = \frac{16905}{30} = 563.5$$

c. Standard deviation

$$S = \sqrt{S^2} = \sqrt{563.5} = 23.74$$

d. Relative standard deviation

$$CV = \frac{standard\ deviation}{mean} = \frac{23.74}{77.5} = 0.306$$

$$RSD = CV \times 100\ (percent) = 0.306 \times 100 = 30.6$$

3. Final examination results for a pharmacokinetics course (Table 5.8):

   a. Range: Highest - lowest grade = 98 - 60 = 38 percent

   b. Median: Value between 16th and 17th observation = 84 percent

Table 5.8 Examination Results Ranked
in Descending Order

98	87	84	77
96	86	83	77
95	86	82	76
92	85	80	75
90	85	80	72
90	85	79	70
88	84	78	69
87	84	78	60

c. Sample mean

$$\overline{X} = \frac{\Sigma x}{n} = \frac{85 + 79 + 98 + ... 85 + 80}{32} = 82.4 \ percent$$

d. Sample variance

$$S^2 = \frac{(85 - 82.4)^2 + (79 - 82.4)^2 + ...(80 - 82.4)^2}{31} = 67.16$$

e. Sample standard deviation

$$S = \sqrt{S^2} = \sqrt{67.16} = 8.19 \ percent$$

4. Clinical trials data with possible skewed data (Table 5.9):

a. Median = 1.51 hours

b. Arithmetic mean

$$\overline{X} = \frac{\Sigma x}{n} = \frac{24.84}{15} = 1.66 \ hours$$

c. Geometric mean

$$\overline{X_G} = \sqrt[n]{product \ of \ all \ data}$$

Table 5.9 t_{max} Results in Ascending Order

Subject	t_{max}	Subject	t_{max}
G	0.78	K	1.62
O	0.91	B	1.81
E	1.09	F	1.96
L	1.15	M	2.03
I	1.18	N	2.21
D	1.37	J	2.56
A	1.41	C	3.25
H	1.51	$\Sigma =$	24.84

$$\overline{X_G} = \sqrt[15]{0.78 \, x \, 0.91 \, x \, 1.09 \, x \ldots 3.25} = 1.54$$

It can be assumed that the distribution is positively skewed, because the mean is larger than the median (pulled to the right) and the geometric mean is much closer to the median.

3. Noradrenaline levels obtained during a clinical trial.

x	x^2
2.5	6.25
2.5	6.25
2.3	5.29
2.6	6.76
2.5	6.25
2.7	7.29
2.5	6.25
2.6	6.76
2.3	5.29
2.4	5.76
2.5	6.25
2.8	7.84
2.4	5.76
2.6	6.76
2.2	4.84
$\Sigma x = 37.4$	$93.60 = \Sigma x^2$

Mean

$$\overline{X} = \frac{\Sigma x}{n} = \frac{37.4}{15} = 2.49 \, nmol/L$$

Variance

$$S^2 = \frac{n(\Sigma X^2) - (\Sigma X)^2}{n(n-1)} = \frac{15(93.6) - (37.4)^2}{(15)(14)} = 0.025$$

Standard Deviation

$$S = \sqrt{S^2} = \sqrt{0.025} = 0.158 \, nmol \, / \, L$$

6. Prolactin levels obtained during a clinical trial.

	$\underline{x}$	$\underline{x^2}$	
	9.4	88.36	
	8.6	73.96	
	7.0	49.00	
	6.8	46.24	
	7.6	57.76	
	10.6	112.36	
	6.3	39.69	
	8.9	79.21	
	6.7	44.89	
	9.4	88.36	
$\Sigma x =$	81.3	679.83	$= \Sigma x^2$

Mean

$$\overline{X} = \frac{\Sigma x}{n} = \frac{81.3}{10} = 8.13 \, ng/L$$

Variance

$$S^2 = \frac{\Sigma(x_i - \overline{X})^2}{n-1}$$

$$S^2 = \frac{(9.4 - 8.13)^2 + (8.6 - 8.13)^2 \ldots + (9.4 - 8.13)^2}{9} = 2.096$$

Standard deviation

$$S = \sqrt{S^2} = \sqrt{2.096} = 1.45\, ng\, /\, L$$

7. Randall-Selitto paw pressure test and the following results (in grams) were observed.

$$\Sigma x = 3{,}810 \qquad \Sigma x^2 = 972{,}800 \qquad n = 15$$

Sample mean

$$\overline{X} = \frac{\Sigma x}{n} = \frac{3810}{15} = 254\ grams$$

Sample variance

$$S^2 = \frac{n(\Sigma X^2) - (\Sigma X)^2}{n(n-1)} = \frac{15(972{,}800) - (3{,}810)^2}{15(14)} = 361.4$$

Sample standard deviation

$$S = \sqrt{S^2} = \sqrt{361.4} = 19.0\ grams$$

Median = eighth response in rank order = 250 grams

6

The Normal Distribution and Confidence Intervals

Described as a "bell shaped" curve, the normal distribution is a symmetrical distribution which is one of the most commonly occurring outcomes in nature and its presence is assumed in several of the most commonly used statistical tests. Properties of the normal distribution have a very important role in the statistical theory of drawing inferences about population parameters (estimating confidence intervals) based on samples drawn from that population.

The Normal Distribution

The normal distribution is the most important distribution in statistics. This curve is a special frequency distribution that describes the population distribution of many continuously distributed biological traits. The normal distribution is often referred to as the **Gaussian distribution**, after the mathematician Carl Friedreich Gauss, even though it was first discovered by the French mathematician Abraham DeMoivre (Porter, 1986).

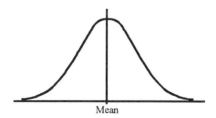

Mean

It is critical at this point to realize that we are focusing our initial discussion on the *total population, not a sample*. As mentioned in the previous chapter, in the population, the mean is expressed as μ and standard deviation as σ.

The characteristics of a normal distribution are as follows. First, the normal distribution is continuous and the curve is symmetrical about the mean. Second, the mode, median, and mean are equal and represent the middle of the distribution. Third, since the mean and median are the same, the 50th percentile is at the mean with an equal amount of area under the curve, above and below the mean. Fourth, the probability of all possible outcomes is equal to 1.0, therefore, the total area under the curve is equal to 1.0. Since the mean is the 50th percentle, the area to left or right of the mean equals 0.5. Fifth, by definition, the area under the curve between one standard deviation above and one standard deviation below the mean contains an area equal to approximately 68% of the total area under the curve. At two standard deviations this area is approximately 95%. Sixth, as distance from the mean (in the positive or negative direction) approaches infinity, the frequency of occurrences approaches zero. This last point illustrates the fact that most observations cluster around the center of the distribution and very few occur at the extremes of the distribution. Also, if the curve is infinite in its bounds we cannot set absolute external limits on the distribution.

The frequency distribution (curve) for a normal distribution is defined as follows:

$$f_i = \frac{1}{\sigma\sqrt{2\pi}} e^{-(x_i-\mu)^2/2\sigma^2} \qquad \text{Eq. 6.1}$$

where: π (pi) = 3.14159 and e = 2.71828 (the base of natural logarithms).

In a normal distribution, the area under the curve between the mean and one standard deviation is approximately 34%. Because of the symmetry of the distribution, 68% of the curve would be divided equally above and below the mean. Why 34%? Why not a nice round number like 35%, 30%, or even better 25%? The standard deviation is that point of inflection on the normal curve where the frequency distribution stops its descent to the baseline and begins to pull parallel with the x-axis. Areas or proportions of the normal distribution associated with various standard deviations are seen in Figure 6.1.

The term "*the* bell-shaped curve" is a misnomer since there are many bell-shaped curves, ranging from those which are extremely peaked with very small ranges to those which are much flatter with wide distributions (Figure 6.2). A normal distribution is completely dependent on its parameters of μ and σ. A

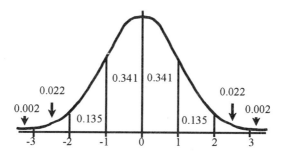

Figure 6.1 Proportions between various standard deviations under a normal distribution.

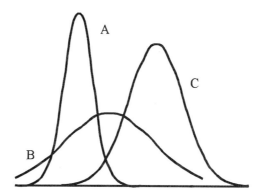

Figure 6.2 Example of three normal distributions with different means and different standard deviations.

standardized normal distribution has been created to compare and compute variations in such a distribution regardless of center or spread from the center. In this standard normal distribution the mean equals 0 (Figure 6.3). The spread of the distribution is also standardized by setting one standard deviation equal to +1 or -1, and two standard deviations equal to +2 or –2 (Figure 6.4).

As seen previously, the area between +2 and -2 is approximately 95%. Additionally, fractions of a standard deviation are calculated and their equivalent areas presented. If such a distribution can be created (with a mean equal to zero and standard deviation equal to one) then the equation for the frequency distribution can be simplified to:

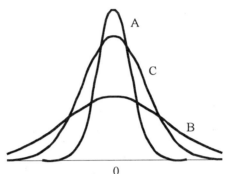

Figure 6.3 Example of three normal distributions with the same mean and different standard deviations.

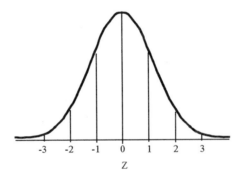

Figure 6.4 Standard normal distribution.

$$f_i = \frac{1}{\sqrt{2\pi}} e^{-(x_i)^2/2}$$

$$f_i = \frac{1}{2.5066272} 2.71828^{-(x_i)^2/2}$$

$$f_i = 1.0844371^{-(x_i)^2/2} \qquad \text{Eq. 6.2}$$

Table 6.1 is an abbreviation of a Standard Normal Distribution (a more complete distribution is presented in Table B2 in Appendix B, where every hundredth of the z-distribution is defined between 0.01 to 3.09). An important

Table 6.1 Selected Areas of a Normal Standardized Distribution (Proportion of the Curve Between 0 and z)

z	Area	z	Area	z	Area
.00	.0000	1.00	.3413	2.00	.4772
.05	.0199	1.05	.3531	2.05	.4798
.10	.0398	1.10	.3543	2.10	.4821
.15	.0596	1.15	.3749	2.15	.4842
.20	.0793	1.20	.3849	2.20	.4861
.25	.0987	1.25	.3944	2.25	.4878
.30	.1179	1.30	.4032	2.30	.4893
.35	.1368	1.35	.4115	2.35	.4906
.40	.1554	1.40	.4192	2.40	.4918
.45	.1736	1.45	.4265	2.45	.4929
.50	.1915	1.50	.4332	2.50	.4938
.55	.2088	1.55	.4394	2.55	.4946
.60	.2257	1.60	.4452	2.60	.4953
.65	.2422	1.65	.4505	2.65	.4960
.70	.2580	1.70	.4554	2.70	.4965
.75	.2734	1.75	.4599	2.75	.4970
.80	.2881	1.80	.4641	2.80	.4974
.85	.3023	1.85	.4678	2.85	.4978
.90	.3159	1.90	.4713	2.90	.4981
.95	.3289	1.95	.4744	2.95	.4984

feature of the standard normal distribution is that the number of standard deviations away from the population mean can be expressed as a given percent or proportion of the area of the curve. The symbol z, by convention, symbolizes the number of standard deviations away from the population mean. The numbers in these tables represent the area of the curve which falls between the mean ($z = 0$) and that point on the distribution <u>above</u> the mean (i.e., $z = +1.5$, would be the point at 1.5 standard deviations above the mean). Since the mean is the 50th percentile, the area of the curve that falls below the mean (or below zero) is .5000. Because a normal distribution is symmetrical, this table could also represent the various areas below the mean. For example, for $z = -1.5$ (or 1.5 standard deviations below the mean), z represents the same area from 0 to -1.5, as the area from 0 to +1.5. A z-value tells us how far above and below the mean any given score is in units of the standard deviation.

Using the information in Table 6.1, the area under the curve that falls below +2 would be the area between +2 and 0, plus the area below 0.

Area (<+2) = Area (between 0 and +2) + Area (below 0)
Area (<+2) = .4772 + .5000 = .9772

These probabilities can be summed because of the addition theorem discussed in Chapter 2.

All possible events would fall within this standard normal distribution ($p\Sigma(x) = 1.00$). Since the probability of all events equals 1.00 and the total area under the curve equals 1, then various areas within a normalized standard distribution can also represent probabilities of certain outcomes. In the above example, the area under the curve below two standard deviations (represented as +2) was .9972. This can also be thought of as the probability of an outcome being less than two standard deviations above the mean. Conversely, the probability of being two or more standard deviations above the mean would be 1.0000 - .9772 or .0228.

Between three standard deviations above and below the mean, approximately 99.8% of the observations will occur. Therefore, assuming a normal distribution, a quick method for roughly approximating the standard deviation is to divide the range of the observations by six, since almost all observations will fall within these six intervals. For example, consider the data in Table 4.3. The true standard deviation for this data is 16.8 mcg. The range of 86 mcg, divided by six would give a rough approximation of 14.3 mcg.

It is possible to calculate the probability of any particular outcome within a normal distribution. The areas within specified portions of our curve represent the probability of the values of interest lying between the vertical lines. To illustrate this, consider a large container of tablets (representing a total population) which is expected to be normally distributed with respect to the tablet weight. What is the probability of randomly sampling a tablet that weighs within 1.5 standard deviations of the mean?

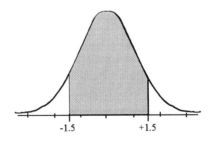

Because weight is a continuous variable, we are concerned with p(>-1.5 or <+1.5). From Table 6.1:

p(z<+1.5) = Area between 0 and +1.5 =   .4332
p(z>-1.5) = Area between 0 and -1.5 =   .4332
p(z -1.5 to +1.5) =   .8664

There is a probability of .8664 (or 87% chance) of sampling a tablet within 1.5 standard deviations of the mean. What is the probability of sampling a tablet greater than 2.25 standard deviations above the mean?

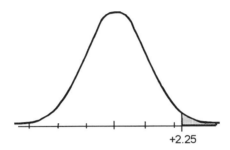

+2.25

First, we know that the total area above the mean is .5000. By reading Table 6.1, the area between 2.25 standard deviations (z = 2.25) and the mean is .4878 (the area between 0 and +2.25). Therefore the probability of sampling a tablet weighing more than 2.25 standard deviations above the mean weight is:

$$p(z>+2.25) \ = \ .5000 - .4878 \ = \ .0122$$

If we wish to know the probability of a tablet being less than 2.25 standard deviations above the mean, the complement probability of being less than a z-value of +2.25 is:

$$p(z<+2.25) = 1 - p(z>+2.25) = 1.000 - .0122 = .9878$$

Also calculated as:

$$p(z<+2.25) = p(z<0) + p(z<2.25) = .5000 + .4878 = .9878$$

If the mean and standard deviation of a population are known, the exact location (z above or below the mean) for any observation can be calculated using the following formula:

$$z = \frac{x - \mu}{\sigma}$$ Eq. 6.3

Because values in a normal distribution are on a continuous scale and are handled as continuous variables, we must correct for continuity. Values for *x* would be as follows:

Likelihood of being: greater then 185 mg =   p(>185.5);
less than 200 mg =   p(<199.5);
200 mg or greater =   p(>199.5); and
between and including 185 and 200 mg =   p(>184.5 and <200.5).

To examine this, consider a sample from a known population with expected population parameters (previous estimates of the population mean and standard deviation, for example based on prior production runs). With an expected population mean assay of 750 mg and a population standard deviation of 60 mg, what is the probability of sampling a capsule with an assay greater than 850 mg?

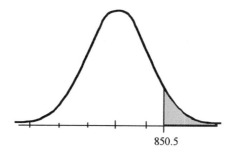

850.5

As a continuous variable, the p(>850 mg) is actually p(>850.5 mg) when corrected for continuity.

$$z = \frac{x - \mu}{\sigma} = \frac{850.5 - 750}{60} = \frac{100.5}{60} = +1.68$$

p(z>+1.68)   = .5000 - p(z<1.68)
            = .5000 - .4535 = .0465

Given the same population as above, what is the probability of randomly sampling a capsule with an assay between 700 and 825 mg?

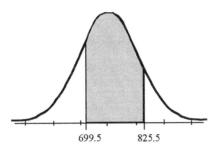

699.5   825.5

Once again correcting for continuity, p(<825 mg) is rewritten as p(<825.5 mg) and p(>700 mg) is really p(>699.5 mg).

$$z = \frac{x-\mu}{\sigma} = \frac{825.5-750}{60} = \frac{75.5}{60} = +1.26$$

$$z = \frac{x-\mu}{\sigma} = \frac{699.5-750}{60} = \frac{-50.5}{60} = -0.84$$

$$
\begin{aligned}
p(\text{between } 699.5 \text{ and } 825.5) &= p(z<+1.26) + p(z>-0.84) \\
&= .3962 + .2995 = .6957
\end{aligned}
$$

Given the same population, what is the probability of randomly sampling a capsule with an assay less than 600 mg?

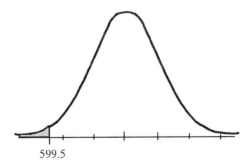

599.5

As a continuous variable, p(<600 mg) is p(>599.5 mg):

$$z = \frac{x-\mu}{\sigma} = \frac{599.5-750}{60} = \frac{-150.5}{60} = -2.5$$

$$p(z<-2.5) = .5000 - p(z<2.5)$$
$$= .5000 - .4938 = .0062$$

Thus, in these examples with the given population mean and standard deviation, the likelihood of randomly sampling a capsule greater than 850 mg is approximately 5%, a capsule less than 600 mg is less than 1%, and a capsule between 700 and 825 mg is almost 70%.

Lastly, the probability of obtaining any one particular value is zero, but we can determine probabilities for specific ranges. Correcting for continuity, the value 750 (the mean) actually represents an infinite number of possible values between 749.5 and 750.5 mg. The area under the curve between the center and the upper limit would be

$$z = \frac{x - \mu}{\sigma} = \frac{750.5 - 750}{60} = \frac{0.5}{60} = 0.01$$

$$p(z<0.01) = .004$$

Since there would be an identical area between 749.5 and the mean, the total proportion associated with 750 mg would be

$$p(750 \text{ mg}) = .008$$

In the previous examples we knew both the population mean (μ) and the population standard deviation (σ). However, in most statistical investigations this information is not available and formulas must be employed that use estimates of these parameters based on the sample results.

Important z-values related to other areas under the curve for a normal distribution include:

$$90\% \quad -1.64 < z < +1.64$$
$$95\% \quad -1.96 < z < +1.96$$
$$99\% \quad -2.57 < z < +2.57$$

Determining if the Distribution is Normal

The sample selected is our best guess at the composition of the population: the center, the dispersion, and the shape of the distribution. Therefore, the appearance of the sample is our best estimate if the population is normally distributed. In the absence of any information which would disprove normality, it is assumed that a normal distribution exists (i.e., initial sample results look extremely skewed or bimodal).

One quick method to determine if the population is normally distributed is to determine if the sample mean and median are approximately equal. If they are about the same (similar in value) then the population probably has a normal distribution. If the mean is substantially greater than the median, the population is probably positively skewed and if the mean is substantially less than the median, a negatively skewed population probably exists. Other methods for determining normality would be to: 1) plot the distribution on graph paper; 2) plot histogram cumulative frequencies on probability paper; or 3) do a chi square goodness-of-fit test (described in Chapter 15).

Simple visual methods to determine if sample data is consistent with expectations for a normal distribution is to plot a **cumulative frequency curve** or use special graph paper known as **probability paper.** In a cumulative frequency curve, data is arranged in order of increasing size and plotted on normal graph paper:

$$\% \text{ cumulative frequency} = \frac{cumulative\ frequency}{n} \times 100$$

If the data came from a normally distributed population, the result will be an S-shaped curve.

Probability paper has a unique non-linear scale (i.e., National #12-083 or Keuffel and Esser #46-8000) on the cumulative frequency axis which will convert the S-shaped curve to a straight line. If a straight line can be drawn through the percent cumulative frequency data points, the estimated population is normally distributed. If the curvilinearly relationship exists, the population is skewed.

Sampling Distribution

If we have a population and withdraw a random sample of observations from that population, we could calculate a sample mean and a sample standard deviation. As mentioned previously, this information would be our best estimate of the true population parameters.

$$\overline{X}_{sample} \approx \mu_{population}$$
$$S_{sample} \approx \sigma_{population}$$

The characteristics of dispersion or variability are not unique to samples alone. Individual samples can also vary around the population mean. Just by chance, or luck, we could have sampled from the upper or lower ends of the population distribution and calculated a sample mean that was too high or too low. Through no fault of our own, our estimate of the population mean would be erroneous.

To illustrate this point, let us return to the pharmacokinetic data used in Chapter 4. From this example, we will assume that the data in Table 4.3 represented the *entire population* of pharmacokinetic studies ever conducted on this drug. Due to budgetary restraints or time, we were only able to analyze five samples from this population. How many possible ways could five samples be randomly selected from this data? Based on the combination formula (Eq. 2.11) there would be

$$\binom{125}{5} = \frac{125!}{5!\,120!} = 234,531,275$$

possible ways. Thus, it is possible to sample these 125 values in over 234 million different ways and because they are sampled at random, each possible combination has an equal likelihood of being selected. Therefore, by chance alone we could sample the smallest five values in our population (Sample A) or the largest five (Sample D) or any combination in between these extremes (Table 6.2). Samples B and C were generated using the Random Numbers Table B1 in Appendix B.

The mean is a more efficient estimate measure of the center, because with repeated samples of the same size from a given population, the mean will show less variation than either the mode or the median. Statisticians have defined this outcome as the central limit theorem and its derivation is beyond the scope of this book. However, there are three important characteristics that will be utilized in future statistical tests.

1. The mean of all possible sample means is equal to the mean of the original population from which they were sampled.

$$\overline{X_{\bar{x}}} = \mu \qquad\qquad \text{Eq. 6.4}$$

If we averaged all 234,531,275 possible sample means, this grand mean or **mean of the mean** would equal the population mean ($\mu = 752.4$ mcg for $N = 125$) from which they were sampled.

Table 6.2 Possible Samples from Population Presented as Table 4.3

	Sample A	Sample B	Sample C	Sample D
	706	731	724	778
	714	760	752	785
	718	752	762	788
	720	736	734	790
	724	785	775	793
Mean =	716.4	752.8	749.4	786.8
S.D. =	6.8	21.5	20.6	5.7

2. The standard deviation for all possible sample means is equal to the population standard deviation divided by the square root of the sample size.

$$\sigma_{\bar{x}} = \frac{\sigma}{\sqrt{n}} \qquad \text{Eq. 6.5}$$

Similar to the mean of the sample means, the standard deviation for all the possible means would equal the population standard deviation divided by the square root of the sample size. The standard deviation for the means is referred to as the **standard error of the mean** or **SEM**.

3. Regardless of whether the population is normally distributed or skewed, if we plot all the possible sample means, the frequency distribution will approximate that of a normal distribution, based on the **central limit theorem**. This theorem is critical to many statistical formulas because it justifies the assumption of normality. The sampling distribution will approximate a normal distribution, regardless of the distribution of the original population, when the sample size is relatively large. However, a sample size as small as n=30 will often result in a near normal sampling distribution (Kachigan, 1991).

If all 234,531,275 possible means were plotted, they would produce a frequency distribution which is normally distributed. Because the sample means are normally distributed, values in the normal standardized distribution (z distribution), will also apply to the distribution of sample means. For example, of all the possible sample means:

68% fall within + or - 1.00 SEM
90% fall within + or - 1.64 SEM
95% fall within + or - 1.96 SEM
99% fall within + or - 2.57 SEM

The distribution of the mean will be a probability distribution, consisting of various values and their associated probabilities, and if we sample from any population, the resultant means will be distributed on a normal bell shaped curve. Most will be near the center and 5% will be outside 1.96 standard deviations of the distribution.

Standard Error of the Mean versus the Standard Deviation

As seen in the previous section, in a sampling distribution, the overall mean of the means would be equal to the population mean and the dispersion would depend on the amount of variance in the population. Obviously, the more we know about our population (the larger the sample size), the better our estimate of the population center. The best estimate of the population standard deviation is the sample standard deviation, which can be used to replace the σ in Eq. 6.5 to produce a standard error of the mean based on sample data:

$$S_{\bar{x}} = \frac{S}{\sqrt{n}} = SEM \qquad\qquad \text{Eq. 6.6}$$

The standard deviation (S or SD) describes the variability within a sample; whereas, the standard error of the mean (SEM) represents the possible variability of the mean itself. The SEM is sometimes referred to as the **standard error** (SE) and describes the variation of all possible sample means and equals the SD of the sample data divided by the square root of the sample size. As can be seen by the formula, the distribution of sample means (the standard error of the mean) will always be smaller than the dispersion of the sample (the standard deviation).

Authors may erroneously present the distribution of sample results by using the SEM to represent information because there appears to be less variability. This may be misleading since the SEM has a different meaning than the SD. The SEM is smaller than the SD and the intentional presentation of the SEM instead of the larger SD is a manipulation to make data look more precise. The SEM is extremely important in the estimation of a true population mean, based on sample results. However, because it is disproportionately low, it should never be used as a measure of the distribution of sample results. For example, the SEM from our previous example of liquid fill volumes (Table 5.1) is much smaller (by a factor of almost six) than the calculated standard deviation:

$$SEM = \frac{0.835}{\sqrt{30}} = 0.152$$

By convention, the term standard error refers to the variability of a sampling distribution. However, authors still use the standard error of the mean to present sample distributions, because the SEM is much smaller than the SD and presents a much smaller variation of the results. An even more troublesome occurrence is the failure of authors to indicate in reports or publications whether a result represents a SD or a SEM. For example, the reporting of 456.1 ± 1.3, with no indication of what the term to the right of the signs represents. Is this a very tight SD? Is it the SEM? Could it even be the RSD?

Standard error of the mean can be considered as a measure of precision. Obviously, the smaller the SEM, the more confident we can be that our sample mean is closer to the true population mean. However, at the same time, large increases in sample size produce relatively small changes in this measure of precision. For example, using a constant sample SD of 21.5 for sample B, presented above, the measure of SEM changes very little as sample sizes increase past 30 (Figure 6.5). A general rule of thumb is that with samples of 30 or more observations, it is safe to use the sample standard deviation as an estimate of population standard deviation.

Confidence Intervals

As discussed in Chapter 5, using a random sample and independent measures, one can calculate measures of central tendency ($\overline{X}$ and S). The result represents only one sample that belongs to a distribution of many possible sample means. Because we are dealing with a sample and in most cases don't know the true population parameters, we often must make a statistical "guess" at these parameters. For example, the previous samples A through D all have calculated means, any of which could be the true mean for the population from which they were randomly sampled. In order to define the true population mean, we need to allow for a range of possible means based on our estimate:

$$\begin{array}{c} Population \\ Mean \end{array} = \begin{array}{c} Estimate \\ Sample\ Mean \end{array} \pm \begin{array}{c} "Fudge" \\ Factor \end{array}$$

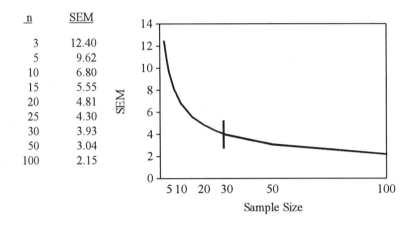

n	SEM
3	12.40
5	9.62
10	6.80
15	5.55
20	4.81
25	4.30
30	3.93
50	3.04
100	2.15

Figure 6.5 Variation in standard error of the means by sample size.

This single estimate of the population mean (based on the sample) can be referred to as a **point estimate**. The result is a range of possible outcomes defined as **boundary values** or **confidence limits**. At the same time, we would like to have a certain amount of confidence in our statement that the population mean falls within these boundary values. For example, we may want to be 95% certain that we are correct, or 99% certain. Note again that because it is a sample, not an entire population, we cannot be 100% certain of our prediction. The only way to be 100% certain would be to measure every item in the population and in most cases that is either impractical or impossible to accomplish. Therefore, in order to have a certain confidence in our decision (i.e., 95% or 99% certain) we need to add to our equation a factor to allow us this confidence:

$$\frac{Population}{Mean} = \frac{Estimate}{Sample\,Mean} \pm \frac{Reliability}{Coefficient} \; x \; \frac{Standard}{Error} \qquad \text{Eq. 6.7}$$

This reliability coefficient can be obtained from the normal standardized distribution. For example if we want to be certain 95% of the time, we will allow an error 5% of the time. We could error to the high side or low side and if we wanted our error divided equally between the two extremes, we would allow a 2.5% error of being too high in our estimation and 2.5% of being too low in our estimate of the true population mean. In Table B2 of Appendix B we find that 95% of the area under the curve falls between -1.96 z and +1.96 z. This follows the theory of the normal distribution where 95% of the values, or in this case sample means, fall within 1.96 standard deviations of the mean. The actual calculation for the 95% confidence interval would be:

$$\mu = \overline{X} \pm Z_{(1-\alpha/2)} \; x \; \frac{\sigma}{\sqrt{n}} \qquad \text{Eq. 6.8}$$

or in the case of a 95% confidence interval:

$$\mu = \overline{X} \pm (1.96)\frac{\sigma}{\sqrt{n}}$$

The standard error term or standard error of the mean term, is calculated based on the population standard deviation and specific sample size. If the confidence interval were to change to 99% or 90%, the reliability coefficient would change to 2.57 and 1.64 respectively (based on values in Table B1 where 0.99 and 0.90 of the area fall under the curve). In creating a range of possible outcomes instead of one specific measure "it is better to be approximately correct, than precisely wrong" (Kachigan, 1991, p.99).

Many of the following chapters will deal with the area of confidence intervals and tests involved in this area. But at this point let us assume that we know the population standard deviation (σ), possibly through historical data or previous tests. In the case of the pharmacokinetic data (Table 4.3), the population standard deviation is known to be 16.8, based on the raw data, and was calculated using the formula to calculate a population standard deviation (Eq. 5.5 and 5.6). Using the four samples in Table 6.2 it is possible to estimate the population mean based on data for each sample. For example, with Sample A:

$$\mu = 716.4 \pm 1.96\frac{16.8}{\sqrt{5}} = 716.4 \pm 14.7$$

$$701.7 < \mu < 731.1 \; mcg.$$

The best estimate of the population mean (for the researcher using Sample A) would be between 701.7 and 731.1 mcg. Note that the "fudge factor" would remain the same for all four samples since the reliability coefficient will remain constant (1.96) and error term (the population standard deviation divided by square root of the sample size) does not change. Therefore the results for the other three samples would be:

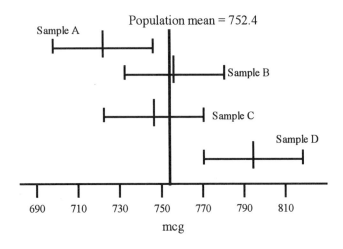

Figure 6.6 Sample results compared with the population mean.

Sample B:	$\mu = 752.8 \pm 14.7$
	$738.1 < \mu < 767.5$ mcg
Sample C:	$\mu = 749.4 \pm 14.7$
	$734.7 < \mu < 764.1$ mcg
Sample D:	$\mu = 786.8 \pm 14.7$
	$772.1 < \mu < 801.5$ mcg

From our previous discussion of presentation mode, the true population mean for these 125 data points is a C_{max} of 752.4 mcg. In the case of samples B and C, the true population mean did fall within the 95% confidence interval and we were correct in our prediction of this mean. However, with the extreme samples (A and D), the population mean falls outside the confidence interval (Figure 6.6). With over 234 million possible samples and using the reliability coefficient (95%), almost 12 million possible samples will give us erroneous results.

Adjusting the confidence interval can increase the likelihood of predicting the correct population mean. One more sample was drawn consisting of five outcomes and the calculated mean is 768.4. If a 95% confidence interval is calculated, the population mean falls outside the interval.

$$\mu = 768.4 \pm 1.96 \frac{16.8}{\sqrt{5}} = 768.4 \pm 14.7$$

$$753.7 < \mu < 783.1 \, mcg$$

However, if we decrease our confidence to 90%, the true population mean falls even further outside the interval.

$$\mu = 768.4 \pm 1.64 \frac{16.8}{\sqrt{5}} = 768.4 \pm 12.4$$

$$756.0 < \mu < 780.8 \, mcg$$

Similarly, if we increase our confidence to 99%, the true population mean will be found within the predicted limits.

$$\mu = 768.4 \pm 2.57 \frac{16.8}{\sqrt{5}} = 768.4 \pm 19.3$$

$$749.1 < \mu < 787.7 \, mcg$$

As seen in Figure 6.7, as the percentage of confidence increases, the width of the confidence interval increases. Creation and adjustment of the confidence intervals is the basis upon which statistical analysis and hypothesis testing is based.

What we have accomplished is our first inferential statistic; to make a statement about a population parameter based on a subset of that population. The z-test is the oldest of the statistical tests and was often called the **critical ratio** in early statistical literature. The **interval estimate** is our best guess, with a certain degree of confidence, where the actual parameter exists. We must allow for a certain amount of error (i.e., 5% or 1%) since we do not know the entire population. As shown in Figure 6.7, as our error decreases the width of our interval estimate will increase. In order to be 100% confident, our estimate of the interval would be from $-\infty$ to $+\infty$ (negative to positive infinity). Also as can be seen in the formula for the confidence interval estimate, with a large sample size, the standard error term will decrease and our interval width will decrease. Relating back to terms defined in Chapter 3, we can relate confidence interval in terms of precision and the confidence level is what we establish as our reliability.

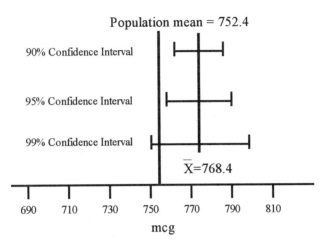

Figure 6.7. Sample results with different confidence levels compared with the true population mean.

As we shall see in future chapters, a basic assumption for many statistical tests (i.e., student t-test, F-test, correlation) is that populations from which the samples are selected are composed of random outcomes that approximate a normal distribution. If this is true, then we know many characteristics about our population with respect to its mean and standard deviation.

The one troublesome feature of Eq. 6.8 is the fact that it is highly unlikely that we will know a population standard deviation (σ). An example of an exception might be a quality control situation where a measurement has been repeated many times and is based on historical data. As will be shown in the next section, one could make a reasonable guess of what σ should be based on past outcomes. However, in Chapter 8 we will find an alternative test for creating a confidence interval when the population standard deviation is unknown or cannot be approximated.

Statistical Control Charts

Quality control charts represent an example of the application of confidence intervals using σ or an approximation of the population standard deviation. Traditionally, control charts have been used during manufacturing to monitor production runs and insure the quality of the finished product. More recently these charts have been used to monitor the quality of health care systems, along with techniques such as cause-and-effect diagrams, quality-function deployment and process flow analysis (Laffel, 1989; Wadsworth,

1985). Our discussion of control charts will focus on production issues, but the process could be easily applied to the monitoring of quality performance indicators in the provision of health services.

Statistical quality control is the process of assessing the status of a specific characteristic or characteristics, over a period of time, with respect to some target value or goal. During the production process, control charts provide a visual method for evaluating an intermediate or the final product during the ongoing process. They can be used to identify problems during production and document the history of a specific batch or run.

The use of control charts is one of the most common applications of statistics to the process of pharmaceutical quality control. The design of such charts were originally developed by Walter Shewhart in 1934 (Taylor, 1987, p.121). Over the years, modifications have been made, but most of the original characteristics of the **Shewhart control chart** continue today. Control charts assess and monitor the variability of a specific characteristic, which is assumed to exist under relatively homogeneous and stable conditions. There are generally two type of control charts: 1) measuring consistency of the production run (**property chart**) around a target value and 2) measuring the variability of the samples (**precision chart**).

To assess and monitor a given characteristic during a production, we periodically sample items (i.e., tablets, vials) using random or selected sampling and measuring the specific variable (i.e., weight, fill rate). The results are plotted on a graph with an x- and y-axis. The x-axis is a "time-ordered" sequence. The outcomes or changes are plotted on the y-axis over this time period to determine if the process is under control.

A **sampling plan** is developed to determine times, at equal intervals, during which samples are selected. In the case of a selected sampling process (i.e., every 15 minutes samples are selected from a production line), it is assumed that individual samples are withdrawn at random. How often should a sample be selected? The length of time between samples is dependent on the stability of the process being measured. A relatively stable process (for example, weights of finished tablets in a production run), may require only occasional monitoring, (i.e., every 30 minutes). A more volatile product or one with potential for large deviations from the target outcome may require more frequent sampling. When drawing samples for control charts, the time intervals should be consistent (every 30 minutes, every 60 minutes, etc.) and the sample sizes should be equal. The size and frequency of the sample is dependent on the nature of the control process and desired precision. Sample sizes as small as four or five observations have been recommended (Bolton, 1997, p. 447).

The creation of a quality control chart is a relatively simple process. Time intervals are located on the x-axis and outcomes for the variable of interest (or property) is measured on the y-axis. The "property" chart uses either a single

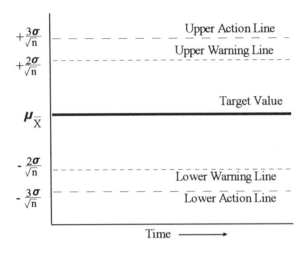

Figure 6.8   Traditional quality control chart.

measurement (sometime referred to as an **x-chart**) or the mean of several measurements (a **mean chart**) of a selected variable (i.e., capsule weight, tablet hardness, fill volume of a liquid into a bottle). The mean chart ($\overline{X}$ chart) would be preferable to a simple x-chart because it is less sensitive to extreme results because these would offset the remainder of the measures that are averaged. Also, the x-chart consists of a series of single measures and does not provide any information about the variance of outcomes at specific time periods.

Control charts contain a **central line** running through the chart parallel to the x-axis. This central line represents the "target" or "ideal" goal and is often based on historical data from scale up through initial full-scale runs. Also referred to as the **average line**, the central line defines the target for the variable being plotted. This is seen as the center line in Figure 6.8. In an ideal world, if a process is under control all results should fall on the central line. Unfortunately most outcomes will be observed to fall above or below the line, due to simple random error. The distance from the central line and the actual point is a measure of variability. Thus, in addition to identifying a central line it is important to determine acceptable limits, above and below this line, within which observations should fall.

There are two types of variability that can be seen in statistical control charts: 1) common cause variability and 2) assignable cause variability. **Common cause variation** is due to random· error or normal variability attributed to the sampling process. This type of error is due to natural chance error or error inherent in the process. **Assignable cause variation** is systematic error or bias that occurs in excess of the common-cause variability of the process. Also called **special cause variation,** it is the responsibility of the person controlling the process to identify the cause of this variation, correct it and maintain a process that is under control. When the control chart shows excessive variation from the ideal outcome the process is said to be "out of statistical control". Thus, the required measures for constructing a statistical quality control chart are: 1) a sampling plan (size and length of time interval); 2) a target value; and 3) an estimate of the random error, which as we shall see is based on either expected standard deviations or ranges.

How much deviation from the central line is acceptable? The original Shewhart format utilized the population standard deviation (σ) and created **action lines** at three standard deviations above and below the target value. These lines were referred to as the three-sigma limits or the upper and lower control limits (UCL and LCL).

$$UCL = target + \frac{3\sigma}{\sqrt{n}}$$ Eq. 6.9

$$LCL = target - \frac{3\sigma}{\sqrt{n}}$$ Eq. 6.10

These are the boundaries within which essentially all of the sample data should fall if the process is under statistical control. In order to create these upper and lower action lines we need to be able to estimate the population standard deviation. This could be based on historical data about a particular product or process, or it can be estimated from previous samples.

One method for estimating σ is to calculate an average or "pooled" sample standard deviation. Also call **process capability**, this can be calculated by averaging standard deviations from previous runs:

$$S_p = \frac{S_1 + S_2 + S_3 + ... S_k}{k}$$ Eq. 6.11

The square of this process is sometimes referred to as the **within sample estimate of variance** or random error:

$$\sigma^2_{WSE} = \frac{\sum S^2}{k}$$ Eq. 6.12

This pooling the sample variances (or standard deviations) for many subgroups can provide a good estimate of the true population standard deviation.

More recent control charts incorporate additional limits called warning lines. This method involves establishing two sets of lines; warning lines at two sigmas and action lines at three sigmas (see Figure 6.8). Because they only involve two standard deviations above and below the target line, the warning limits are always narrower and do not demand the immediate intervention seen with the action lines. The warning lines would be calculated as follows:

$$\mu_w = \mu_0 \pm \frac{2\sigma}{\sqrt{n}} \qquad \text{Eq. 6.13}$$

and the action lines are:

$$\mu_a = \mu_0 \pm \frac{3\sigma}{\sqrt{n}} \qquad \text{Eq. 6.14}$$

Some control charting systems even evaluate observations falling outside one standard deviation beyond the central line. As discussed, virtually all samples will fall between ±3-sigma, 95% will be located within ±2-sigma and approximately 2/3 are contained within ±1-sigma. Therefore, deviations outside any of these three parameters can be used to monitor production. Possible indicators of a process becoming "out-of-control" would be two successive samples outside the 2-sigma limit or four successive samples outside the 1-sigma limit or any systematic trends (several samples in the same direction) up or down from the central line (Taylor, 1987, p.135-6).

As mentioned previously, two components that can influence a control chart are: 1) the variable or property of interest (systematic or assignable cause variability) and 2) the precision of the measurement (random or common-cause variability). The center, warning and action lines monitor a given property in a quality control chart. However, we are also concerned about the precision or variability of our sample (the random variability). Standard deviations and ranges can be used as a measure of consistency of the samples. Variations in these measures are not seen in as simple Shewhart chart. A precision chart measures the amount of random error and consists of a plotting of the sample standard deviation (or the sample range) in parallel with the control chart for the sample means.

In addition to creating a control chart based on the standard deviation, a similar chart can be produced using the easiest of all measures of dispersion, the range. The central line for a range chart is calculated similar to the line used for the property chart. An average range is computed based on past observations.

$$\overline{R} = \frac{R_1 + R_2 + R_3 + ... R_k}{k} \qquad\qquad \text{Eq. 6.15}$$

Obviously the range is easier to calculate and is as efficient as the standard deviation to measure deviations from the central line if the sample size is greater than five (Mason, 1989, p.66). Also, to calculate $\overline{R}$, there should be at least eight observations and preferably at least 15 for any given time period (Taylor, 1987, p.140).

An alternative method for calculating the action lines around the target value utilized $\overline{R}$ and an A-value from Table 6.3.

$$AL = \overline{X} \pm A\overline{R} \qquad\qquad \text{Eq. 6.16}$$

Using the above formula will produce action lines almost identical to those created using Eq. 6.14.

To calculate the action lines for variations in the range, as a measure of dispersion, a value similar to the reliability coefficient portion of Eq. 6.8 is selected from Table 6.3. The D_L and D_U-values from the table for the lower and upper limits, respectively, are used in the following formula:

$$Upper\ Action\ Line = D_U \overline{R} \qquad\qquad \text{Eq. 6.17}$$

$$Lower\ Action\ Line = D_L \overline{R} \qquad\qquad \text{Eq. 6.18}$$

Note as more is known about the total population (i.e., larger sample sizes), the values in Table 6.3 become smaller and the action line becomes closer together. Also, based on the values in the table, the lines around the average range will not be symmetrical and the upper action line will always be further from the central, target range. By presenting these two plots in parallel, it is possible to monitor both the variability of the characteristic being measured, as well as the precision of the measurements at each specific time period.

As an example of the use of a quality control chart, consider the intermediate step of producing a core table which will eventual become enteric coated. Periodically during the pressing of these core tablets, samples of ten tablets are randomly sampled. The ideal target weight for the individual tablets is 200 mg or a mass weight of 2,000 mg for all ten tablets. Based on historical data from previous runs, the expected average range should be 6.2 mg. Using the range as our measure of dispersion, the action lines are determined using the A-values taken from Table 6.3 for n = 10 (A=0.31):

Table 6.3   Factors for Determining Upper and Lower 3σ Limits for Mean and Range Quality Control Charts

Sample Size of subgroup, N	A: Factor for X chart	Factors for range chart	
		D_L for lower limit	D_U for upper limit
2	1.88	0	3.27
3	1.02	0	2.57
4	0.73	0	2.28
5	0.58	0	2.11
6	0.48	0	2.00
7	0.42	0.08	1.92
8	0.37	0.14	1.86
9	0.34	0.18	1.82
10	0.31	0.22	1.78
15	0.22	0.35	1.65
20	0.18	0.41	1.59

From: Bolton, S. (1997). Pharmaceutical Statistics: Practical and Clinical Applications, Marcel Dekker, Inc., New York, p. 658. Reproduced with permission of the publisher.

Table 6.4. Sample Weights (mg) During a Production Run

Date	Time	Mean	Range
9/6	9:00	200.4	6.7
	9:30	199.4	4.4
	10:00	201.2	7.3
	10:30	200.0	6.9
	11:00	200.6	5.5
	11:30	201.0	8.1
	12:00	201.3	9.2
	12:30	200.2	6.5
	13:00	199.8	5.0
	13:30	199.6	7.2
	14:00	199.3	3.5
	14:30	199.0	6.4

$$AL = \overline{X} \pm A\overline{R} = 200 \pm 0.31(6.2) = 200 \pm 1.92$$

$$A_U L = 201.92 \qquad A_L L = 198.08$$

The mean range $(\overline{R})$ is 6.2 and using the DU and DL-values from Table 6.3, the following action lines for our measures of precision are:

$$D_U \overline{R} = 1.78(6.2) = 11.04$$

$$D_L \overline{R} = 0.22(6.2) = 1.36$$

During production, with sampling done every thirty minutes, creates the results presented in Table 6.4. Plotting of the results of this run appears in Figure 6.9. Note that there is no significant change in the variability of the samples, as seen in the plotting of the ranges. However, there appears to be a downward trend in the mean weights of the tablets and the operator should make adjustments in the process to return the weight back to the target mean.

    A second type of control chart is the **cumulative sum** or **CUSUM** charting technique. It is considered more sensitive than are Shewhart control charts to modest changes in the characteristic being monitoring (Mason, 1989, p.66). The name CUSUM is from the fact that successive deviations are accumulated from a fixed reference point in the process. There is evidence of a special-cause variation when the cumulative sum of the deviations is extremely large or extremely small. Further information on CUSUM charts can be found in Mason's book (Mason, 1989, pp. 67-70).

References

Bolton, S. (1997). Pharmaceutical Statistics: Practical and Clinical Applications, Marcel Dekker, Inc. New York, pp. 444-489.

Kachigan, S.K. (1991). Multivariate Statistical Analysis, Second edition, Radius Press, New York, pp. 89-90

Laffel, G. and Blumenthal, D. (1989). "The case for using industral quality management science in health care organizations," Journal of the American Medical Association 262:2869-2873.

Mason, R.L., Gunst, R.F. and Hess, J.L. (1989). Statistical Design and Analysis of Experiments with Applications to Engineering and Science, John Wiley and Sons,

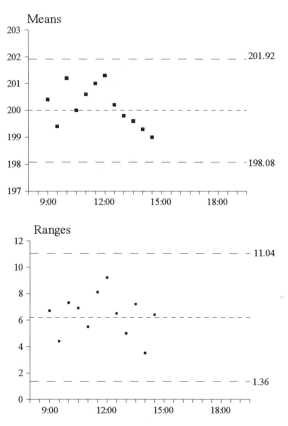

Figure 6.9 Quality control charts for the means and ranges of the data presented in Table 6.4.

New York.

Porter, T.M. (1986). The Rise of Statistical Thinking, Princeton University Press, p. 93.

Taylor, J.K. (1987). Quality Assurance of Chemical Measurements, Lewis Publications, Chelsea, MI.

Wadsworth, H.M., Stephens, K.S. and Godfrey, A.B. (1986). Modern Methods for Quality Control and Improvement, John Wiley and Sons, New York.

Suggested Supplemental Readings

Bolton, S. (1997). Pharmaceutical Statistics: Practical and Clinical Applications, Marcel Dekker, Inc. New York, pp. 444-489.

Cheremisinoff, N.P. (1987). Practical Statistics for Engineers and Scientists, Technomic Publishing, Lancaster, PA, pp. 41-50.

Mason, R.L., Gunst, R.F. and Hess, J.L. (1989). Statistical Design and Analysis of Experiments with Applications to Engineering and Science, John Wiley and Sons, New York, pp 62-70.

Taylor, J.K. (1987). Quality Assurance of Chemical Measurements, Lewis Publications, Chelsea, MI, p.129-146.

Example Problems

1. Assume that three assays are selected at random from the following results:

Tablet Number	Assay (mg.)	Tablet Number	Assay (mg.)	Tablet Number	Assay (mg.)
1	75	11	73	21	80
2	74	12	77	22	75
3	72	13	75	23	76
4	78	14	74	24	73
5	78	15	72	25	79
6	74	16	74	26	76
7	75	17	77	27	73
8	77	18	76	28	75
9	76	19	74	29	76
10	78	20	77	30	75

The resultant sample is tablet 05, 16 and 27.

a. Based on this one sample and assuming that the population standard deviation (σ) is known to be 2.01, calculate 95% confidence intervals for the population mean.

b. Again, based on this one sample, calculate the 90% and 99% confidence intervals for the population mean. How do these results compare to the 95% confidence interval for the same sample in the previous example?

c. Assuming the true population mean (μ) is 75.47 for all 30 data points, did our one sample create confidence intervals at the 90%, 95% and 99% levels which included the population mean?

2. Assuming the true population mean (μ) is 75.47 and the population standard deviation (σ) is 2.01 for the question 1, calculate the following:

a. How many different samples of n=3 can be selected from the above population of 30 data points?

b. What would be the grand mean for all the possible samples of n=3?

c. What would be the standard deviation for all the possible samples of n=3?

3. During scale up and initial production of an intravenous product in a 5 cc vial, it was found that the standard deviation for volume fill was 0.2 cc. Create a Shewhart control chart to monitor the fill rates of the production vials. Monitor the precision assuming the range is 0.6 cc (6 x σ) and the each sample size is 10 vials.

4. During the production of a specific solid dosage form it is expected that the standard deviation (σ) for the specific strength will be approximately 3.5 mg, based of experience with the product. Twenty tablets are sampled at random from Batch #1234 and found to have a mean assay of 48.3 mg. With 95% confidence, does this sample come from a batch with the correct strength (50 mg) or is this batch subpotent?

Answers to Problems

1. Results of different samples will vary based on the random numbers selected off the table. Results can vary from the smallest possible mean outcome of 72.3 to the largest possible mean of 79.0. Assume that our sample results for Sample C were tables 05, 16 and 27. The mean assay result would be:

$$\overline{X} = \frac{78 + 74 + 73}{3} = 75 \ mg.$$

a.   The 95% confidence interval would be:

$$\mu = \bar{x} \pm Z_{(1-\alpha/2)} \, x \, \frac{\sigma}{\sqrt{n}}$$

$$\mu = 75 \pm 1.96 \, x \frac{2.01}{\sqrt{3}} = 75 \pm 2.27$$

$$72.73 < \mu < 77.27 \, mg.$$

b.   Using the above sample the 90% and 99% confidence intervals for the population mean would be:

$$90\% \, CI: \qquad \mu = 75 \pm 1.64 \, x \frac{2.01}{\sqrt{3}}$$

$$73.10 < \mu < 76.90 \, mg.$$

$$99\% \, CI: \qquad \mu = 75 \pm 2.57 \, x \frac{2.01}{\sqrt{3}}$$

$$72.02 < \mu < 77.98 \, mg.$$

As expected the interval becomes much wider (includes more possible results) when we wish to be 99% certain and becomes smaller as we accept a greater amount of error.

c.   Since the true population mean (μ) is 75.47 mg., this would represent the most frequent outcome, but very few samples if any will produce 75.47. Instead we would see a clustering of means around that center point for the population.

2.   With $\mu = 75.47$, $\sigma = 2.01$ and N=30

a.   There are a possible 4,060 different samples of n=3:

$$\binom{n}{x} = \frac{n!}{x!(n-x)!} = \frac{30!}{3!\,27!} = 4060$$

b. The grand mean for all 4,060 possible sample means is 75.47 mg.:

$$\mu_{\overline{X}} = \mu = 75.47 \; mg.$$

c. The standard deviation for all 4,060 possible sample means is 1.16 mg.:

$$\sigma_{\overline{X}} = \frac{\sigma}{\sqrt{n}} = \frac{2.01}{\sqrt{3}} = 1.16 \; mg.$$

3. Creation of a quality control chart with the target $\mu = 5$ cc, $\sigma = 0.2$ cc and $n = 10$:

Warning lines:

$$\mu_w = \mu_0 \pm \frac{2\sigma}{\sqrt{n}} = 5 \pm \frac{2(0.2)}{\sqrt{10}} = 5 \pm 0.13$$

$$\mu_w = 5.13 \; and \; 4.87$$

Action lines:

$$\mu_a = \mu_0 \pm \frac{3\sigma}{\sqrt{n}} = 5 \pm \frac{3(0.2)}{\sqrt{10}} = 5 \pm 0.19$$

$$\mu_a = 5.19 \; and \; 4.81$$

Action lines using range formulas:

$$AL = \overline{X} \pm A\overline{R} = 5 \pm 0.31(0.6) = 5 \pm 0.19$$

$$A_U L = 5.19 \qquad\qquad A_L L = 4.81$$

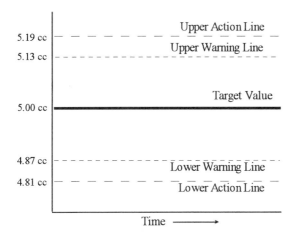

Range action lines:

$$Upper\ Action\ Line = D_U\ \overline{R} = 1.78(0.6) = 1.07$$

$$Lower\ Action\ Line = D_L\ \overline{R} = 0.22(0.6) = 0.13$$

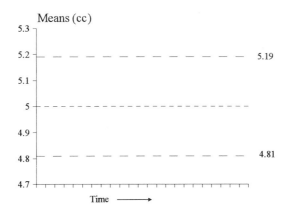

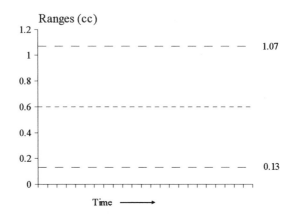

4. Creation of a 95% confidence interval where $\overline{X}$ = 48.3, σ = 3.5 and n = 20:

$$\mu = \overline{x} \pm Z_{(1-\alpha/2)} \times \frac{\sigma}{\sqrt{n}}$$

$$\mu = 48.3 \pm 1.96 \cdot \frac{3.5}{\sqrt{20}} = 48.3 \pm 1.53$$

$$44.77 < \mu < 49.83$$

Based on a sample of only 20 tablets, there is 95% certainty that the true population mean (strength) is between 44.77 and 49.83 mg. The goal of 50 mg does not fall within this confidence interval; therefore, it is assumed that Batch #1234 is subpotent.

7

Hypothesis Testing

Hypothesis testing is the process of inferring from a sample whether or not to accept a certain statement about a population or populations. The sample is assumed to be a small representative proportion of the total population. Two errors can occur, rejection of a true hypothesis or failing to reject a false hypothesis.

As mentioned in the beginning of Chapter 1, inferential statistical tests are intended to answer questions confronting the researcher. Statistical analysis is based on hypotheses that are formulated and then tested. Often in published articles, these hypotheses or questions are described as an "objective" or "purpose" of the study.

Hypothesis Testing

Sometimes referred to as **significance testing**, hypothesis testing is the process of inferring from a sample whether or not to accept a certain statement about the population from which the sample was taken.

> Hypothesis: Fact A
> Alternative: Fact A is false

Researchers must carefully define the population about which they plan to make inferences and then randomly select samples or subjects that should be representative of this population. For example, if 100 capsules were drawn at random from a particular batch of a medication and some analytical procedure was performed on the sample, this measurement could be considered indicative of the population. In this case, the population is only those capsules in that specific batch and cannot be generalized to other batches of the same medication. Similarly, pharmacokinetic results from a Phase I clinical trial performed only on healthy male volunteers between 18 and 55 years old, are not necessarily reflective of the responses expected in females, children, geriatric patients or even individuals with the specific illness for which the drug is intended to treat.

In addition, with any inferential statistical test it is assumed that the individual measurements are independent of one another and any one measurement will not influence the outcome of any other member of the sample. Also, the stated hypotheses should be free from apparent prejudgment or bias. Lastly, the hypotheses should be well-defined and clearly stated. Thus, the results of the statistical test will determine which hypothesis is correct.

The hypothesis may be rejected, meaning the evidence from the sample casts enough doubt on the hypothesis for us to say with some degree of certainty that the hypothesis is false. On the other hand, the hypothesis may not be rejected if we are unable to statistically contradict it. Using an inferential statistic there are two possible outcomes:

H_0: Hypothesis Under Test (Null Hypothesis)
H_1: Alternative Hypothesis (Research Hypothesis)

By convention, the **null hypothesis** is stated as no real differences in the outcomes. For example, if we are comparing three levels of a discrete independent variable (μ_1, μ_2, μ_3), the null hypothesis would be stated $\mu_1 = \mu_2 = \mu_3$. The evaluation then attempts to nullify the hypothesis of no significant difference in favor of an alternative research hypothesis. The type of null hypothesis will depend upon the type of variables and the outcomes the researcher is interested in measuring. These two hypotheses are mutually exclusive and exhaustive:

H_0: Hypothesis A
H_1: Hypothesis A is false

They cannot both occur and they include all possible outcomes. The sample values, if they are randomly sampled and measured independently, are the best estimate of the population values, therefore, in the case of two levels of a discrete independent variable:

$$\overline{X}_1 \approx \mu_1 \qquad \text{and} \qquad \overline{X}_2 \approx \mu_2$$

With the null hypothesis as a hypothesis of no difference, we are stating that the two populations under the hypothesis are the same:

$$H_0: \mu_1 = \mu_2$$

We are really testing our sample data $\overline{X}_1 = \overline{X}_2$ and inferring that these data are representative of the population $\mu_1 = \mu_2$, allowing for a certain amount of error in our decision. The alternative hypothesis is either accepted or rejected based upon the decision about the hypothesis under test. Thus, an **inference** can be defined as any conclusion that is drawn from a statistical evaluation.

Statistics from our sample provide us with a basis for estimating the probability that some observed difference between samples should be expected due to sampling error. Two approaches could be used: 1) creation of a confidence interval or 2) a comparison with a **critical value**. The former has already been employed in the previous chapter, with the establishment of a confidence interval for a population parameter based on sample results.

$$\begin{array}{c} Population \\ Mean \end{array} = \begin{array}{c} Estimate \\ Sample\,Mean \end{array} \pm \begin{array}{c} Reliability \\ Coefficient \end{array} \; x \; \begin{array}{c} Standard \\ Error \end{array}$$

In the second method we would calculate a "test statistic" (a value based on the manipulation of sample data). This value is compared to a preset "critical" value (usually found in a special table) based on a specific acceptable error rate (i.e., 5%). If the test statistic is extremely rare it will be to the extreme of our critical value and we will reject the hypothesis under test in favor of the research hypothesis, which is the only possible alternative. For example, assume that we are interested in the hypothesis $H_0: \mu_1 = \mu_2$. If we calculate a number (result of the statistical test) to test this hypothesis we would expect our calculated statistic to equal zero if the two populations are identical. As this number becomes larger, or to an extreme of zero (either in the positive or negative direction), it becomes more likely that the two populations are not equal. In other words, as the absolute value of the calculated statistic becomes large, there is a smaller probability that H_0 is true and that this difference is not due to chance error alone. The critical values for most statistical tests indicate an extreme at which we reject H_0 and conclude that H_1 is the true situation (in this case that $\mu_1 \neq \mu_2$).

The statistical test results has only two possible outcomes, either we cannot reject H_0 or we reject H_0 in favor of H_1. At the same time, if all the facts were known (the real world) or we had data for the entire population, the hypothesis

(H_0) is either true or false for the population that the sample represents. This may be represented as follows, where we want our results to fall into either of the two clear areas and the results fall into either of the shaded areas, considered mistakes or errors.

		The Real World	
		H_0 is true	H_0 is false
Results of Statistical Test	Fail to Reject H_0		▨
	Reject H_0	▨	

An analogy to hypothesis testing can be seen in American jurisprudence (Kachigan, 1991). Illustrated below are the possible results from a jury trial.

H_0:   Person is innocent of crime
H_1:   Person is guilty of crime

		All the Facts are Known	
		Person is Innocent	Person is Guilty
Jury's Verdict	Not Guilty		ERROR II
	Guilty	ERROR I	

During the trial, the jury will be presented with data (information, exhibits, testimonies, evidence) which will help, or hinder, their decision making process. The original hypothesis is that the person is innocent until proven guilty. Evidence will conflict and the jury will never know the true situation, but will be required to render a decision. They will find the defendant either guilty or not guilty, when in fact if all the data were known the person is either guilty or innocent. Two errors are possible: 1) sending an innocent person to prison (error I) or 2) freeing a guilty person (error II). For most, the former error would be the more grievous of the two mistakes.

Note that in this analogy, if the jury fails to find the person guilty their decision is not that the person is "innocent." Instead they present a verdict of "not guilty." In a similar vein, the decision is not to accept a null hypothesis, but to <u>fail</u> to reject it. If we cannot reject the null hypothesis, it does not prove that the statement is actually true. It only indicates that there is insufficient evidence to justify rejection. One cannot prove a null hypothesis, only fail to reject it.

It is hoped that outcomes from our court system will end in the clear areas and the innocent are freed and the guilty sent to jail. Similarly, it is hoped that the results of our statistical analysis will not fall into the shaded error regions. Like our system of jurisprudence, a statistical test can only disprove the null hypothesis, it can never prove the hypothesis is true.

Types of Errors

Similar to our jurisprudence example, there are two possible errors associated with hypothesis testing. Type I error is the probability of rejecting a true null hypothesis (H_0) and Type II error is the probability of accepting a false H_0. Type I error is also called the **level of significance** and uses the symbol α or p. Like sending an innocent person to jail, this is the most important error to minimize or control. Fortunately, the researcher has more control over the amount of acceptable Type I error. Alternatively, our level of confidence in our decision, or **confidence level**, is $1-\alpha$ (the probability of all outcomes less Type I error).

Type II error is symbolized using the Greek letter β. The probability of rejecting a false H_0 is called **power** $(1-\beta)$. In hypothesis testing we always want to minimize the α and maximize $1-\beta$. Continuing with our previous example of two populations being equal or not equal, the hypotheses are

$$H_0: \mu_1 = \mu_2$$
$$H_1: \mu_1 \neq \mu_2$$

with the four potential outcomes being:

$1-\alpha$: Do not reject H_0 when in fact $\mu_1 = \mu_2$ is true
α: Reject H_0 when in fact $\mu_1 = \mu_2$ is true
$1-\beta$: Reject H_0 when in fact $\mu_1 = \mu_2$ is false
β: Do not reject H_0 when in fact $\mu_1 = \mu_2$ is false

		The Real World	
		H_0 is true	H_0 is false
Results of Statistical Test	Fail to Reject H_0	$1-\alpha$	β
	Reject H_0	α	$1-\beta$

In Chapter 3 we discussed the different types of error in research (random and systematic). Statistics allow us to estimate the extent of our random errors or establish acceptable levels of random error. Systematic error is controlled through the experimental design use in the study (including random sampling and independence). In many cases systematic errors are predictable and often unidirectional. Random errors are unpredictable and relate to sample deviations that were discussed in the previous chapter.

Type I Error

The Type I error rate should be established before making statistical computations. By convention, a probability of less than five percent ($p < 0.05$ or a 1/20 chance) is usually considered an unlikely event. However, we may wish to establish more stringent criteria (i.e., 0.01, 0.001) or a less demanding level (i.e., 0.10, 0.20) depending on the type of experiment and impact of erroneous decisions. For the purposes of this book, the error rates will usually be established at either 0.05 or 0.01. The term "statistically significant" is used to indicate that the sample data is incompatible with the null hypothesis for the proposed population and that it is rejected in favor of the alternate hypothesis.

If Type I error must be chosen before the data is gathered, it prevents the researcher from choosing a significance level to fit the p values resulting from statistical testing of the data. A **decision rule** is established, which is a statement in hypothesis testing that determines whether or not the hypothesis under test should be rejected; for example, "with $\alpha = .05$, reject H_0 if ... ."

In the previous illustration of pharmacokinetic data (Table 4.3), we found that there were over 234 million possible samples (n=5) which produced a normally distributed array of possible outcomes. Using any one of these samples it is possible to estimate the population mean (Eq. 6.8):

$$\mu = \overline{X} \pm Z_{(1-\alpha/2)} \, x \, \frac{\sigma}{\sqrt{n}}$$

Using this equation we can predict a range of possible values within which the true population would fall. If we set the reliability coefficient to α=.05, then 95% of the possible samples would create intervals which correctly include the population mean (μ) based on the sample mean ($\overline{X}$). Unfortunately, 5% of the potential samples produce estimated ranges that do not include the true population mean.

As will be shown in the next chapter, the reverse of this procedure is to use a statistical formula, calculate a "test statistic" and then compare it to a critical number from a specific table in Appendix B. If the "statistic" is to the extreme of the table value, H_0 is rejected. Again, if we allow for a 5% Type I error rate, 95% of the time our results should be correct. However, through sampling distribution and random error, we could still be wrong 5% (α) of the time due to chance error in sampling.

The **acceptance region** is that area in a statistical distribution where the outcomes will not lead to a rejection of the hypothesis under test. In contrast, the **rejection region**, or **critical region**, represents outcomes in a statistical distribution, which lead to the rejection of the hypothesis under test and acceptance of the alternative hypothesis. In other words, outcomes in the acceptance region could occur as a result of random or chance error. However, the likelihood of an occurrence falling in the critical region is so rare that this result cannot be attributed to chance alone.

The critical value is that value in a statistical test that divides the range of all possible values into an acceptance and a rejection region for the purposes of hypothesis testing. For example:

$$\text{With } \alpha = .05, \text{ reject } H_0 \text{ if } F > F_{3,120}(.95) = 2.68$$

In this particular case, if "F" (which is calculated through a mathematical procedure) is greater than "$F_{3,120}(.95)$" (which is found in a statistical table), then the null hypothesis is rejected in favor of the alternative.

To illustrate the above discussion, assume we are testing the fact that two samples come from different populations ($\mu_A \neq \mu_B$). Our null hypothesis would be that the two populations are equal and, if mutually exclusive and exhaustive, the only alternate hypothesis would be that they are not the same.

$$H_0: \quad \mu_A = \mu_B$$
$$H_1: \quad \mu_A \neq \mu_B$$

The best, and only, estimate of the population(s) are the two sample means ($\overline{X}_A$, $\overline{X}_B$). Based on the discussion in the previous chapter on sampling distributions, we know that sample means can vary and this variability is the standard error of the mean. Obviously, if the two sample means are the same we cannot reject the null hypothesis. But what if one is 10% larger than the other? Or 20%? Or even 100%? Where do we "draw the line" and establish a point at which we must reject the null hypothesis of equality? At what point can the difference no longer be attributed to random error alone? As illustrated in Figure 7.1, this point is our critical value. If we exceed this point there is a significant difference. If the sample difference is zero or less than the critical value, then this difference could be attributed to chance error due to the potential distribution associated with samples.

Statistics provides us with tools for making statements about our certainty that there are real differences, as opposed to only chance differences between populations based on sample observations. The decision rule, with assistance from tables in Appendix B, establishes the critical value. The numerical manipulations presented in the following chapters will produce the test statistic. If we fail to reject the null hypothesis, then there is insufficient evidence available to conclude that H_0 is false.

Our hypothesis can be bi-directional or unidirectional. For example, assume we are not making a prediction that one outcome is better or worse than the other. Using the previous example:

$$H_0: \quad \mu_A = \mu_B$$
$$H_1: \quad \mu_A \neq \mu_B$$

In this case the alternate hypothesis only measures that there is a difference, μ_A could be significantly larger or smaller than μ_B. If $\alpha = .05$, then we need to

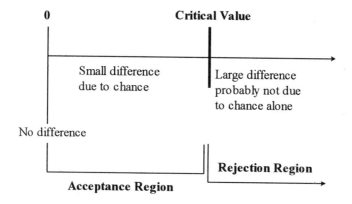

Figure 7.1 The critical value.

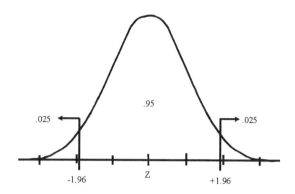

Figure 7.2 Two-tailed 95% confidence interval.

divide it equally between the two extremes of our sampling distribution of outcomes and create two rejection regions (Figure 7.2). We then demarcate finite regions of their distribution. The range of these demarcations define the limits beyond which will reject the null hypothesis.

An alternative would be to create a **directional hypothesis** where we predict that one population is larger or smaller than the other:

$$H_0: \quad \mu_A \leq \mu_B$$
$$H_1: \quad \mu_A > \mu_B$$

In this case, if we reject H_0 we would conclude that population A is significantly larger than population B (Figure 7.3). Also referred to as

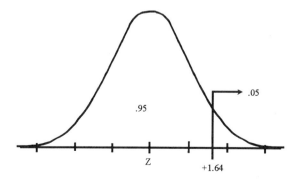

Figure 7.3 One-tailed 95% confidence interval.

truncated, curtailed or **one-sided hypotheses** we must be absolutely certain, usually on logical grounds, that the third omitted outcome ($\mu_A < \mu_B$) has a zero probability of occurring. The one-tailed test should never be used unless there is a specific reason for being directional.

Type II Error and Power

Type II error and power are closely associated with sample size and the amount of difference the researcher wishes to detect. We are primarily interested in power, which is the complement of Type II error (β). Symbolized as *1-β*, **power** is the ability of a statistical test to show if a significant difference truly exists. It is the probability that a statistical test will reveal a true difference when one exists. It is dependent on several factors including the size of the groups as well as the size of the difference in outcomes. In hypothesis testing, it is important to have a sizable sample to allow statistical tests to show significant differences where they exist.

Power is more difficult to understand than Type I error, where we simply select from a statistical table the amount of error we will tolerate in rejecting the null hypotheses. We are concerned with the ability to reject a false H_0. In the simplest example (H_0: $\mu_1 = \mu_2$), we need the ability to reject this hypothesis if it is false and accept the alternative hypothesis (H_1: $\mu_1 \neq \mu_2$).

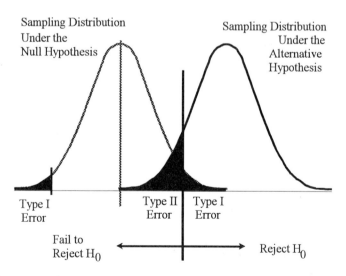

Figure 7.4 Comparisons of sampling distributions under H_0 and H_1.

Let us assume for the moment that we know, or can approximate the population variance as a measure of dispersion. We could estimate our Type II error using the following equation:

$$z_\beta = \frac{\delta}{\sqrt{\dfrac{2\sigma^2}{n}}} - z_{\alpha/2} \qquad \text{Eq. 7.1}$$

In this equation, σ^2 represents the variance of the population (assuming the two samples are the same ($\mu_1 = \mu_2$), then the dispersion will be the same for μ_1 and μ_2); δ is the detectable difference we want to be able to identify if $\mu_1 \neq \mu_2$; n is the sample size for each level of the independent variable (assuming equal n); and $z_{\alpha/2}$ is the amount of Type I error pre-selected for our analysis. $z_{\alpha/2}$ is expressed a z-value from the normal standardized distribution (Table B2 in Appendix B). Obviously, z_β represents the amount of Type II error, again expressed as a value in the normalized standard distribution and reporting the probability (β) of being greater than z_β. The complement of our calculated β would be the power associated with our statistical test $(1-\beta)$.

As seen in Eq. 7.1, Type II error is a one-tailed distribution (z_β); whereas the Type I error rate may be set either unidirectional (z_α) or bi-directional ($z_{\alpha/2}$). This can be explained through using the simplest hypothesis (H_0: $\mu_1 - \mu_2 = 0$), where we want to be able to reject this hypothesis if there is a true difference and accept the alternative hypothesis (H_0: $\mu_1 - \mu_2 \neq 0$). The question that needs to be asked is how large should the difference be in order to accept this alternative hypothesis? Figure 7.4 illustrates the relationship between Type I and II errors. In this figure, Type I error is divided equally between the two tails of our null hypothesis and the Type II errors to the left side of the distribution for the alternative hypothesis (if it is true). Notice the common point where both types of errors end, which becomes our decision point to accept or reject the null hypothesis.

To illustrate this point, assume we are comparing samples from two tablet production runs (batches) and are concerned that there might be a difference in the average weights of the tablets. Based on historical data for the production of this dosage form, we expect a standard deviation of approximately 8 mg ($\sigma^2 = 64$). If the two runs are not the same with respect to tablet weight ($\mu_1 \neq \mu_2$), we want to be able to identify true population differences as small as a 10 mg (δ). At the same time, we would like to be 95% confident in our decision ($z_{\alpha/2} = 1.96$). We sample 6 tablets from each batch. The Type II error calculation is as follows:

$$z_\beta = \frac{\delta}{\sqrt{\frac{2\sigma^2}{n}}} - z_{\alpha/2}$$

$$z_\beta = \frac{10}{\sqrt{\frac{2(8)^2}{6}}} - 1.96$$

$$z_\beta = 2.17 - 1.96 = 0.21$$

The value z_β represents the a point on a normal distribution, below which the β proportion of the curve falls. In other word the probability of being below this point is the Type II error. Looking at the normal standardize distribution table we see that the proportion of the curve between 0 and z = 0.21 is .0832. The area below the curve, representing the Type II error, is .4168 (.5000-.0832). Thus, for this particular problem we have power less than 60% (1-.4168) to detect a 10 mg difference, if such a difference exists.

As will be discussed later, if we can increase our sample size we will increase our power. Let's assume that we double our sample, collecting 12 tablets from each batch, then z_β would be:

$$z_\beta = \frac{10}{\sqrt{\frac{2(8)^2}{12}}} - 1.96 = 3.06 - 1.96 = 1.10$$

Once again referring to the normal standardize distribution table, we see that the proportion of the curve between 0 and z = 1.10 is .3643. In this case the area below the curve, representing the Type II error, is .1357 (.5000-.3643). In this second case, by doubling the sample size we produce power greater than 86% (1-.1357) to detect a 10 mg difference, if such a difference exists.

We can modify Eq. 7.1 slightly to identify the sample size required to produce a given power.

$$n \geq \frac{2\sigma^2}{\delta^2}(z_{\alpha/2} + z_\beta)^2 \qquad \text{Eq. 7.2}$$

Using the same example, assume that we still wish to be able to detect a 10 mg difference between the two batches with 95% confidence ($z_{\alpha/2} = 1.96$). In this case, we also wish to have at least 80% power (the ability to reject H_0 when H_0 is false). Therefore β (1-power) is the point on our normal standardize distribution below which 20% (or 0.20 proportion of the area of the curve) falls. At the same time 0.30 will fall between that point and 0 (.50-.20). Once again looking at Table B2 in Appendix B we find that proportion (.2995) to be located at a z-value of 0.84. Note in Figure 7.4 that the critical values are based on $\alpha/2$ (two-tailed) and 1-β (one-tailed).

$$n \geq \frac{2\sigma^2}{\delta^2}(z_{\alpha/2} + z_\beta)^2$$

$$n \geq \frac{2(64)}{(10)^2}(1.96 + 0.84)^2$$

$$n \geq (1.28)(2.80)^2 = 10.03 \approx 10 \text{ samples}$$

Therefore, to insure a power of at least 80% we should have 11 samples.

Four characteristics are considered regarding power: 1) sample size; 2) the dispersion of the sample(s); 3) amount of Type I error; and 4) the amount of difference to be detected.

$$Type\ II\ Error = \frac{Detectable\ Difference}{\sqrt{\dfrac{Dispersion}{n}}} + Type\ I\ Error \qquad \text{Eq. 7.3}$$

Using Eq. 7.1, it is possible to modify one of the four factors affecting power to detect differences: 1) as the detectable difference increases the power will increase; 2) as sample size increases the denominator decreases and the power once again increases; 3) as the dispersion increases the denominator increases and the power decreases; and 4) as the amount of Type I error decreases it will result in a decreased power. These are graphically illustrated in the following series of figures (Figures 7.5 through 7.8).

The only way to reduce both types of error is to increase the sample size. Thus, for a given level of significance (α), larger sample sizes will result in greater power. Using data from the previous example, Figure 7.5 illustrates the importance of sample size. With α and the dispersion remaining the same, note that as we increase the sample size, the Type II error decreases and the power increases. Therefore, small sample sizes generally lack statistical power and are more likely to fail to identify important differences because the test

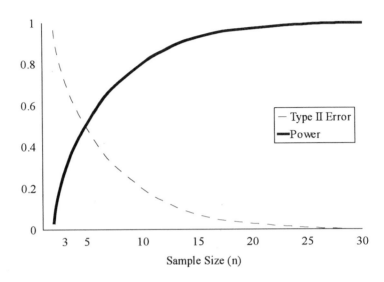

Figure 7.5 Effect of changes in sample size on statistical power (constants δ = 10, σ^2 = 68, α = 0.05).

results will be statistically insignificant.

Obviously, it's easier to detect large differences than very small ones. The importance of detectable differences is seen in Figure 7.6 where the sample size is constant (n=10), the estimated variance is 64 and α remains constant at 0.05. The only change is the amount of difference we wish to detect. As difference increases, power also increases. If we are interested in detecting a difference between two populations, obviously the larger the difference, the easier it is to detect. Again, the question we must ask ourselves is how small a difference do we want to be able to detect or how small should a difference be to be worth detecting?

As seen in Eq. 7.1, the amount of dispersion or variance can also influence power. Figure 7.7 displays the decrease in power that is associated with greater variance in the sample data. Conversely, as the variance within the population decreases, the power of the test to detect a fixed difference (δ) will increase.

Generally Type II error is neither known nor specified in an experimental design. Both types of error are related inversely to each other. If we lower α without changing the sample size, we will increase the probability of having a Type II error and consequently decrease the power ($1-\beta$). Figure 7.8

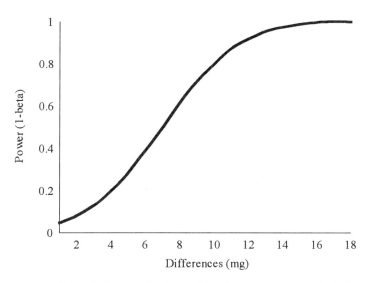

Figure 7.6 Effect of changes in detectable differences on statistical power (constants n $=10$, $\sigma^2 = 64$, $\alpha = 0.05$).

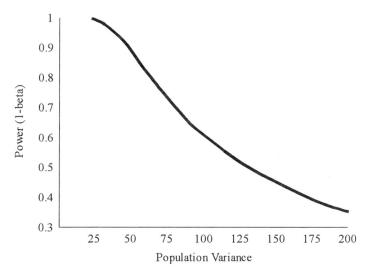

Figure 7.7 Effect of changes in variance on statistical power (constants n $= 10$, $\delta = 10$, $\alpha = 0.05$).

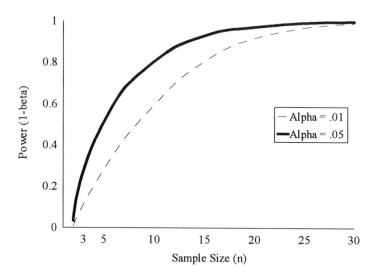

Figure 7.8 Effect of changes in sample sizes on statistical power for two levels of type I error (constants $\delta = 10$, $\sigma^2 = 68$).

illustrates changes in power for two different levels of Type I error with increasing sample sizes. As we increase our confidence that there is a difference (making α smaller), we also increase the chance of missing a true difference, increasing β or decreasing power.

In addition to the above four factors, the number of treatment levels must also be factored in when considering designs that are more complicated than comparing two levels of discrete independent variables.

The size of the sample, or number of observations, is extremely important to statistical research design. We can increase the power of a statistical test without sacrificing our confidence level ($1-\alpha$) solely by increasing our sample size. Unfortunately, sometimes the sample sizes required to satisfy the desired power are extremely large with respect to time and cost considerations. The ways to reduce the required sample size are to increase the precision of the test, or instrument or to increase the level of the minimal acceptable level of detectable differences. Even though it is important to have a large enough sample size to be able to detect important differences; having too large a sample size may result in a significant finding even though for all practical purposes the difference is unimportant. Thus producing results that are statistically significant but have clinically insignificant differences.

The problem with the previous example is that the formula is limited to only two levels of discrete independent variables. Also, we must know the population variance. Therefore, Eq. 7.1 represents only one unique method of determining Type II error (specifically for the alternative hypothesis that two population means are not equal). Numerous formulas exist which can be used to calculate the appropriate sample size under different criteria. These include power curves presented by Kirk (1968), based on α, $1-\beta$ and the number of levels of the independent variable; and Young's nomograms (1983) for sample size determination (an excellent reference for many of these methods is presented by Zar). Listed in Table 7.1 are pages from Zar's book for power and sample size determination for many of the statistical tests presented in the remainder of this book. A discussion of power and sample size with the binomial tests was given by Bolton (1997).

Power is often calculated after the experiment has been completed. In these *post hoc* cases the sample standard deviation can be substituted for σ. In general, Type II error is neither known or specified in an experimental design. For a given sample size, α and β are inversely proportional. If we lower α without changing the sample size, we will increase the probability of a Type II error and consequently decrease the power ($1-\beta$). The more "powerful" the test, the better the chances are that the null hypothesis will be rejected, when the

Table 7.1 Formulas for Determination of Statistical Power and Sample Size Selection

Chapter	Statistical Test	Page(s) in Zar
8	One-sample t-test	110-111
8	Two-sample t-test	134-136
8	Paired t-test	153
9	One-way Analysis of Variance	171-176
11	Two-way Analysis of Variance	227-228
12	Correlation	312
13	Linear regression	283
14	Z-test of Proportions	397-400

From: Zar, J.H. (1984). Biostatistical Analysis, 2nd ed., Prentice Hall, Englewood Cliffs, NJ.

null hypothesis is in fact false. The greater the power, the more sensitive the statistical test.

One of the advantages of statistical analysis and hypothesis testing is that its principles are general and applicable to data from any field of study (i.e., biological, physical or behavioral). All of the tests presented apply to data regardless of the source of the information or the branch of science or academia from which it was derived. As mentioned in Chapter 1 and seen in Appendix A, the most important first step, in selecting the most appropriate statistic is to identify the independent and dependent variables and define them as discrete or continuous.

References

Bolton, S. (1997). Pharmaceutical Statistics: Practical and Clinical Applications, Marcel Dekker, Inc., New York, 1984, pp. 199-207.

Kachigan, S.K. (1991). Multivariate Statistical Analysis, Radius Press, New York, p.112-3.

Kirk, R.E. (1968). Experimental Design: Procedures for the Behavioral Science, Brooks/Cole Publishing Co., Belmont, CA, pp.9-11, 540-546.

Young, M.J., et al. (1983). Sample size nomograms for interpreting negative clinical studies. Annals of Internal Medicine 99:248-251.

Suggested Supplemental Readings

Daniel, W.W. (1991). Biostatistics: A Foundation for Analysis in the Health Sciences, John Wiley and Sons, New York, pp. 191-233.

Kachigan, S.K. (1991). Multivariate Statistical Analysis, Radius Press, New York, p.104-116.

Snedecor, G.W. and Cochran W.G. (1989). Statistical Methods, Iowa State University Press, Ames, IA, pp.64-82.

Example Problems

1. Write the alternate hypothesis for each of the following null hypotheses:

    a. $\mu_A = \mu_B$

    b. $\mu_H \geq \mu_L$

    c. $\mu_1 = \mu_2 = \mu_3 = \mu_4 = \mu_5 = \mu_6$

    d. $\mu_A \leq \mu_B$

    e. $\mu = 125$

    f.   populations C, D, E, F and G are the same

    g.   both samples come from the same population

2. If power is calculated to be 85%, with Type I error rate of 5%, what are the percentages associated with the four possible outcomes associated with hypothesis testing? What if the power was only 72%?

Answers to Problems

1. The null hypothesis and alternative hypothesis must create mutually exclusive and exhaustive statements.

    a. H_0: $\mu_A = \mu_B$
              H_1: $\mu_A \neq \mu_B$

    b. H_0: $\mu_H \geq \mu_L$
              H_1: $\mu_H < \mu_L$

    c. H_0: $\mu_1 = \mu_2 = \mu_3 = \mu_4 = \mu_5 = \mu_6$
              H_1: H_0 is false
       (As will be discussed in Chapter 8, traditional tests do not allow us to immediately identify which population means are different, only that at least two of the six means are significantly different. Further testing is required to determine the exact source of the difference(s).)

d. H_0: $\quad \mu_A \leq \mu_B$

   H_1: $\quad \mu_A > \mu_B$

e. H_0: $\quad \mu = 125$

   H_1: $\quad \mu \neq 125$

f. H_0: $\quad$ Populations C, D, E, F and G are the same

   H_1: $\quad$ Populations C, D, E, F and G are not the same

   (Similar to c above, we do not identify the specific difference(s).)

g. H_0: $\quad$ Both samples come from the same population

   H_1: $\quad$ Both samples do not come from the same population

2. In the first part of the question: α (Type I error) = 0.05; confidence level $(1-\alpha)$ = 0.95; power $(1-\beta)$ = 85%; therefore, β (Type II error) = 0.15. If the power happens to be only 72% or 0.72, then the other outcomes in our test of null hypotheses are: β (Type II error) = 1-0.72 = 0.28; α (Type I error) = 0.05; confidence level $(1-\alpha)$ = 0.95. Note that α and $1-\alpha$ did not change because the researcher would have set these parameters prior to the statistical test.

8

t-tests

The initial seven chapters of this book focused on the "threads" associated with the statistical tests which will be discussed in the following ten chapters. The order of presentation of these statistical tests are based on the types of variables (continuous or discrete) which researchers may encounter in the their design of experiments. As noted in Chapter 1, in this book independent variables are defined as those which the researcher can control (i.e., assignment to a control or experimental group); whereas, dependent variables fall outside the control of the researcher and are measured as outcomes or responses (i.e., pharmacokinetic responses). It should be noted that other authors may use the terms factors or predictor variables to describe what we've defined as an independent variables or response variable to describe the dependent variable. We will continue to use the terms used in the preceding seven chapters.

Chapters 8 through 11 (t-tests, one-way analysis of variance, post hoc procedures and factorial designs) are concerned with independent variables that are discrete and outcomes measured on some continuum (dependent variable). Chapters 12 and 13 present tests where both the dependent and independent variables are presented on continuous scales (i.e., correlation and regression). Chapters 14, 15 and 16 (z-test of proportions and chi square tests) continue the presentation of tests concerned with discrete independent variables, but in these chapters the dependent variable is measured as a discrete outcome (i.e., pass or fail, live or die). Chapter 17 provides nonparametric or distribution-free statistics for evaluating data which does not meet the criteria required for many of the tests presented in Chapters 8 through 16.

Parametric Procedures

The parametric procedures include such tests as the t-tests, analysis of variance (ANOVAs or F-tests), correlation and linear regression; Chapters 8, 9, 12 and 13 respectively. In addition to the requirements that the samples must be randomly selected from their population and independently measured, two additional "parameters" must be met. First, it must be assumed that the sample is drawn from a population whose distribution approximates that of a normal distribution. Second, when two or more distributions are being compared, there must be **homogeneity of variance** or **homoscedasticity** (sample variances must be approximately equal). A rule of thumb is that if the largest variance divided by the smallest variance is less than two, then homogeneity may be assumed. A more specific test for homoscedasticity will be discussed in the next chapter. With both the t-tests and F-tests there is an independent discrete variable containing one or more levels and a dependent variable that is measured on a continuous scale. Three types of parametric tests are presented in this chapter: 1) one-sample t-test; 2) two-sample t-test; and 3) paired t-test. In each case, the independent variable is discrete and the dependent variable represents continuously distributed data.

The t-distribution

In Chapter 6, discussion focused on the standardized normal distribution, the standard error of the mean and the use of the z-test to create a confidence interval. This interval is the researchers "best guess" of a range of scores within which the true population mean will fall (Eq. 6.8):

$$\mu = \overline{X} \pm (1.96)\frac{\sigma}{\sqrt{n}}$$

The disadvantage with this formula is the requirement that the population standard deviation (σ) must be known. In most research, the population standard deviation is unknown or at best a rough estimate can be made based from previous research (i.e., initial clinical trials or previous production runs). As seen in Figure 6.5, the larger the sample size the more constant the value of the standard error of the mean; therefore, the z-test is accurate only for large samples. From this it would seem logical that the researcher should produce a more conservative statistic as sample sizes become smaller and less information is known about the true population variance. This was noted and rationalized by William S. Gossett in an excellent 1908 article (Student, 1908). He published this work under the pseudonym "student." At least two stories exist regarding the pseudonym: 1) he was a graduate student and at the time only professors were allowed to publish such theses; and 2) he worked for Guinness Brewing Company and could not be published because of his commercial association. Regardless of which story is correct, the distribution became known as the Student t-distribution and subsequent tests are called Student t-tests or t-tests.

The t-tests, and their associated frequency distributions, are used 1) to compare one sample to a known population or value or 2) to compare two samples to each other and make inferences to their populations. These are the most commonly used tests to compare two samples because in most cases the population variances are unknown. To correct for this, the t-tables are used which adjust the z-values of a normal distribution to account for sample sizes. Note in the abbreviated t-table below (Table 8.1), that any t-value at infinity degrees of freedom is equal to the corresponding z-value for a given Type I error (α). In other words, the t-table is nothing more than a normal standardized distribution (z-table) which corrects for the number of observations per sample.

Like the normal distribution, the shape of the Student t-distribution is symmetrical and the mean value is zero. The exact shape of the curve depends on the degrees of freedom. As the sample sizes get smaller, the amplitude of the curve becomes shorter and the range becomes wider (Figure 8.1). A more complete table of t-values is presented in Table B3 in Appendix B. Note in Table 8.1 that this is a table designed for two-tailed bi-directional tests. The Type I error rate is divided in half ($\alpha/2$). In the case of 95% confidence, there is a 2.5% chance of being wrong to the high side of the distribution and 2.5% chance of error to the lower tail of the distribution. Therefore, allowing for 5% error divided in half and subtracted from all possible outcomes ($1-\alpha/2$) the

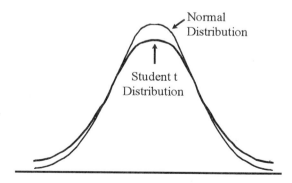

Figure 8.1 Comparison of curves for a t-distribution and z-distribution.

Table 8.1 Selected Values for the t-distribution for (1-α/2)

d.f. degrees of freedom	t.95 90%	t.975 95%	t.995 99%
5	2.015	2.570	4.032
10	1.812	2.228	3.169
20	1.724	2.086	2.845
30	1.697	2.042	2.750
60	1.670	2.000	2.660
120	1.657	1.979	2.617
∞	1.645	1.960	2.576

symbol of $t_{.975}$ presented in the second column of Table 8.1 represents the column for 95% confidence. Reviewing the table, the first column is degrees of freedom ($n-1$), the second column represents critical values for 90% confidence levels, the third for 95% and the last for 99% confidence intervals. As the number of observations decreases, the Student t-value increases and the spread of the distribution increases to give a more conservative estimate, because less information is known about the population variance.

One-tailed vs. Two-tailed Tests

There are two ways in which the type I error (α) can be distributed. In a **two-tailed test** the rejection region is equally divided between the two ends of the sampling distribution ($\alpha/2$) as described above. For example, assume we are comparing a new drug to a traditional therapeutic approach. With a two-tailed test we are not predicting that one drug is superior to the other.

$$H_0: \qquad \mu_{new\ drug} = \mu_{old\ drug}$$
$$H_1: \qquad \mu_{new\ drug} \neq \mu_{old\ drug}$$

Assuming we would like to be 95% confident in our decision, the sampling error could result in a sample that is too high (2.5%) or too low (2.5%) based on chance sampling error. This would represent a total error rate of 5%. The rejection region for a two-tailed test where p<0.05 and df = ∞ is illustrated as Figure 8.2.

In contrast, a **one-tailed test** is a test of hypothesis in which the rejection region is placed entirely at one end of the sampling distribution. In our current example, assume we want to prove that the new drug is superior to traditional therapy:

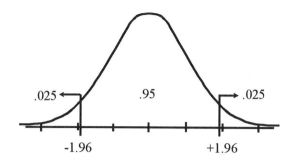

Figure 8.2 Graphic representation of a two-tailed test.

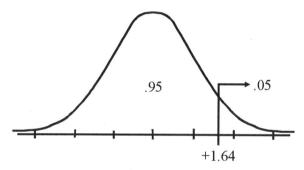

Figure 8.3 Graphic representation of a one-tailed test.

$$H_0: \quad \mu_{\text{new drug}} \leq \mu_{\text{old drug}}$$
$$H_1: \quad \mu_{\text{new drug}} > \mu_{\text{old drug}}$$

If a one-tailed test is used, all the α is loaded on one side of the equation:

$$H_0: \mu_1 \leq \mu_2$$
$$H_1: \mu_1 > \mu_2$$

and the decision rule with $\alpha = 0.05$, would be to reject H_0 if $t > t_{df}(1-\alpha)$. Once again we would like to be 95% confident in our decision. The rejection region for a one-tailed test where $p<.05$ and df $= \infty$ is seen in Figure 8.3. In our example, what if our drug was truly inferior to the older drug. Using a one-tailed test we would not be able to prove this result. For that reason, the one-tailed test should never be used unless there is a specific justification for being directional. Table B4 in Appendix B provides critical t-values for both one-tailed and two-tailed tests.

Failure to reject the null hypothesis does not mean that this hypothesis is accepted as truth. Much like the jurisprudence example, the defendant is acquitted as "not guilty," as contrasted to "innocent." Thus, we fail to reject the null hypothesis, we do not prove that the null hypothesis is true. Insufficient evidence is available to conclude that H_0 is false.

One-Sample t-tests

The one-sample case can be used to either estimate the population mean or compare the sample mean to an expected population mean. In the first method, a sample is taken on some measurable data and the researcher wishes to "guess" at the true population mean. In a previous chapter, 30 bottles of a cough syrup are randomly sampled from a production line (Table 5.1). From this information, it was found that the sample mean equaled 120.05 ml with a standard deviation of 0.84 ml. This data could be used to predict the mean for the entire population of cough syrup in this production lot. With 95% certainty, the confidence interval would be:

$$\mu = \overline{X} \pm t_{n-1}(1-\alpha/2) \cdot \frac{S}{\sqrt{n}} \qquad \text{Eq. 8.1}$$

Notice that the population standard deviation in the error term portion of the z-test (Eq. 6.8) has been replaced with the sample standard deviation. The expression $t_{n-1}(1-\alpha/2)$ is the t-value in Tables B3 or B4 in Appendix B for 29 observations or n-1 degrees of freedom[1].

$$\mu = 120.05 \pm (2.045) \cdot \frac{0.84}{\sqrt{30}} = 120.05 \pm 0.31$$

$$119.74 < \mu < 120.36$$

The value 2.045 is an interpolation of the t-value between 30 and 25 degrees of freedom in Table B3. Therefore, based on our sample of 30 bottles, it is

---

[1] Note that exactly 29 degrees of freedom are not listed in Tables 3A or 4A, but the value can be interpolation from a comparison values for 25 and 30 df. The difference between 25 and 30 df is equivalent to 0.017 (2.059-2.042).

$$1/5 = x/0.017 \qquad x = 0.003$$

Therefore, $t_{29}(.975) = 2.042 + 0.003 = 2.045$

estimated with 95% confidence that the true population (all bottles in the production lot) is between 119.74 and 120.34 ml.

With 99% confidence the values would be calculated as follows:

$$\mu = 120.05 \pm (2.757) \frac{0.84}{\sqrt{30}} = 120.05 \pm 0.42$$

where 2.757 represents an interpolated value off Table B3 or B4 for 29 degrees of freedom at $\alpha = 0.01$.

$$119.63 < \mu < 120.47$$

Note that in order to express greater confidence in our decision regarding the population mean, the range of our estimate increases. If it were acceptable to be less confident (90% or 80% certain that the population mean was within the estimated range) the width of the interval would decrease.

One method for decreasing the size of the confidence interval is to increase the sample size. As seen in Equation 8.1, an increase in sample size will not only result in a smaller value for $t_{n-1}(1-\alpha/2)$, but the denominator (square root of n) will increase causing a decrease in the standard error portion of the equation. To illustrate this, assume the sample standard deviation remains constant for Sample B in the example of C_{max} presented in Chapter 6 (Table 6.2), where the $\overline{X} = 752.8$, S = 21.5 and n = 5. With $t_4(.975) = 2.78$, our best guess of the population mean would be:

$$\mu = \overline{X} \pm t_{n-1}(1-\alpha/2) \frac{S}{\sqrt{n}}$$

$$\mu = 752.8 \pm (2.78) \frac{21.5}{\sqrt{5}} = 752.8 \pm 26.73$$

$$726.07 < \mu < 779.53$$

If the sample size were increased to 25, where $t_{24}(.975) \approx 2.06$, the new confidence interval would be:

$$\mu = 752.8 \pm (2.06) \frac{21.5}{\sqrt{25}} = 752.8 \pm 8.86$$

$$743.94 < \mu < 761.66$$

If we had the ability, funds and time to have another five-fold increase to 125 samples, where $t_{124}(.975) \approx 1.98$, the confidence interval would shrink to the following size:

$$\mu = 752.8 \pm (1.98)\ \frac{21.5}{\sqrt{125}} = 752.8 \pm 3.81$$

$$748.99 < \mu < 756.61$$

This "shrinking" in the size of the confidence interval can be graphically seen in Figure 8.4. Obviously, the more we know about the population, as reflected by a large sample size, the more precisely we can estimate the population mean.

Two-Sample t-tests

A two-sample t-test compares two levels of a discrete independent variable to determine, based on the sample statistics, if their respective populations are the same or different. Two approaches can be taken in performing a two-sample t-test: 1) establish a confidence interval for the population differences or 2) compare test results to a critical value. Either method will produce the same results and the same decision will be made with respect to the null hypothesis.

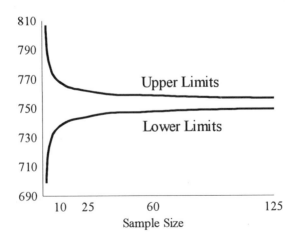

Figure 8.4 Effect of sample size on width of confidence intervals.

A two-sample t-test will be used to illustrate these two methods of hypothesis testing. The hypotheses could be written in two similar, but not identical statements.

	Confidence Interval	Critical Value
The population means are the same:	H_0: $\mu_1 - \mu_2 = 0$	H_0: $\mu_1 = \mu_2$
The population means are different:	H_1: $\mu_1 - \mu_2 \neq 0$	H_1: $\mu_1 \neq \mu_2$

The first case is an extension of the methodology used in performing a one-sample t-test. An interval is established based upon the estimated centers of the distributions (sample means), their respective standard error of the means and a selected reliability coefficient to reflect how confident we wish to be in our final decision (Eq. 6.7).

$$\frac{Population}{Difference} = \frac{Sample}{Difference} \pm \frac{Reliability}{Coefficient} \ x \ \frac{Standard}{Error}$$

The statistical formula compares the central tendencies of two different samples and based on the results determines whether or not their respective populations are equal or not. If they are equal, H_0: $\mu_1 - \mu_2 = 0$, then a zero difference must fall within the confidence interval. If they are not equal, H_1: $\mu_1 - \mu_2 \neq 0$, then zero does not fall within the estimated population interval and the difference cannot be attributed only to random error.

In the one-sample t-test the standard deviation (or variance) was critical to the calculation of the error term in Equation 6.7. In the two-sample case, the variances should be close together (homogeneity of variance requirement), but more than likely they will not be identical. The simplest way to calculate a central variance term would be to average the two variances:

$$S^2_{average} = \frac{S^2_1 + S^2_2}{2} \qquad \text{Eq. 8.2}$$

Unfortunately the number of observations per level may not be the same; therefore, it's necessary to "pool" these two variances and weigh them by the number of observations per discrete level of the independent variable.

$$S^2_p = \frac{(n_1 - 1)S^2_1 + (n_2 - 1)S^2_2}{n_1 + n_2 - 2} \qquad \text{Eq. 8.3}$$

Using this latter equation, differences in sample sizes are accounted for by producing a **pooled variance** (S_p^2).

The confidence interval for the difference between the population means, based on the sample means, is calculated using the following equation:

$$\mu_1 - \mu_2 = (\overline{X}_1 - \overline{X}_2) \pm t_{n_1+n_2-2}(1 - \alpha/2) \sqrt{\frac{s_p^2}{n_1} + \frac{s_p^2}{n_2}} \qquad \text{Eq. 8.4}$$

Obviously, $\overline{X}_1$ and $\overline{X}_2$ represent the two sample means and n_1 and n_2 are the respective sample sizes. The expression ($\overline{X}_1 - \overline{X}_2$) serves as our best estimate of the true population difference ($\mu_1 - \mu_2$).

The second, alternative method for testing the hypothesis is to create a statistical ratio and compare this to the critical value for a particular level of confidence. We can think of this t-test as a ratio:

$$t = \frac{\textit{difference between the means}}{\textit{distribution of the means}} \qquad \text{Eq. 8.5}$$

Obviously, if the difference between the samples is zero, the numerator would be zero, the resultant t-value would also be zero and the researcher would conclude no significant difference. As the difference between the sample mean becomes larger, the numerator increases, the t-value increases and there is a greater likelihood that the difference is not due to chance error alone. Looking at the illustrations in Figure 8.5, it is more likely that the groups to the left are significantly different because the numerator will be large; whereas the pair to the right will have a larger denominator because of the large overlap of the spreads of the distributions. But how far to the extreme does the calculated

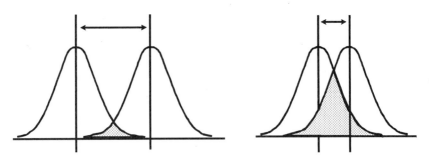

Figure 8.5 Comparison of two different means with similar dispersions.

$t_{obt} > t_{crit} \rightarrow reject\ H_0$

$t_{obt} > 63.93$

2.5^+

t-value in Equation 8.5 need to be in order to be significant? Greater than 1? Or 2? Or 50? The critical value is selected off the Student t-table (Table B3, Appendix B) based on the number of degrees of freedom. In the case of a two-sample t-test the degrees of freedom are n_1-1 plus n_2-1, or more commonly written n_1+n_2-2.

$$df = n_1 + n_2 - 2 = (n_1 - 1) + (n_2 - 1)$$

The variance also influences the calculated t-value. As observations cluster closer together, it is likely that smaller differences between means may be significant. With respect to Equation 8.5, as the variance becomes smaller the denominator in the ratio becomes smaller and the t-value will increase. If the t-value is to the extreme of the critical value then the null hypothesis will be rejected in favor of the alternative hypothesis. Once again the pooled variance (Eq. 8.3) is used to calculate this t-value:

$$t = \frac{\overline{X_1} - \overline{X_2}}{\sqrt{\dfrac{S_P^2}{n_1} + \dfrac{S_P^2}{n_2}}} \qquad \text{Eq. 8.6}$$

As discussed in the next section, the t-test can be either one-tailed or two tailed. For the moment we shall focus only on two-tailed tests:

$$H_0: \mu_1 = \mu_2$$
$$H_1: \mu_1 \neq \mu_2$$

and no prediction is made whether μ_1 or μ_2 is larger. In this case the decision rule is, with α equal to a set value (usually 0.05), reject H_0 if $t > t_{df}(1-\alpha/2)$ or if $t < -t_{df}(1-\alpha/2)$. Note that the calculated t-value can be either positive or negative depending on which sample mean is considered first. Thus, the resultant t-value can be either positive or negative. Again, if the value resulting from Equation 8.6. is to the extreme (farther from zero to the positive or negative direction) than the critical value there is sufficient reason to reject the null hypothesis and conclude that this difference cannot be explained by chance error alone.

The use of these two different approaches for using the t-test in hypothesis testing is presented in the following example. An investigator used a two period cross over study to compare two formulations of a drug to determine the time to maximum concentration (C_{max}). Is there a significant difference between the two formulations (Table 8.2)? The first approach is to establish a

Table 8.2 C$_{max}$ Values for Two Formulations of the Same Drug

Formulation A						Formulation B					
125	130	135	126	140	135	130	128	127	149	151	130
128	121	123	126	121	133	141	145	132	132	141	129
131	129	120	117	126	127	133	136	138	142	130	122
119	133	125	120	136	122	129	150	148	136	138	140
Mean (ng/ml)		127.00				Mean (ng/ml)		136.54			
Standard deviation		6.14				Standard deviation		8.09			
Subjects		24				Subjects		24			

confidence interval where the hypotheses are:

$$H_0: \ \mu_A - \mu_B = 0$$
$$H_1: \ \mu_A - \mu_B \neq 0$$

The test statistic is Equation 8.4 and the decision rule is, with $\alpha = .05$, reject H_0 if zero does not fall within the confidence interval. The computations involve first calculating the pooled variance and then the confidence interval with 95% confidence:

$$S_p^2 = \frac{23(6.14)^2 + 23(8.09)^2}{24 + 24 - 2} = \frac{2372.40}{46} = 51.57$$

$$\mu_A - \mu_B = (127.00 - 136.54) \pm 2.01 \ \sqrt{\frac{51.57}{24} + \frac{51.57}{24}}$$

$$\mu_A - \mu_B = -9.54 \pm 2.01(2.07) = -9.54.36 \pm 4.16$$

$$-13.70 < \mu_A - \mu_B < -5.38$$

Thus, since zero is not within the C.I., reject H_0 and conclude that there is a significant difference, with formulation A requiring a smaller for C$_{max}$. A zero outcome (H_0) is not a possible outcome with 95% confidence.

The second approach is to compare a calculated t-value to its corresponding critical value on the t-table (Table B3), where the hypotheses are the same:

$$H_0: \mu_A = \mu_B$$
$$H_1: \mu_A \neq \mu_B$$

The test statistic is Equation 8.6 and the decision rule is, with $\alpha = .05$, reject H_0 if $t > t_{46}(.025)$ or $t < -t_{46}(.025)$. In this case with 46 degrees of freedom reject H_0 if $t > 2.01$ or $t < -2.01$. The computations are as follows:

$$S_p^2 = \frac{(n_A-1)S_A^2+(n_B-1)S_B^2}{n_A+n_B-2} = 51.57$$

$$t = \frac{127.0-136.54}{\sqrt{\dfrac{51.57}{24}+\dfrac{51.57}{24}}} = \frac{-9.54}{2.07} = -4.61$$

The results show that the calculated t-value is smaller than (to the extreme negative side of) the critical-t of -2.01. Therefore, we would reject H_0, conclude that there is a significant difference, with formulation B reaching a significantly higher C_{max}. In both cases, the results of the statistical test were identical, the rejection of the null hypothesis. With only two formulas being compared, the initial data can be looked at and the results can state that there were was significant difference between the two formulations, and that with 95% confidence ($\alpha=.05$) Formula B has a significantly higher C_{max}.

One-sample t-test Revisited for Critical Values

The one-sample t-test can also use an established critical value as a method for testing the null hypothesis that a sample is taken from a certain population. Using the previous sample of 30 bottles of cough syrup (Table 5.1), assume that we expect this particular syrup to have a fill volume of 120.0 ml. In this case our expected population center (μ_0) is 120 ml. Is this sample taken from that population?

$$H_0: \mu = \mu_0 = 120.0$$
$$H_1: \mu \neq \mu_0$$

The null hypothesis is that the samples come from a given population and that any difference has arisen simply by chance. The one-sample t-test enables us to determine the likelihood of this hypothesis. The test statistic is:

$$t = \frac{\overline{X} - \mu_0}{\dfrac{S}{\sqrt{n}}}$$ Eq. 8.7

The decision rule can be established based on the researcher's desired confidence (acceptable amount of Type I error) in the outcome of the hypothesis testing. With 1-α equal to 0.95 (95% confidence) the decision rule is, reject H_0 if t > $t_{29}(1-\alpha/2)$ or if t < $-t_{29}(1-\alpha/2)$, where $t_{29}(1-\alpha/2)$ is 2.04. For 99% confidence, the decision rule would be, with α = .01, reject H_0 if t > +2.75 or if t < -2.75. Therefore if the t-value we calculate is to the extreme of 2.04 (positive or negative) H_0 can be rejected with 95% confidence in the decision. If the result is to the extreme of 2.75, H_0 is rejected with 99% confidence. The calculation of the t-value or t-statistic is:

$$t = \frac{120.05 - 120.00}{\dfrac{0.84}{\sqrt{30}}} = \frac{0.05}{0.15} = 0.33$$

Similar to both the 95% and 99% confidence interval created in a previous section, where 120.0 fell within the interval, we cannot reject the hypothesis that the sample is equal to the expected population mean of 120 ml. Stated differently, we cannot reject the hypothesis that our sample is taken from a population with a mean of 120 ml.

Matched Pair t-Test (Difference t-Test)

The matched pair, or **paired t-test**, is used when complete independence does not exist between the two samples, two time periods or repeated measures. For example, in a pretest-posttest design, where the same individual takes both tests, it is assumed that his/her results on the posttest will be affected (not independent) by the pretest. The individual actually serves as his/her own control. Therefore the test statistic is not concerned with differences between groups, but actual individual subject differences. The hypotheses are associated with the mean difference in the samples:

$$H_0: \ \mu_d = 0$$
$$H_1: \ \mu_d \neq 0$$

To perform the test a table showing the differences must be created and used to calculate the mean difference and the standard deviation of the difference between the two sample measurements.

Before	After	d (After-Before)	d^2
x_1	x'_1	$d_1 = (x'_1 - x_1)$	d_1^2
x_2	x'_2	$d_2 = (x'_2 - x_2)$	d_2^2
x_3	x'_3	$d_3 = (x'_3 - x_3)$	d_3^2
...	...	...	...
x_n	x'_n	$d_n = (x'_n - x_n)$	d_n^2
		Σd	Σd^2

Each row represents an individual's score or response. The first two columns are the actual outcomes. The third column is the difference between the first two columns per individual. Traditionally the first measure (before) is subtracted from the second measurement (after). Therefore a positive difference represents a larger outcome on the second measure. The mean difference is calculated:

$$\overline{X}_d = \frac{\Sigma d}{n} \qquad \text{Eq. 8.8}$$

and the standard deviation of the difference is the square root of the variance difference:

$$S_d^2 = \frac{n(\Sigma d^2) - (\Sigma d)^2}{n(n-1)} \qquad \text{Eq. 8.9}$$

$$S_d = \sqrt{S_d^2} \qquad \text{Eq. 8.10}$$

The t-value calculations are as follows, depending on use of confidence intervals or critical values:

$$\mu_d = \overline{X}_d \pm t_{n-1}(\alpha/2) \cdot \frac{S_d}{\sqrt{n}} \qquad \text{Eq. 8.11}$$

Similar to the two-sample t-test, if zero falls within the confidence interval, a zero outcome is possible and we fail to reject the H_0. Alternatively, if all the possible values in the confidence interval are positive or all are negative, we reject the null hypothesis and conclude that there is a significant difference. The second method for hypothesis testing would be to: 1) establish a decision rule based on a critical t-value from Tables B3 or B4; 2) calculate a t-value based on the ratio of the difference divided by the distribution; and 3) reject the hypothesis under tests if the t-value that is calculated is greater than the critical value off the table. Similar to previous tests, our estimator is in the numerator and an error term in the denominator:

$$t = \frac{\overline{X_d}}{\frac{S_d}{\sqrt{n}}}$$ Eq. 8.12

Like the decision rules for hypothesis testing with the two-sample case, the test can be either one-tailed or two-tailed. In the one-tailed paired t-test the hypotheses would be either:

$$H_0: \mu_d \leq 0 \qquad \text{or} \qquad H_0: \mu_d \geq 0$$
$$H_1: \mu_d > 0 \qquad\qquad\quad H_1: \mu_d < 0$$

and the decision rule would be, with $\alpha = 0.05$, reject H_0 if $t > t_{df}(1-\alpha)$. In the two-tailed test we again split the Type I error between the two tails with our hypotheses being:

$$H_0: \mu_d = 0$$
$$H_1: \mu_d \neq 0$$

the decision rule with $\alpha = 0.05$, is to reject H_0 if $t > t_{df}(1-\alpha/2)$ or if $t < -t_{df}(1-\alpha/2)$.

Because we are interested in differences in each individual, with the matched-paired t-test the degrees of freedom (df) is concerned with the number of pairs rather than the number of individual observations.

$$df = n\text{-}1 \text{ (number of pairs)}$$

The following illustrates the use of a one-tailed matched paired t-test. A preliminary study was conducted to determine if a new antihypertensive agent could lower the diastolic blood pressure in normal individuals. Initial clinical results are presented in the first two columns of Table 8.3. Because this is a one-tailed test (did the new drug lower the blood pressure, indicating a desired direction for the alternate hypothesis) the hypotheses are as follows:

Table 8.3 Diastolic Blood Pressure Before and After Administration of a New Antihypertensive

Subject	Before	After	d(after-before)	d^2
1	68	66	-2	4
2	83	80	-3	9
3	72	67	-5	25
4	75	74	-1	1
5	79	70	-9	81
6	71	77	+6	36
7	65	64	-1	1
8	76	70	-6	36
9	78	76	-2	4
10	68	66	-2	4
11	85	81	-4	16
12	74	68	-6	36
		$\Sigma =$	-35	253

$$H_0: \mu_d \geq 0$$
$$H_1: \mu_d < 0$$

In this case a rise in blood pressure or no change in blood pressure would result in a failure to reject H_0. Only if there was a significant decrease in the blood pressure would we reject H_0 in favor of the alternative hypothesis.

In this first example we will first establish a critical t-value, where the test statistic (Eq. 8.12) is:

$$t = \frac{\overline{X_d}}{\dfrac{S_d}{\sqrt{n}}}$$

The decision rule would be, with $\alpha = .05$, reject H_0 if $t < -t_{11}(.95)$, which is 1.795 in Table B3 (note that this is a one-tailed test; therefore, the critical value comes from the third column, t_{95}). In this case we have set up our experiment to determine if there is a significant decrease in blood pressure and the difference we record is based on the second measure (after) minus the original results (before). Therefore a "good" or "desirable" response would be a negative number. If the ratio we calculate using the t-test is a negative value to the extreme of the critical value we can reject the H_0. Because we are performing a one-tailed test we need to be extremely careful about the signs (positive or negative).

The calculations for the mean difference and standard deviation of the difference are as follows:

$$\overline{X}_d = \frac{\Sigma d}{n} = \frac{-35}{12} = -2.92$$

$$S_d^2 = \frac{n(\Sigma d^2) - (\Sigma d)^2}{n(n-1)} = \frac{12(253) - (-35)^2}{12(11)} = 13.72$$

$$S_d = \sqrt{S_d^2} = \sqrt{13.72} = 3.70$$

The calculation of the t-value would be:

$$t = \frac{-2.92}{\dfrac{3.70}{\sqrt{12}}} = \frac{-2.92}{1.07} = -2.73$$

Therefore, based on a computed t-value less than the critical t-value of -1.795, the decision is to reject H_0 and conclude that there was a significant decrease in the diastolic blood pressure.

Using this same example, it is possible to calculate a confidence interval with $\alpha = 0.05$. If zero falls within the confidence interval, then zero difference between the two measures is a possible outcome and the null hypothesis cannot be rejected. From the previous example we know that $\overline{X}_d = -2.92$, $S_d = 3.70$ and $n = 12$. From Table B4 in Appendix B the reliability coefficient for 11 degrees of freedom $(n-1)$ is $t_{11}(1-\frac{\alpha}{2}) = \text{1.795}$ at 95% confidence. Calculation of the confidence interval is

$$\mu_d = \overline{X}_d \pm t_{n-1}(\alpha - 1/2) \frac{S_d}{\sqrt{n}}$$

$$\mu_d = -2.92 \pm (1.795) \frac{3.70}{\sqrt{12}} = -2.92 \pm 1.92$$

$$-4.84 < \mu_d < -1.00$$

Since zero does not fall within the interval and in fact all possible outcomes are in the negative direction, it could be concluded with 95% certainty that there was a significant decrease in blood pressure. The results are exactly the same as found when the t-ratio was calculated the first time.

Reference

Student (1908). "The probable error of a mean" Biometrika 6(1):1-25.

Suggested Supplemental Readings

Bolton, S. (1997). Pharmaceutical Statistics: Practical and Clinical Applications, Marcel Dekker, New York, pp. 141-148, 151-158.

Daniel, W.W. (1991). Biostatistics: A Foundation for Analysis in the Health Sciences, John Wiley and Sons, New York, pp. 138-148, 209-213.

Snedecor, G.W. and Cochran W.G. (1989). Statistical Methods, Iowa State University Press, Ames, IA, pp.83-105.

Example Problems

1. An examination evaluating cognitive knowledge in basic pharmacology was mailed to a random sample of all pharmacists in a particular state. Those responding were classified as either hospital or community pharmacists. The examination results were:

	Hospital Pharmacists	Community Pharmacists
Mean Score	82.1	79.9
Variance	151.29	210.25
Respondents	129	142

   Assuming that these respondents are representative of their particular populations, is there any significant difference between the types of practice based on the examination results?

2. Twelve subjects in a clinical trial to evaluate the effectiveness of a new bronchodilator were assessed for changes in their pulmonary function. Forced expiratory volume in one second (FEV_1) measurements were taken before and three hours after drug administration.

Subject Number	Before Administration	FEV_1 Three Hours Past Administration
1	3.0	3.1
2	3.6	3.9
3	3.5	3.7
4	3.8	3.8
5	3.3	3.2
6	3.9	3.8
7	3.1	3.4
8	3.2	3.3
9	3.5	3.6
10	3.4	3.4
11	3.5	3.7
12	3.6	3.5

a.   What is $t_{(1-\alpha/2)}$ for $\alpha = 0.05$?

b.   Construct a 95% confidence interval for the difference between population means.

c.   Use a t-test to compare the two groups.

3.   Calculate the mean, standard deviation, relative standard deviation and 95% confidence interval for each of the time periods presented in the following dissolution profile (percentage of label claim):

		Time (minutes)			
Sample	10	20	30	45	60
1	60.3	95.7	97.6	98.6	98.7
2	53.9	95.6	97.5	98.6	98.7
3	70.4	95.1	96.8	97.9	98.0
4	61.7	95.3	97.2	98.0	98.2
5	64.4	92.8	95.0	95.8	96.0
6	59.3	96.3	98.3	99.1	99.2

4.   A first-time in man clinical trial was conducted to determine the pharmacokinetic parameters for a new calcium channel blocker. The study involved 20 healthy adult males and yielded the following C_{max} data (maximum serum concentration in ng/ml):

715, 728, 735, 716, 706, 715, 712, 717, 731, 709,
722, 701, 698, 741, 723, 718, 726, 716, 720, 721

Compute a 95% confidence interval for the population mean for this pharmacokinetic parameter.

5. Following training on content uniformity testing, comparisons are made between the analytical result of the newly trained chemist with those of a senior chemist. Samples of four different drugs (compressed tablets) are selected from different batches and assayed by both individuals. These results are listed below:

Sample Drug, Batch	New Chemist	Senior Chemist
A,42	99.8	99.9
A,43	99.6	99.8
A,44	101.5	100.7
B,96	99.5	100.1
B,97	99.2	98.9
C,112	100.8	101.0
C,113	98.7	97.9
D,21	100.1	99.9
D,22	99.0	99.3
D,23	99.1	99.2

6. Two groups of physical therapy patients are subjected to two different treatment regimens. At the end of the study period, patients are evaluated on specific criteria to measure percent of desired range of motion. Do the results listed below indicate a significant difference between the two therapies at the 95% confidence level?

Group 1		Group 2	
78	82	75	91
87	87	88	79
75	65	93	81
88	80	86	86
91		84	89
		71	

7. A study was undertaken to determine the cost effectiveness of a new treatment procedure for peritoneal adhesiolysis. Twelve pairs of individuals who did not have complications were used in the study, and each pair was

matched on degree of illness, laboratory values, sex, and age. One member of each pair was randomly assigned to receive the conventional treatment, while the other member of the pair received the new therapeutic intervention. Based on the following data, is there sufficient data to conclude at a 5% level of significance that the new therapy is more cost effective than the standard?

Cost in Dollars

Pair	New	Conventional
1	11,813	13,112
2	6,112	8,762
3	13,276	14,762
4	11,335	10,605
5	8,415	6,430
6	12,762	11,990
7	7,501	9,650
8	3,610	7,519
9	9,337	11,754
10	6,538	8,985
11	5,097	4,228
12	10,410	12,667

8. Samples are taken from a specific batch of drug and randomly divided into two groups of tablets. One group is assayed by the manufacturer's own quality control laboratories. The second group of tablets is sent to a contract laboratory for identical analysis.

Percentage of labeled amount of Drug

Manufacturer	Contract Lab
101.1	97.5
100.6	101.1
98.8	99.1
99.0	98.7
100.8	97.8
98.7	99.5

Is there a significant difference between the results generated by the two labs?

a. What is $t_{(1-\alpha/2)}$ for $\alpha = 0.05$?

b. Construct a 95% confidence interval for the difference between population means.

c. Use a t-test to compare the two groups.

9. In a major cooperative of hospitals the average length of stay for kidney transplant patients is 21.6 days. In one particular hospital the average time for 51 patients was only 18.2 days with a standard deviation of 8.3 days. From the data available, is the length of stay at this particular hospital significantly less than expected for all the hospitals in the cooperative?

Answers to Problems

1. Evaluating cognitive knowledge between hospital and community pharmacists.

Independent variable:	hospital vs. community (discrete)
Dependent variable:	knowledge score (continuous)
Statistical test:	two-sample t-test

	Hospital Pharmacists	Community Pharmacists
Mean Score	82.1	79.9
Variance	151.29	210.25
Respondents	129	142

Hypotheses: H_0: $\mu_h = \mu_c$
$\qquad\qquad\quad$ H_1: $\mu_h \neq \mu_c$

Test statistic:

$$t = \frac{\overline{X}_h - \overline{X}_c}{\sqrt{\dfrac{S_P^2}{n_h} + \dfrac{S_P^2}{n_c}}}$$

Decision rule: With $\alpha = .05$, reject H_0 if $t > t_{269}(.025)$ or $< -t_{269}(.025)$.
$\qquad\qquad\qquad$ With $\alpha = .05$, reject H_0 if $t > 1.96$ or $t < -1.96$.

Computation:

$$S_p^2 = \frac{(n_h - 1)S_h^2 + (n_c - 1)S_c^2}{n_h + n_c - 2}$$

$$S_p^2 = \frac{128(151.29) + 141(210.25)}{129 + 142 - 2} = \frac{49010.37}{269} = 182.2$$

$$t = \frac{82.1 - 79.9}{\sqrt{\dfrac{182.2}{129} + \dfrac{182.2}{142}}} = \frac{2.2}{1.64} = 1.34$$

Decision: With t < 1.96 and > -1.96, do not reject H_0, conclude that a significant difference between the populations of pharmacists could not be found.

2. Clinical trial to evaluate the effectiveness of a new bronchodilator
Independent variable: two time periods (patient serves as own control)
Dependent variable: forced expiratory volume (continuous)
Test statistic: paired t-test

Subject Number	Before Administration	FEV$_1$ Three Hours Past Administration	d	d^2
1	3.0	3.1	+0.1	0.01
2	3.6	3.9	+0.3	0.09
3	3.5	3.7	+0.2	0.04
4	3.8	3.8	0	0
5	3.3	3.2	-0.1	0.01
6	3.9	3.8	-0.1	0.01
7	3.1	3.4	+0.3	0.09
8	3.2	3.3	+0.1	0.01
9	3.5	3.6	+0.1	0.01
10	3.4	3.4	0	0
11	3.5	3.7	+0.2	0.04
12	3.6	3.5	-0.1	0.01
		$\Sigma =$	+1.0	0.32

Mean difference and standard deviation difference:

$$\overline{X}_d = \frac{\Sigma d}{n} = \frac{+1.0}{12} = 0.083$$

$$S_d^2 = \frac{n(\Sigma d^2) - (\Sigma d)^2}{n(n-1)} = \frac{12(0.32) - (1.0)^2}{12(11)} = 0.022$$

$$S_d = \sqrt{S_d^2} = \sqrt{0.022} = 0.148$$

a. What is $t_{(1-\alpha/2)}$ for $\alpha = 0.05$? $t_{11}(.975) = 2.201$

b. Construct a 95% confidence interval for the difference between population means.

$$\mu_d = \overline{X_d} \pm t_{n-1}(1-\alpha/2)\frac{S_d}{\sqrt{n}}$$

$$\mu_d = + 0.083 \pm 2.201\frac{0.148}{\sqrt{12}} = + 0.083 \pm 0.094$$

$$-0.011 < \mu_d < + 0.177 \quad \underline{not \; significant}$$

c. Use a t-test to compare the two groups.

$$t = \frac{\overline{X_d}}{\frac{S_d}{\sqrt{n}}}$$

$$t = \frac{0.083}{\frac{0.148}{\sqrt{12}}} = 1.94$$

Decision: With t < 2.20, fail to reject H_0, fail to show a significant difference between the two time periods.

3. Calculattion of measures of central tendency and 95% confidence interval.
Independent variable: 5 time periods (discrete)
Dependent variable: percent active ingredient (continuous)
Test statistic: one-sample t-test

Sample	Time (minutes)				
	10	20	30	45	60
1	60.3	95.7	97.6	98.6	98.7
2	53.9	95.6	97.5	98.6	98.7
3	70.4	95.1	96.8	97.9	98.0
4	61.7	95.3	97.2	98.0	98.2
5	64.4	92.8	95.0	95.8	96.0
6	59.3	96.3	98.3	99.1	99.2

Example of the first (10 minute) time period:

Sample mean

$$\overline{X} = \frac{\Sigma x}{n} = \frac{60.3 + 53.9 + 70.4 + 61.7 + 64.4 + 59.3}{6} = 61.67\%$$

Sample variance/standard deviation

$$S^2 = \frac{\Sigma (x_i - \overline{X})^2}{n-1}$$

$$S^2 = \frac{(60.3 - 61.67)^2 + ...(59.3 - 61.67)^2}{5} = 30.305$$

$$S = \sqrt{S^2} = \sqrt{30.305} = 5.505\%$$

Relative standard deviation

$$C.V. = \frac{S}{\overline{X}} = \frac{5.505}{61.67} = 0.089267$$

$$RSD = C.V. \times 100 = 0.08927 \times 100 = 8.927\%$$

95% Confidence interval: $\overline{X} = 61.67$, $S = 5.505$, $n = 6$

$$\mu = \overline{X} \pm t_{1-\alpha/2} \times \frac{S}{\sqrt{n}}$$

$$\mu = 61.67 \pm 2.57 \cdot \frac{5.505}{\sqrt{6}} = 61.67 \pm 5.78$$

$$55.89 < \mu < 67.45 \quad 95\% \, C.I.$$

Results for all five time periods:

Sample	Time (minutes)				
	<u>10</u>	<u>20</u>	<u>30</u>	<u>45</u>	<u>60</u>
1	60.3	95.7	97.6	98.6	98.7
2	53.9	95.6	97.5	98.6	98.7
3	70.4	95.1	96.8	97.9	98.0
4	61.7	95.3	97.2	98.0	98.2
5	64.4	92.8	95.0	95.8	96.0
6	59.3	96.3	98.3	99.1	99.2
Mean	61.67	95.13	97.07	98.00	98.13
SD	5.505	1.214	1.127	1.164	1.127
RSD	8.927	1.276	1.161	1.188	1.148
95% Confidence Interval					
Upper Limit	67.45	96.40	98.25	99.22	99.31
Lower Limit	55.89	93.86	95.89	96.78	96.95

4. First-time in humans clinical trial
   Independent variable: volunteer assignment
   Dependent variable: C_{max} (continuous)
   Test statistic: one-sample t-test

Results: $\overline{X} = 718.5$ $S^2 = 114.6$ $S = 10.7$ $n = 20$

Calculation:

$$\mu = \overline{X} \pm t_{(1-\alpha/2)} \frac{S}{\sqrt{n}}$$

$$\mu = 718.5 \pm 2.09 \frac{10.7}{\sqrt{20}} = 718.5 \pm 5.00$$

$$713.5 < \mu_{C_{max}} < 723.5 \, ng/ml$$

Conclusion, with 95% confidence, the true population C_{max} is between 713.5 and 723.5 ng/ml.

5. Comparisons between the analytical result of the newly trained chemist and senior chemist.
   Independent variable: two time periods (each sample serves as own control)
   Dependent variable: assay results (continuous)
   Test statistic: paired t-test

Sample Drug, Batch	New Chemist	Senior Chemist	d	d²
A,42	99.8	99.9	0.1	0.01
A,43	99.6	99.8	0.2	0.04
A,44	101.5	100.7	-0.8	0.64
B,96	99.5	100.1	0.6	0.36
B,97	99.2	98.9	-0.3	0.09
C,112	100.8	101.0	0.2	0.04
C,113	98.7	97.9	-0.8	0.64
D,21	100.1	99.9	-0.2	0.04
D,22	99.0	99.3	0.3	0.09
D,23	99.1	99.2	0.1	0.01
		$\Sigma =$	-0.6	1.96

Confidence interval:

$$\overline{X}_d = \frac{-0.6}{10} = -0.06$$

$$S_d^2 = \frac{10(1.96) - (-0.6)^2}{10(9)} = 0.214$$

$$S_d = \sqrt{0.214} = 0.463$$

$$\mu_d = -0.06 \pm 2.262 \frac{0.463}{\sqrt{10}} = -0.06 \pm 0.33$$

$$-0.39 < \mu_d < +0.27$$

Use a t-test to compare the two measures.

$$\overline{X}_d = -0.06$$
$$S_d = 0.466$$

Hypotheses: $H_0: \mu_h = \mu_c$
$H_1: \mu_h \neq \mu_c$

Test statistic:

$$t = \frac{\overline{X}_d}{\dfrac{S_d}{\sqrt{n}}}$$

Decision rule: With $\alpha = .05$, reject H_0 if $t > t_9(.025)$ or $< -t_9(.025)$.
With $\alpha = .05$, reject H_0 if $t > 2.26$ or $t < -2.26$.

Calculations:

$$t = \frac{-0.06}{\dfrac{.463}{\sqrt{10}}} = \frac{-0.06}{.146} = 0.41$$

Decision: With $t < 2.26$, fail to reject H_0, fail to show a significant difference assay results for the two scientists.

6. Comparison of two groups of physical therapy patients.
    Independent variable: group 1 vs. group 2 (discrete)
    Dependent variable: percent range of motion (continuous)
    Statistical test: two-sample t-test

	Group 1	Group 2
Mean =	81.44	83.91
S.D. =	8.08	6.80
n =	9	11

Hypotheses: H_0: $\mu_1 = \mu_2$

H_1: $\mu_1 \neq \mu_2$

Decision rule: With $\alpha = .05$, reject H_0 if $t > t_{18}(.025)$ or $t < -t_{18}(.025)$.
With $\alpha = .05$, reject H_0 if $t > 2.12$ or $t < -2.12$.

$$S_p^2 = \frac{(n_1 - 1)S_1^2 + (n_2 - 1)S_2^2}{n_1 + n_2 - 2} = \frac{8(8.08)^2 + 10(6.80)^2}{9 + 11 - 2} = 54.70$$

$$t = \frac{\overline{X}_1 - \overline{X}_2}{\sqrt{\dfrac{S_p^2}{n_1} + \dfrac{S_p^2}{n_2}}} = \frac{81.44 - 83.91}{\sqrt{\dfrac{54.7}{9} + \dfrac{54.7}{11}}} = \frac{-2.47}{3.32} = -0.74$$

Decision: With $t > -2.12$ cannot reject H_0, conclude that there is no significant difference between the two type of treatment regimens.

7. Study evaluating cost effectiveness of a new treatment for peritoneal adhesiolysis.

Independent variable: treatment received
(each pair serves as its own control)

Dependent variable: costs (continuous)

Test statistic: paired t-test (one-tailed)

Cost in Dollars

Pair	New	Conventional	(conventional-new)	d^2
1	11,813	13,112	+1,299	1,687,401
2	6,112	8,762	+2,650	7,022,500
3	13,276	14,762	+1,486	2,208,196
4	11,335	10,605	-730	532,900
5	8,415	6,430	-1,985	3,940,225
6	12,762	11,990	-772	595,984
7	7,501	9,650	+2,149	4,618,201
8	3,610	7,519	+3,909	15,280,281
9	9,337	11,754	+2,417	5,841,889
10	6,538	8,985	+2,447	5,987,809
11	5,097	4,228	-869	755,161
12	10,410	12,667	+2,257	5,094,049
		$\Sigma =$	+14,258	53,564,596

Hypotheses: H_0: $\mu_d \neq 0$
                H_1: $\mu_d > 0$

Decision Rule: With $\alpha = .05$, reject H_0 if $t > t_{11}(.05) = 1.795$.

$$\overline{X}_d = \frac{\Sigma d}{n} = \frac{+14,258}{12} = +1,188.17$$

$$S_d^2 = \frac{n(\Sigma d^2)-(\Sigma d)^2}{n(n-1)} = \frac{12(53,564,596)-(14,258)^2}{12(11)} = 3,329,428.697$$

$$S_d = \sqrt{S_d^2} = \sqrt{3,329,428.697} = 1,824.67$$

$$t = \frac{\overline{X}_d}{\dfrac{S_d}{\sqrt{n}}} = \frac{+1,188.17}{\dfrac{1,824.67}{\sqrt{12}}} = \frac{+1,188.17}{526.74} = +2.26$$

Decision: With $t > 1.795$, reject H_0, conclude that the new treatment is more cost effective than the conventional one.

8. Comparison of results from a contract laboratory and manufacturer's quality control laboratory.
    Independent variable: manufacturer vs. contract laboratory (discrete)
    Dependent variable: assay results (continuous)
    Statistical test: two-sample t-test

Percentage of labeled amount of Drug

Manufacturer		Contract Lab	
101.1		97.5	
100.6	$\overline{X} = 99.83$	101.1	$\overline{X} = 98.95$
98.8		99.1	
99.0	S = 1.11	98.7	S = 1.30
100.8		97.8	
98.7	n = 6	99.5	n = 6

a. What is $t_{(1-\alpha/2)}$ for $\alpha = 0.05$?   Critical $t = t_{10}(.975) = 2.228$

b. Construct a 95% confidence interval for the difference between population means.

$$S_p^2 = \frac{(n_1 - 1)S_1^2 + (n_2 - 1)S_2^2}{n_1 + n_2 - 2} = \frac{5(1.11)^2 + 5(1.30)^2}{6 + 6 - 2} = 1.46$$

$$\mu_1 - \mu_2 = (\overline{X}_1 - \overline{X}_2) \pm t_{n_1+n_2-2}(1-\alpha/2)\sqrt{\frac{S_P^2}{n_1} + \frac{S_P^2}{n_2}}$$

$$\mu_1 - \mu_2 = (99.83 - 98.95) \pm 2.228\sqrt{\frac{1.46}{6} + \frac{1.46}{6}}$$

$$\mu_1 - \mu_2 = (0.88) \pm 2.228(0.698) = 0.88 \pm 1.55$$

$$-0.67 < \mu_1 - \mu_2 < +2.43$$

Zero falls within the confidence interval; therefore assume there is a significant difference between the results from the two laboratories.

c. Use a t-test to compare the two groups.

Hypotheses: H_0: $\mu_m = \mu_c$
H_1: $\mu_m \neq \mu_c$

Test statistic:

$$t = \frac{\overline{X}_h - \overline{X}_c}{\sqrt{\frac{S_P^2}{n_h} + \frac{S_P^2}{n_c}}}$$

Decision Rule: With $\alpha = .05$, reject H_0 if $t > t_{10}(.025)$ or $< -t_{10}(.025)$.
With $\alpha = .05$, reject H_0 if $t > 2.228$ or $t < -2.228$.

Computation:

$$t = \frac{\overline{X_1} - \overline{X_2}}{\sqrt{\dfrac{S_P^2}{n_1} + \dfrac{S_P^2}{n_2}}} = \frac{0.88}{\sqrt{\dfrac{1.46}{6} + \dfrac{1.46}{6}}} = \frac{0.88}{0.698} = 1.26$$

Decision: With t < 2.228, fail to reject H_0, fail to show a significant difference between the results from the two laboratories.

9. Evaluation of the average length of stay for kidney transplant patients in a particular hospital.
    Independent variable: hospital
    Dependent variable: length of stay (continuous)
    Test statistic: one-sample t-test (one-tailed)

Hypotheses:
    H_0: $\mu_A \neq 21.6$
    H_1: $\mu_A < 21.6$

Decision rule: With $\alpha = .05$, reject H_0 if $t < -t_{50}(.95) = -1.675$.

Calculations:

$$t = \frac{\overline{X} - \mu_0}{\dfrac{S}{\sqrt{n}}}$$

$$t = \frac{18.2 - 21.6}{\dfrac{8.3}{\sqrt{51}}} = \frac{-3.4}{1.16} = -2.93$$

Decision: With t < -1.675, reject H_0 and assume that the lengths of stay for kidney transplant patients at Hospital A is significantly less than the other facilities.

Creating a confidence interval (5% error to estimate the upper limits of the interval):

$$\mu_{upper\ limit} = \overline{X} + t_{n-1}(1 - \alpha/2) \cdot \frac{S}{\sqrt{n}}$$

$$\mu_U = 18.2 + (1.675)\ \frac{8.3}{\sqrt{51}} = 18.2 + 1.95$$

$$\mu_U < 20.15$$

Decision: The mean for all the hospitals, 21.6 days, does not fall within the upper limits of the confidence interval; therefore, Hospital A is significantly different and their patients appear to have shorter length of stays.

9

One-way Analysis of Variance (ANOVA)

Where the t-test was appropriate for the one or two sample cases (one or two levels of the discrete independent variable), the F-test or one-way analysis of variance can be expanded to k levels of the independent variable. The calculation involves an *analysis of variance* of the individual sample means around a central grand mean. Like the t-test, the dependent variable represents data that is in continuous distribution. The analysis of variance is also referred to as the F-test, after R.A. Fisher, a British statistician who developed this test (Snedecor and Cochran, 1989, p.223). The hypotheses associated with the one-way analysis of variance, often abbreviated with the acronym ANOVA, can be expanded to any number (*k*) levels of the discrete variable.

$$H_0: \mu_1 = \mu_2 = \mu_3 \ldots = \mu_k$$
$$H_1: H_0 \text{ is false}$$

The ANOVA represents a variety of techniques used to identify and measure sources of variation within a collection of observations, hence the name analysis of variance. The one-way ANOVA is nothing more than an expansion of the t-test to more than two levels of the discrete independent variable. Therefore, the same assumptions for the t-test hold true for this procedure, namely normality and homogeneity of variance. If *n* (cell size) for each sample is approximately equal, it increases the validity of assuming homogeneity. The null hypothesis states that there is no differences among the population means, and that any fluctuations in the sample means is due to chance error only.

Note that the alternative hypothesis does not say that all samples are unequal, nor does it tell where any inequalities exist. The test results merely identify that a difference does occur somewhere among the population means. In order to find where this difference is, some form of post hoc procedure should be performed once the null hypothesis is rejected (Chapter 10).

The F-distribution

A full discussion of the derivation of the sampling distribution associated with the analysis of variance is beyond the scope of this text. A more complete description can be found in Daniel (1991) or Kachigan (1991). The simplest approach would be to consider the ratio of variances for two samples randomly selected from a normally distributed population. The ratio of the variances, based on sample sizes of n_1 and n_2 would be:

$$F = \frac{S_1^2}{S_2^2}$$

Assuming the sample was taken from the same population, the ratio of the variances would be:

$$E(F) = E\left(\frac{S_1^2}{S_2^2}\right) = \frac{\sigma^2}{\sigma^2} = 1$$

However, due to the variations in sampling distributions (Chapter 6), some variation from $E(F)=1$ would be expected by chance alone due to expected difference between the two sample variances. Based on previous discussions in Chapter 6 it would be expected that the variation of the sampling distribution of S^2 should depend on the sample size n and the larger the sample size, the smaller that variation. Thus, sample size is important to calculating the various F-distributions.

As will be shown in the next section, the F-test will create such a ratio comparing the variation the levels of the independent variable and the variation within the samples. Curves have been developed that provide values that can be exceeded only 5% or 1% of the time by chance alone (Figure 9.1). Obviously if the calculated F-value is much larger than one and exceeds the critical value indicated below, it is most likely not due to random error. Because of the mathematical manipulations discussed later in this chapter the calculated F-

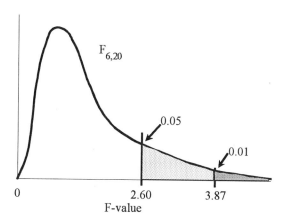

Figure 9.1 Example of an F-distribution.

statistic must be positive. Therefore, unlike the t-test, we are only interested in positive values to the extreme of our critical value. Similar to the t-distribution, the F-distribution is a series of curves, whose shape differs based on the degrees of freedom. As will be seen later in the chapter, the decision to accept or reject the null hypothesis, based on the shape of the F-distribution, is dependent on both the total sample size and the number of levels associated with the discrete independent variable. As the number of degrees of freedom get larger, the F-distribution will approach the shape of a normal distribution. A listing of the critical F-values (F_c) is given in Table B5 of Appendix B.

Test Statistic

The analysis of variance involves determining if the observed values belong to the same population, regardless of the level of the discrete variable (group), or whether the observations in at least one of these groups come from a different population.

$$H_0: \mu_1 = \mu_2 = \mu_3 \ldots = \mu_k = \mu$$

To obtain an F-value we need two estimates of the population variance. It is necessary to examine the variability (analysis of variance) of observations within groups as well as between groups. With the t-test, we computed a t-statistic by calculating the ratio of the difference between the two means over the distribution of the means (represented by the pooled variance). The F-statistic is computed using a simplified ratio similar to the t-test.

$$F = \frac{\textit{difference between the means}}{\textit{standard error of the difference of the means}} \qquad \text{Eq. 9.1}$$

The actual calculation of the F-statistic is as follows:

$$F = \frac{MS_B}{MS_W} \qquad \text{Eq. 9.2}$$

This formula shows the overall variability between the samples means (**MS$_B$** or **mean squared between**) and at the same time it corrects for the dispersion of data points within each sample (**MS$_W$** or **mean squared within**). The actual calculations for the MS$_B$ and MS$_W$ will be discussed in the following two sections. Obviously, the greater the differences between the sample means (the numerator), the less likely that all the samples were selected from the same population (all the samples represent population that are the same or are equal). If all the sample means are equal, the numerator measuring the differences between the means will be zero and the corresponding F-statistics also will be zero. As the F-statistic increases it becomes likely that a significant difference exists. Like the t-test, it is necessary to determine if the calculated F-value is large enough to represent a true difference between the populations sampled or due to chance error or sampling variation. The decision rule to reject the null hypothesis of equality is stated as follows:

with $\alpha = 0.05$, reject H$_0$ if F > $F_{v1,v2}(1-\alpha)$.

The critical F-value is associated with two separate degrees of freedom. The numerator degrees of freedom (v_1) equals K-1 or the number of treatment levels minus one; and the denominator degrees of freedom (v_2) equals N-K or the total number of observations minus the number of treatment levels (K).

An analogy can be made between the F-distribution and the t-distribution. As will be seen in the following sections, the process involves a squaring of the differences between sample means the total mean for all the sample observations. Values for the F-distribution for two levels of the discrete independent variable will be identical to the corresponding t-distribution value, squared. In other words, with only two levels of the independent variable $F_{1,N-2}$ equals $(t_{N-2})^2$, or $(t_{n1+n2-2})^2$, for the same level of confidence (1-α). This is illustrated in Table 9.1. As might be expected, the outcome for an F-test on data with only two levels of a discrete independent variable will be the same as

Table 9.1 Comparison of Critical Value Between t- and F-distributions

df	t_{N-2}	$\alpha = 0.05$ $(t_{N-2})^2$	$F_{1,N-2}$	t_{N-2}	$\alpha = 0.01$ $(t_{N-2})^2$	$F_{1,N-2}$
15	2.131	4.54	4.54	2.946	8.68	8.68
30	2.042	4.17	4.17	2.750	7.56	7.56
60	2.000	4.00	4.00	2.660	7.08	7.08
120	1.979	3.92	3.92	2.617	6.85	6.85
∞	1.960	3.84	3.84	2.576	6.63	6.63

t- and F- values taken from Table B3 and B5 in Appendix B, respectively.

a t-test performed on the same information.

To calculate the F-statistic for the decision rule either the definitional or computational formulas may be used. With the exception of rounding errors, both methods will produce the same results. In the former case the sample means and standard deviations are used:

$\overline{X}_1, \overline{X}_2, \dots \overline{X}_k$ = sample means
$S_1^2, S_2^2, \dots S_k^2$ = sample variance
$n_1, n_2, \dots n_k$ = sample sized
N = total number of observations
K = number of discrete levels (treatment levels)
    of the independent variable

Whereas, in the computational formula: 1) individual observations; 2) the sum of observations for each level of the discrete independent variable; and 3) the total sum of all observations, are squared and manipulated to produce the same outcome. The analysis of variance is a statistical procedure to analyze the overall dispersion for data in our sample outcomes.

ANOVA Definitional Formula

The denominator of the F-statistic (Eq. 9.2), the **mean square within** (MS$_W$), is calculated in the same way as the pooled variance is calculated for the t-test, except there are k levels instead of only two levels as found in the t-test.

$$MS_W = \frac{(n_1-1)S_1^2 + (n_2-1)S_2^2 + (n_3-1)S_3^2 + \dots + (n_k-1)S_k^2}{N-K}$$ Eq. 9.3

Note the similarity of this formula and the pooled variance for the t-test (Eq. 8.3). Since no single sample variance is a better measure of dispersion than the other sample variances, our best estimate is to pool the variances and create a single estimate for within variation. The mean square within is often referred to as the **mean squared error** (MS_E) or **pooled within group variance** (S_w^2) and these terms are synonymous.

$$MS_W = MS_E = S_w^2$$

The mean squared within is a measure of random variability or random "error" among the measured objects and is not the same as the variability of the total set (N).

In the t-test, the numerator was the difference between the two means (Eq. 8.6), which was easily calculated by subtracting one mean from the other. But how do we calculate a measure of difference when there are more than two means? In the ANOVA, there are k different means, therefore a measure is calculated to represent the variability between the different means. This measure of dispersion of the means is calculated similarily to a previous dispersion term, the variance (Eq. 5.3). First, the center (the grand mean) for all sample observations is calculated. Then the squared differences between each sample mean and the grand central mean are calculated. This measures an analysis of the variance between the individual sample means and the total center for all the sample observations. The **grand mean** or **pooled mean** is computed:

$$\overline{X}_G = \frac{(n_1 \overline{X}_1) + (n_2 \overline{X}_2) + (n_3 \overline{X}_3) + ... + (n_k \overline{X}_k)}{N} \qquad \text{Eq. 9.4}$$

This grand mean represents a weighted combination of all the sample means and an approximation of the center for all the individual sample observation. From it, the mean squared between (MS_B) is calculated similar to a sample variance (Eq. 5.3) by squaring the difference between each sample mean and the grand mean, and multiplying by the number of observations associated with each sample mean:

$$MS_B = \frac{n_1 (\overline{X}_1 - \overline{X}_G)^2 + n_2 (\overline{X}_2 - \overline{X}_G)^2 + ... + n_k (\overline{X}_k - \overline{X}_G)^2}{K - 1} \qquad \text{Eq. 9.5}$$

Finally the F-statistic is based on the ratio of the difference between the means over the distribution of their data points (Eq. 9.2):

$$F = \frac{MS_B}{MS_W}$$

In both the F-test and the t-test, the numerator of the final ratio considers differences between the means and the denominator takes into account how data are distributed around these means. The greater the spread of the sample observations, the larger the denominator and the smaller the calculated statistic, and thus the lesser the likelihood of rejecting H_0. The greater the differences between the means, the larger the numerator, the larger the calculated statistic, and the greater the likelihood of rejecting H_0 in favor of H_1. In other words, as the centers (means) get further apart the calculated F-value will increase and there is a greater likelihood that the difference will be significant. Conversely, as the dispersion becomes larger, the calculated F-value will decrease and the observed difference will more than likely be caused by random error.

To illustrate this method of determining the F-statistic, assume that during the manufacturing of a specific enteric coated tablet, samples were periodically selected from production lines at three different facilities. Weights were taken for fifteen tablets and their average weights are listed in Table 9.2. The research question would be: is there any significant difference in weights of the tablets between the three facilities? The hypotheses would be:

H_0: $\mu_{\text{facility A}} = \mu_{\text{facility B}} = \mu_{\text{facility C}}$
H_1: H_0 is false

Table 9.2   Average Weights in Enteric Coated Tablets (in mg)

Facility A		Facility B		Facility C	
277.3	278.4	271.6	275.5	275.5	272.3
280.3	272.9	274.8	274.0	274.2	273.4
279.1	274.7	271.2	274.9	267.5	275.1
275.2	276.8	277.6	269.2	274.2	273.7
273.6	269.1	274.5	283.2	270.5	268.7
276.7	276.3	275.7	280.6	284.4	275.0
281.7	273.1	276.1	274.6	275.6	268.3
278.7		275.9		277.1	
Mean = 276.26		Mean = 275.29		Mean = 273.70	
S.D. = 3.27		S.D. = 3.46		S.D. = 4.16	

The decision rule is with $\alpha = .05$, reject H_0 if $F > F_{2,42}(.95) = 3.23$. The value is approximated from Table B5 in Appendix B, where 2 is selected from the first column ($K-1$) and 42 approximated from the second column ($N-K$) and the value is selected from the fourth column, ($1-\alpha = .95$) is 3.24 (an interpolation between 3.23 for 40 df and 3.15 for 60 df). The computations are as follows:

$$MS_W = \frac{(n_1-1)S_1^2 + (n_2-1)S_2^2 + (n_3-1)S_3^2 + \ldots (n_k-1)S_k^2}{N-K}$$

$$MS_W = \frac{14(3.27)^2 + 14(3.46)^2 + 14(4.16)^2}{42} = 13.32$$

$$\overline{X_G} = \frac{(n_1\overline{X_1}) + (n_2\overline{X_2}) + (n_3\overline{X_3}) + \ldots (n_k\overline{X_k})}{N}$$

$$\overline{X_G} = \frac{15(276.26) + 15(275.29) + 15(273.70)}{45} = 275.08$$

$$MS_B = \frac{n_1(\overline{X_1} - \overline{X_G})^2 + n_2(\overline{X_2} - \overline{X_G})^2 + n_3(\overline{X_3} - \overline{X_G})^2 + \ldots n_k(\overline{X_k} - \overline{X_G})^2}{K-1}$$

$$MS_B = \frac{15(276.26 - 275.08)^2 + 15(275.29 - 275.08)^2 + 15(273.70 - 275.08)^2}{2}$$

$$MS_B = 25.06$$

$$F = \frac{MS_B}{MS_W} = \frac{25.06}{13.32} = 1.88$$

Thus based on the test results, the decision is with $F < 3.23$, do not reject H_0, and conclude that there is inadequate information to show a significant difference between the three facilities.

ANOVA Computational Formula

The computation technique is an alternative "short cut" which arrives at the same results as the computational method, except the formulas involve the raw data, and the means and standard deviations are neither calculated nor needed in the equations. Using this technique the MS_W and MS_B (also know as the mean sum of squares) are arrived at by two steps. First a sum of the squared deviations are obtained and then these sums are divided by their respective degrees of freedom (i.e., numerator or denominator degrees of freedom). Figure 9.2 illustrates the layout for data treated by the computational formula. This type of mathematical notation will be used with similar formulas in future chapters. In the notation scheme, x_{jk} refers to the jth observation in the kth level of the discrete independent variable, where K varies from 1 to k (the number of groups in the analysis), and j varies from 1 to n_j (the number of observations in the kth group). In addition, the sums for each of the columns are added together ($\sum x_T$), represent the sum total for all the observations (N_K).

A series of intermediate equations are calculated. Intermediate I is the sum of all the squared individual observations.

$$ I = \sum_{k=1}^{K} \sum_{i=1}^{n} x_{jk}^2 = \left(x_{a1} \right)^2 + \left(x_{a2} \right)^2 + ... + \left(x_{kn} \right)^2 \qquad \text{Eq. 9.6} $$

Intermediate II is the square of the total sum of all observations, divided by the total number of observations.

$$ II = \frac{\left[\sum_{k=1}^{K} \sum_{i=1}^{n} x_{jk} \right]^2}{N_k} = \frac{\left(\sum x_T \right)^2}{N_{K'}} \qquad \text{Eq. 9.7} $$

Treatments (levels)

A	B	C	...	K
x_{a1}	x_{b1}	x_{c1}	...	x_{k1}
x_{a2}	x_{b2}	x_{c2}	...	x_{k2}
x_{a3}	x_{b3}	x_{c3}	...	x_{k3}
...	...	...	...	...
x_{an}	x_{bn}	x_{cn}	...	x_{kn}

$\sum x_A$	$\sum x_B$	$\sum x_C$	...	$\sum x_K$

Observations $\sum x_T$ = total sum of
per level = n_A n_B n_C ... n_K observations

Figure 9.2   Data format for the ANOVA computational formula.

Intermediate III involves summing each column (level of the discrete variable), squaring that sum, and dividing by the number of observations in the column. Each column result is then summed.

$$III = \sum_{k=1}^{K} \frac{\left[\sum\limits_{i=1}^{n} x_{jk}\right]^2}{n_K} = \frac{(\sum x_A)^2}{n_A} + \frac{(\sum x_B)^2}{n_B} + ... + \frac{(\sum x_K)^2}{n_k} \qquad \text{Eq. 9.8}$$

These intermediate equations are used to determine the various sums of squares which appear in a traditional ANOVA table:

$$SS_B = III - II \qquad\qquad \text{Eq. 9.9}$$

$$SS_W = I - III \qquad\qquad \text{Eq. 9.10}$$

$$SS_T = I - II \qquad\qquad \text{Eq. 9.11}$$

Note that the sum of squared deviations for the within groups (SS_W) and between groups (SS_B) should add to the total sum of the squares (SS_T) and this relationship can serve as a quick check of our mathematical calculations.

$$SS_B + SS_W = SS_T$$

The ANOVA table is used to calculate the F-statistic. Each sum of squares is divided by their respective degrees of freedom and the resultant mean squares are used in the formula present for determining the F-statistic:

Source	Degrees of Freedom	Sum of Squares	Mean Square	F
Between Groups	K-1	III-II	$\dfrac{\text{III-II}}{\text{K-1}}$	$\dfrac{MS_B}{MS_W}$
Within Groups	N-K	I-III	$\dfrac{\text{I-III}}{\text{N-K}}$	
Total	N-1	I-II		

This method can be applied to the same problem that was used for the definitional formula. The hypotheses, test statistic, decision rule and critical

Table 9.3 Average Weights in Enteric Coated Tablets (in mg)

Facility A	Facility B	Facility C
277.3	271.6	275.5
280.3	274.8	274.2
279.1	271.2	267.5
...	...	...
273.1	274.6	268.3
$\sum x_A = 4143.9$	$\sum x_B = 4129.4$	$\sum x_C = 4105.5$

$$\sum\sum x = 12378.8$$

value ($F_{critical}$ = 3.23) remain the same as the data presented in Table 9.2. In Table 9.3 the same data is presented, but includes the sums of the various columns. The mathematics for the computational formula are as follows:

$$I = \sum\sum x_{jk}^2 = (277.3)^2 + (280.3)^2 + ...(268.3)^2 = 3,405,824.58$$

$$II = \frac{\left[\sum\sum x_{jk}\right]^2}{N_k} = \frac{(12378.8)^2}{45} = 3,405,215.32$$

$$III = \sum \frac{\left[\sum x_{jk}\right]^2}{n_k} = \frac{(4143.9)^2}{15} + \frac{(4129.4)^2}{15} + \frac{(4105.5)^2}{15} = 3,405,265.45$$

$$SS_B = III - II = 3,405,265.45 - 3,405,215.32 = 50.13$$

$$SS_W = I - III = 3,405,824.58 - 3,405,265.45 = 559.13$$

$$SS_T = I - II = 3,405,824.58 - 3,405,215.32 = 609.26$$

$$SS_B + SS_W = SS_T \qquad 609.26 = 559.13 + 50.13$$

The ANOVA table for this example would be:

Source	df	SS	MS	F
Between	2	50.13	25.07	1.88
Within	42	559.13	13.31	
Total	44	609.26		

The decision rule is the same, with F < 3.23, do not reject H_0. Note that the results are identical to those using the definitional formula, with minor rounding differences in the mean square column.

A second example of a one-way analysis of variance, seen below, is a case where C_{max} (maximum concentrations in mcg/ml) were found for four different formulations of a particular drug[1]. The researcher wished to determine if there was a significant difference in the time required to C_{max}.

Cmax in mcg/ml:	Mean	S.D.	n
Formulation A	123.2	12.8	20
Formulation B	105.6	11.6	20
Formulation C	116.4	14.6	19
Formulation D	113.5	10.0	18

In this case the hypotheses are:

H_0: $\mu_A = \mu_B = \mu_C = \mu_D$
H_1: H_0 is false

The hypothesis under test is that the four formulas of the study drug produce the same C_{max}, on the average. If this is rejected then the alternate hypothesis is accepted, namely that some difference exists between the four formulas. Using Equation 9.2, our decision rule is, with $\alpha = .05$, reject H_0 if F > $F_{3,73}(.95)$ = 2.74. This critical value comes from Table B5 in Appendix B, with K-1 or 3 in the first column, N-K or 73 approximated in the second column and 2.74 interpolated from the fourth column (between 60 and 120 df) at 95% confidence.

The computations using the definitional formula would be:

---

[1] It should be noted that in most cases distributions of C_{max} data would be positively skewed and a lognormal transformation be required. However, for our purposes we will assume that the sample data approximates a normal distribution. Also note that the variances, squares of the standard deviations, are similar and we can assume homogeneity of variances. Specific tests for homogeneity are presented in the last section of this chapter.

$$MS_W = \frac{(n_1-1)S_1^2 + (n_2-1)S_2^2 + (n_3-1)S_3^2 + ... (n_k-1)S_k^2}{N-K}$$

$$MS_W = \frac{19(12.8)^2 + 19(11.6)^2 + 18(14.6)^2 + 17(10.0)^2}{73} = 153.51$$

$$\overline{X_G} = \frac{(n_1\overline{X_1}) + (n_2\overline{X_2}) + (n_3\overline{X_3}) + ... (n_k\overline{X_k})}{N}$$

$$\overline{X_G} = \frac{20(123.2) + 20(105.6) + 19(116.4) + 18(113.5)}{77} = 114.68$$

$$MS_B = \frac{n_1(\overline{X_1}-\overline{X_G})^2 + n_2(\overline{X_2}-\overline{X_G})^2 + n_3(\overline{X_3}-\overline{X_G})^2 + ... n_k(\overline{X_k}-\overline{X_G})^2}{K-1}$$

$$MS_B = \frac{20(123.2-114.68)^2 + 20(105.6-114.68)^2 + ... 18(113.5-114.68)^2}{3}$$

$$MS_B = 1060.67$$

$$F = \frac{MS_B}{MS_W} = \frac{1060.67}{153.51} = 6.91$$

The decision based on the sample data is, with F > 2.74, reject H_0 and conclude there is a difference between the various formulations.

This last example shows an important feature of the analysis of variance. In this particular case, H_0 was rejected, therefore $\mu_A = \mu_B = \mu_C = \mu_D$ is not true. However, the results of the statistical test do *not* tell us where the difference or differences between the four population means occur. Looking at the data it appears that Formulation A has a C_{max} which is significantly longer than the other formulations. Yet, at the same time Formulation B has a significantly shorter C_{max}. In fact, all four formulations could be significantly different from each other. The F-value that was calculated does not provide an answer to where the significant differences occur. In order to determine this, some type of *post hoc* procedure needs to be performed.

Randomized Complete Block Design

Whereas the one-way analysis of variance was presented as a logical extension of the t-test to more than two levels of the independent variable, the **randomized complete block design** can be thought of as an expansion of the paired t-test to three or more measures of the same subject or sample. Also known as the **randomized block design**, it represents a two-dimensional design with one observation per cell.

The randomized block design was developed in the 1920's by R. A. Fisher, to evaluate methods for improving agricultural experiments (Fisher, 1926). To eliminate variability between different locations of fields, his research design first divided the land into blocks. The area within each block was assumed to be relatively homogenous. Then each of the blocks were further subdivided into plots and each plot within a given block received one of the treatments under consideration. Therefore, only one plot within each block received a specific treatment and each block contained plots that represented all the treatments.

Using this design, subjects are assigned to blocks in order to reduce variability within each treatment level. The randomized complete block design can be used for a variety of situations where there is a need for homogenous blocks. The observations or subjects within each block are more homogeneous than subjects within the different blocks. For example, assume that age of volunteers may influence the study results and the researcher wants to include all possible age groups with each of the possible treatment levels. Volunteers are divided into groups based on age (i.e., 21-25, 26-30, 31-35, etc.), then one subject from each age group is randomly selected to receive each treatment (Table 9.4). In this randomized complete block design, each age group represents one block and there is only one observation per cell (called **experimental units**). Like Fisher's agricultural experiments, each treatment is administered to each block and each block receives every treatment. The rows represent the blocking effect and the columns show the treatment effect.

As a second example, with three treatment levels (three assay methods), assume that instead of twenty-four tablets randomly sampled from one production run, we sample from eight different runs and give one sample from each run to each of three analytical chemists to assay. In this case we assume that each of our individual production runs are more homogeneous than total mixing of all twenty-four samples across the eight runs. As seen in Figure 9.3 three samples in each row comprise a block from the same production run. Note there is still only one observation per cell. Differences between the means for the columns reflect treatment effects (in this case the difference between the three chemists) and differences between the mean for each row reflect the

Table 9.4 Randomized Block Design

Age	Treatment 1	Treatment 2	Treatment 3
21-25	1 volunteer	1 volunteer	1 volunteer
26-30	1 volunteer	1 volunteer	1 volunteer
31-35	1 volunteer	1 volunteer	1 volunteer
...	...	...	...
61-65	1 volunteer	1 volunteer	1 volunteer

differences between the production runs.

As seen in Figure 9.3 the independent variables are 1) the treatment levels that appear in the columns (main effect) and 2) the blocks seen in the rows which are sub-levels of the data. The assumptions are that: 1) there has been random independent sampling; 2) at each treatment level, the outcomes are normally distributed and variances for groups at different treatment levels are similar (homogeniety of variance); and 3) block and treatment effects are additive (no interaction between the treatments and blocks). The hypotheses are as follows:

$$H_0: \mu_A = \mu_B \qquad \text{for two treatment levels}$$
$$H_1: \mu_A \neq \mu_B$$

$$H_0: \mu_A = \mu_B = ... \mu_K \quad \text{for three or more treatment levels}$$
$$H_1: H_0 \text{ is false}$$

	AC_1	AC_2		AC_k	Sum by Block	Block Means
Block (batch) b_1	x_{11}	x_{12}	...	x_{1k}	$\sum x_{b1}$	$\overline{X}_{b1}$
Block (batch) b_2	x_{21}	x_{22}	...	x_{2k}	$\sum x_{b2}$	$\overline{X}_{b2}$
Block (batch) b_3	x_{31}	x_{32}	...	x_{3k}	$\sum x_{b3}$	$\overline{X}_{b3}$
Block (batch) b_4	x_{41}	x_{42}	...	x_{4k}	$\sum x_{b4}$	$\overline{X}_{b4}$
...	...	...	...	...	...	...
Block (batch) b_8	x_{j1}	x_{j2}	...	x_{jk}	$\sum x_{bj}$	$\overline{X}_{b8}$
Sum by Column	$\sum x_{t1}$	$\sum x_{t2}$	...	$\sum x_{tk}$	$\sum\sum x_{jk}$	
Treatment Means	$\overline{X}_{t1}$	$\overline{X}_{t2}$	$\overline{X}_{t3}$			

Figure 9.3 Data format for a randomized block design.

As seen in the hypotheses, the main interest is in treatment effects and the blocking is used to eliminate any extraneous source of variation. The decision rule is, with $\alpha = 0.05$, reject H_0 if $F > F_{K-1,J-1}(1-\alpha)$. The critical F-value is based on K-1 treatment levels as the numerator degrees of freedom, and J-1 blocks as the denominator degrees of freedom. The data is presented as follows:

		Treatment Levels		
Blocks	$\underline{K_1}$	$\underline{K_2}$	...	$\underline{K_k}$
B_1	x_{11}	x_{21}	...	x_{k1}
B_2	x_{12}	x_{22}	...	x_{k2}
...	...	...	...	...
B_j	x_{1j}	x_{2j}	...	x_{kj}

The formula and ANOVA table are similar to those involved in the computational formula for the one-way ANOVA. In this case there are four intermediate calculations, including one which measures the variability of blocks as well as the column treatment effect. The total sum of squares for the randomized complete block design is composed of the sums of squares attributed to the treatments, the blocks and random error. Similar to the computational formula for the F-statistic, Intermediate I is the sum of all the squared individual observations.

$$I = \sum_{k=1}^{K} \sum_{j=1}^{J} x_{kj}^2 \qquad \text{Eq. 9.12}$$

Intermediate II is the square of the total sum of all observations, divided by the product of the number of treatments (K) time the number of blocks (J).

$$II = \frac{\left[\sum_{k=1}^{K} \sum_{j=1}^{J} x_{kj} \right]^2}{KJ} \qquad \text{Eq. 9.13}$$

Intermediate III for the block effect is the calculated by adding up all the sums (second to the last column in Figure 9.3) for each block and dividing by the number of treatment levels.

$$III_R = \frac{\sum_{k=1}^{K} \left[\sum_{j=1}^{J} x_{kj} \right]^2}{K} \qquad \text{Eq. 9.14}$$

Intermediate III for the treatment effect is the calculated by adding up all the sums second to the last row in Figure 9.3) for each treatment and dividing by the number of blocks.

$$III_C = \frac{\sum\limits_{j=1}^{J} \left[\sum\limits_{k=1}^{K} x_{kj} \right]^2}{J} \qquad \text{Eq. 9.15}$$

The intermediate results are used to calculate each of these various sum of squares:

$$SS_{Total} = SS_T = I - II \qquad \text{Eq. 9.16}$$

$$SS_{Blocks} = SS_B = III_R - II \qquad \text{Eq. 9.17}$$

$$SS_{Treatment} = SS_{Rx} = III_C - II \qquad \text{Eq. 9.18}$$

$$SS_{Error} = SS_{Residual} = SS_T - SS_B - SS_{Rx} \qquad \text{Eq. 9.19}$$

An ANOVA table is constructed and each sum of squares is divided by its corresponding degrees of freedom to produce a mean square.

Source	df	SS	MS	F
Treatment	K-1	SS$_{Rx}$	$\dfrac{SS_{Rx}}{K-1}$	$\dfrac{MS_{Rx}}{MS_R}$
Blocks	J-1	SS$_B$	$\dfrac{SS_B}{J-1}$	
Residual	(K-1)(J-1)	SS$_R$	$\dfrac{SS_R}{(K-1)(J-1)}$	
Total	N-1	SS$_T$		

The F-value is calculated by dividing the mean square for the treatment effect by the mean square error (or **mean square residual**):

$$F = \frac{MS_{Rx}}{MS_R} \qquad \text{Eq. 9.20}$$

If the calculated F-value exceeds the critical value (F_c) for K-1 and J-1 degrees of freedom, H_0 is rejected and it is assumed that there is a significant difference between the treatment effects.

One of the most common uses for the randomized block design involves cross-over clinical drug trials. **Cross-over studies**, are experimental designs in which each patient receives two or more treatments which are being evaluated. The order in which patients receive the various treatments is decide through a random assignment process (for example if only treatments A and B are being evaluated, half the patients would be randomly assigned to receive A first, the other half would receive A second). This design contrasts to two others designs already presented, parallel studies and self-controlled studies. In **parallel studies**, two or more treatments are evaluated concurrently in separate, randomly assigned, groups of patients. An example of a parallel study, would be problem 6 in Chapter 8, where physical therapy patients were assigned (presumably by randomized process) to two different treatment regimens and evaluated (using a two-sample t-test) for outcomes as measured by range of motion. A **self-controlled study**, is one in which only one treatment is evaluated and the same patients are evaluated during treatment and at least one period when no treatment is present. Problem 2 in Chapter 8, offers an example of a self-controlled study in which the same patients were measured before and after treatment with a new brochodilator and their response evaluated using a paired t-test.

The major advantage of the cross-over design is that each patients serves as his or her own control which eliminates subject-to-subject variability in response to the treatments being evaluated. The term "randomized" in the title of this design refers to the order in patients are assigned to the various treatments. With each patient serving as a block in the design there is increased precision, because of decreased random error and a more accurate estimate of true treatment differences. Major disadvantages with cross-over experiments are that: 1) the patient may change over time (the disease state becomes worse, affecting later measurements); 2) with increased time there is a chance for subjects to withdraw or drop out of the study which results in decreased sample size; 3) there may be a carry-over effect of the first treatment affecting subsequent treatments; and 4) the first treatment may introduce a permanent physiological changes affecting later measurements. These latter two problems can be evaluated using a two-way analysis of variance design, discussed in Chapter 11, where two independent variables (treatment and order of treatment) can be assessed concurrently. Additional information about these

Table 9.5 Diastolic Blood Pressure Before and After
Administration of a New Antihypertensive

Blocks (Subject)	Treatment 1 (Before)	Treatment 2 (After)	$\sum$	Mean
1	68	66	134	67
2	83	80	163	81.5
3	72	67	139	69.5
4	75	74	149	74.5
5	79	70	149	74.5
6	71	77	148	74
7	65	64	129	64.5
8	76	70	146	73
9	78	76	154	77
10	68	66	134	67
11	85	81	166	83
12	<u>74</u>	<u>68</u>	<u>142</u>	71
$\sum$ =	894	859	1753	
Mean =	74.50	71.58		

types of experimental designs are presented by Bolton (1997) and Freidman and colleagues (1985).

As mentioned, a paired t-test could be considered a special case of the randomized complete block design with only two treatment levels. For example, the data appearing in the first three columns of Table 8.3 could be considered a randomized complete design (Table 9.5). Each subject represents one of twelve blocks, with two treatment measures (before and after). In this particular case the null hypothesis states that there is no difference between the two treatment periods (before vs. after):

$$H_0: \quad \mu_B = \mu_A$$
$$H_1: \quad \mu_B \neq \mu_A$$

The decision rule is with $\alpha = 0.05$, reject H_0 if $F > F_{1,11}(.95)$ which is 4.90 (interpolated from Table B5). The calculations are as follows:

$$I = \sum_{k=1}^{K} \sum_{j=1}^{J} x_{kj}^2$$

$$I = (68)^2 + (83)^2 + (72)^2 + ...(68)^2 = 128,877$$

$$II = \frac{\left[\sum_{k=1}^{K} \sum_{j=1}^{J} x_{kj} \right]^2}{KJ}$$

$$II = \frac{(1753)^2}{24} = 128,042.0417$$

$$III_R = \frac{\sum_{k=1}^{K} \left[\sum_{j=1}^{J} x_{kj} \right]^2}{K}$$

$$III_R = \frac{(134)^2 + (163)^2 + ...(142)^2}{2} = 128,750.5$$

$$III_C = \frac{\sum_{j=1}^{J} \left[\sum_{k=1}^{K} x_{kj} \right]^2}{J}$$

$$III_C = \frac{(894)^2 + (859)^2}{12} = 128,093.0833$$

$$SS_{Total} = SS_T = I - II$$

$$SS_T = 128,877 - 128,042.0417 = 834.9583$$

$$SS_{Blocks} = SS_B = III_R - II$$

$$SS_B = 128,750.5 - 128,042.0417 = 708.4583$$

$$SS_{Treatment} = SS_{Rx} = III_C - II$$

$$SS_{Rx} = 128,093.0833 - 128,042.0417 = 51.0416$$

$$SS_{Error} = SS_{Residual} = SS_T - SS_B - SS_{Rx}$$

$$SS_{Residual} = 834.9583 - 708.4583 - 51.0416 = 75.4584$$

The ANOVA table is:

Source	df	SS	MS	F
Treatment	1	51.0416	51.0416	7.44
Blocks	11	708.4583	64.4053	
Residual	11	75.4584	6.8599	
Total	23	834.9583		

With the calculated F-value greater than the critical value of 4.90, the decision is to reject H_0 and conclude that there is a significant difference between the before and after measurements with the after measure of diastolic blood pressure significantly lower than that before therapy.

Homogeniety of Variance

It is important that we address the issue of homoscedasticity. One of the criteria required to perform any parametric procedure is that the dispersion within the different levels of the independent discrete variable be approximately equal. Because of the robustness of the F-distribution, differences with variances can be tolerated if sample sizes are equal (Cochran, 1947). However, for samples that are unequal in size, a marked difference in variances can effect the statistical outcomes.

As discussed in the beginning of Chapter 8, a general rule of thumb is that the largest variance divided by the smallest variance should be less than two. Several tests are also available to determine if there is a lack of homogeniety. The simplest is **Hartley's F-max test**. Using this test the following hypotheses of equal variances are tested:

H_0: $\sigma_1^2 = \sigma_2^2 = \sigma_3^2 \ldots = \sigma_k^2$
H_1: H_0 is false

The test statistic is a simple ratio between the largest and smallest variances:

$$F_{max} = \frac{S^2_{largest}}{S^2_{smallest}}$$ Eq. 9.21

The resultant F_{max} value is compared to a critical value from Table B6 (Appendix B) for k levels of the discrete independent variable and n-1 degrees of freedom, based on n observations per level of the independent variable (equal cell size). If F_{max} exceeds the critical value, H_0 is rejected and the researcher cannot assume that there is homogeneity. For example, consider the previous example comparing the weights of tablets from three different facilities (Table 9.2). The largest variance is from facility C at 17.31 (4.16^2) and the smallest from Facility A is 10.69 (3.27^2). Can the investigator assume that there is homogeneity of variance?

H_0: $\sigma_A^2 = \sigma_B^2 = \sigma_C^2$
H_1: H_0 is false

With α = 0.05, H_0 would be rejected if F_{max} exceeds the critical $F_{3,14}$, which is approximately 3.75. Calculation of the test statistic is:

$$F_{max} = \frac{S^2_{largest}}{S^2_{smallest}} = \frac{17.31}{10.69} = 1.62$$

With F_{max} less than 3.75 the research would fail to reject the null hypothesis with 95% confidence and would assume that the sample variances are all equal.

A second procedure that can be used for unequal cell sizes (differing numbers of observations per level of the independent variable) would be **Cochran's C test**, which compares the ratio of the largest sample variance with the sum of all variances:

$$C = \frac{S^2_{largest}}{\Sigma S^2_k}$$ Eq. 9.22

Once again a table of critical values is required (Table B7, Appendix B). The calculated C ratio is compared to a critical value from Table B7 for k levels of the independent variable in the samples and n-1 observations per sample. If C exceeds the critical value, H_0 is rejected and the researcher cannot assume that there is homogeneity. Using the same example as above, with α = 0.05, H_0 would be rejected if C exceeds the critical C-value, which is approximately 0.5666. Calculation of the test statistic is:

$$C = \frac{S_{largest}^2}{\sum S_k^2} = \frac{(4.16\,)^2}{(3.27\,)^2 + (3.46\,)^2 + (4.16\,)^2} = \frac{17.31}{39.97} = 0.4331$$

With C less than 0.5666 the exact same result occurs as was found with the F_{max} results.

If the cell size differs slightly, the largest of the n's can be used to determine the degrees of freedom. Consider the second ANOVA example with four different formulations (A,B,C and D) and cell sizes of 20,20,19 and 18, respectively. In this case n=20, n-1=19 and the critical values for C by interpolation would be 0.4355. The test statistic would be:

$$C = \frac{(14.6\,)^2}{(12.8\,)^2 + (11.6\,)^2 + (14.6\,)^2 + (10.0\,)^2} = 0.3486$$

In both cases, the statistics are less than the critical values, the researcher fails to reject H_0 and assume that there is homogeneity of variance.

An alternative procedure that involves more complex calculations is **Bartlett's test** and is described in Kirk's book. Because the F-distribution, upon which the F-test is based, is so robust regarding violations of the assumption of homogeneity of variance, these tests of homogeneity are usually not required.

References

Bolton, S. (1997). Pharmaceutical Statistics: Practical and Clinical Applications, Marcel Dekker, Inc., New York, pp. 397-425.

Cochran, W.G. (1947). Some consequences when the assumptions of analysis of variance are not satisfied. Biometrics 3:22-38.

Daniel, W.W. (1991). Biostatistics: A Foundation for Analysis in the Health Sciences, Second Edition, John Wiley and Sons, New York, pp. 163-167.

Fisher, R.A. (1926). "The arrangement of field experiments," Journal of Ministry of Agriculture 33:503-513.

Friedman, L.M., Furberg, C.D. and DeMets, D.L. (1985). Fundamentals of Clinical Trials, PSG Publishing Company, Inc., Littleton, MA, pp. 33-47.

Kachigan, S.K. (1991). Multivariate Statistical Analysis, Second Edition, Radius Press, New York, pp. 195-197.

Kirk, R.E. (1968). Experimental Design: Procedures for the Behavioral Sciences, Brooks/Cole, Belmont, CA, pp. 61-62.

Snedecor, G.W. and Cochran, W.G. (1989). Statistical Methods, Iowa State University Press, Ames, IA, p. 223.

Suggested Supplemental Readings

Bolton, S. (1997). Pharmaceutical Statistics: Practical and Clinical Applications, Marcel Dekker, Inc., New York, pp. 265-273.

Daniel, W.W. (1991). Biostatistics: A Foundation for Analysis in the Health Sciences, John Wiley and Sons, New York, pp. 297-305.

Kirk, R.E. (1968). Experimental Design: Procedures for the Behavioral Sciences, Brooks/Cole, Belmont, CA, pp. 104-109, 131-134.

Example Problems

1. Three physicians were selected for a study to evaluate the length of stay for patients undergoing a major surgical procedure. All procedures occurred in the same hospital and were without complications. Eight records were randomly selected from patients treated over the past twelve months. Was there a significant difference, by physician, in the length of stay for these patients?

	Days in the Hospital	
Physician A	Physician B	Physician C
9	10	8
12	6	9
10	7	12
7	10	10
11	11	14
13	9	10
8	9	8

Physician A	Physician B	Physician C
Mean = 10.38	Mean = 9.13	Mean = 10.75
S.D. = 2.26	S.D. = 1.81	S.D. = 2.66

2. In a collaborative trial, four laboratories were sent samples from a reservoir and requested to perform ten assays and report the results based on percentage of labeled amount of drug. Were there any significant differences based on the laboratory performing the analysis?

Lab(A)	Lab(B)	Lab(C)	Lab(D)
100.0	99.5	99.6	99.8
99.8	100.0	99.3	100.5
99.5	99.3	99.5	100.0
100.1	99.9	99.1	100.1
99.7	100.3	99.7	99.4
99.9	99.5	99.6	99.6
100.4	99.6	99.4	100.2
100.0	98.9	99.5	99.9
99.7	99.8	99.5	100.4
99.9	100.1	99.9	100.1

3. Acme Chemical and Dye received from the same raw material supplier three batches of oil from three different production sites. Samples were drawn from drums at each location and compared to determine if the viscosity was the same for each batch. Are the viscosities the same regardless of the batch?

Viscosity Batch A	Viscosity Batch B	Viscosity Batch C
10.23	10.24	10.25
10.33	10.28	10.20
10.28	10.20	10.21
10.27	10.21	10.18
10.30	10.26	10.22

4. To evaluate the responsiveness of individuals receiving various commercially available benzodiazepines, volunteers were administered these drugs and subjected to a computer-simulated driving test. Twelve volunteers were randomly divided into four groups, each receiving one of three benzodiazepines or a placebo. At two week intervals they were crossed over to other agents and retested, until each volunteer had received each active drug and the placebo. Driving abilities were measured two hours after the drug administration (at approximately the C_{max} for the benzodiazepines). The higher the score, the greater the number of driving

errors. The following results were observed:

Benzo(A)	Benzo(B)	Benzo(C)	Placebo
58	62	53	50
54	55	45	51
52	58	48	53
62	56	46	57
51	60	58	61
55	48	61	49
45	73	52	50
63	57	51	60
56	64	55	40
57	51	48	47
50	68	62	46
60	69	49	43

Is there a significant difference in the driving scores based on the drug or placebo received?

5. During a clinical trial, Acme Chemical wants to compare two possible generic formulations to the currently available brand product (reference standard). Based on the following results, is there a significant difference between the two Acme formulations and the reference standard?

	Plasma Elimination Half-life (in minutes)		
	Formulation A	Formulation B	Reference Standard
Subject 001	206	207	208
Subject 002	212	218	217
Subject 003	203	199	204
Subject 004	211	210	213
Subject 005	205	209	209
Subject 006	209	205	209
Subject 007	217	213	225
Subject 008	197	203	196
Subject 009	208	207	212
Subject 010	199	195	202
Subject 011	208	208	210
Subject 012	214	222	219

6. Replicate measures were made on samples from various batches of a specific biological product. The researcher was concerned that the first measure would influence the outcome on the second measure. Using a complete randomized block design, is there independence (no effect) between the first and second replicate measures?

Treatment (% recovered)

	Replicate 1	Replicate 2
Batch A	93.502	92.319
Batch C	91.177	92.230
Batch D	87.304	87.496
Batch D2	81.275	80.564
Batch G	79.865	79.259
Batch G2	81.722	80.931

Answers to Problems

1. Evaluation of length of stay for patients of three physicians.
   Independent variable: physicians (discrete, 3 levels)
   Dependent variable: length of patient stays (continuous)
   Statistical test: ANOVA (example of the definitional formula)

Physician A	Physician B	Physician C
Mean = 10.38	Mean = 9.13	Mean = 10.75
S.D. = 2.26	S.D. = 1.81	S.D. = 2.66
n = 8	n = 8	n = 8

Hypothesis: H_0: $\mu_{physician\ A} = \mu_{physician\ B} = \mu_{physician\ C}$
          H_1: H_0 is false

Test statistic:

$$F = \frac{MS_B}{MS_W}$$

Decision rule: With $\alpha = .05$, reject H_0 if $F > F_{2,21}(.95) \approx 3.48$.

Calculations:

$$MS_W = \frac{(n_1-1)S_1^2 + (n_2-1)S_2^2 + (n_3-1)S_3^2 + \dots (n_k-1)S_k^2}{N-K}$$

$$MS_W = \frac{7(2.26)^2 + 7(1.81)^2 + 7(2.66)^2}{21} = 5.15$$

$$\overline{X}_G = \frac{(n_1\overline{X}_1) + (n_2\overline{X}_2) + (n_3\overline{X}_3) + \dots (n_k\overline{X}_k)}{N}$$

$$\overline{X}_G = \frac{8(10.38) + 8(9.13) + 8(10.75)}{24} = 10.09$$

$$MS_B = \frac{n_1(\overline{X}_1-\overline{X}_G)^2 + n_2(\overline{X}_2-\overline{X}_G)^2 + n_3(\overline{X}_3-\overline{X}_G)^2 + \dots n_k(\overline{X}_k-\overline{X}_G)^2}{K-1}$$

$$MS_B = \frac{8(10.38-10.09)^2 + 8(9.13-10.09)^2 + 8(10.75-10.09)^2}{2}$$

$$MS_B = 5.77$$

$$F = \frac{MS_B}{MS_W} = \frac{5.77}{5.15} = 1.12$$

Decision: With $F < 3.48$, do not reject H_0, conclude that

$\mu_{\text{physician A}} = \mu_{\text{physician B}} = \mu_{\text{physician C}}$.

2. Collaborative trial with assays from four laboratories (Table 9.6)
   Independent variable: laboratories (discrete, 4 levels)
   Dependent variable: viscosity (continuous)
   Statistical test: ANOVA (example of the computational formula)

Hypotheses: H_0: $\mu_A = \mu_B = \mu_C = \mu_D$
            H_1: H_0 is false

Decision rule: With $\alpha = .05$, reject H_0 if $F > F_{3,36}(.95) \approx 2.87$.

Table 9.6 Data from Four Different Laboratories

Lab(A)	Lab(B)	Lab(C)	Lab(D)
100.0	99.5	99.6	99.8
99.8	100.0	99.3	100.5
99.5	99.3	99.5	100.0
100.1	99.9	99.1	100.1
99.7	100.3	99.7	99.4
99.9	99.5	99.6	99.6
100.4	99.6	99.4	100.2
100.0	98.9	99.5	99.9
99.7	99.8	99.5	100.4
99.9	100.1	99.9	100.1
Σ = 999.0	996.9	995.1	1000.0

Calculations:

$$I = \sum_{k=1}^{K} \sum_{i=1}^{n} x_{jk}^2 = (100)^2 + (99.8)^2 + \ldots (100.1)^2 = 398,207.04$$

$$II = \frac{\left[\sum_{k=1}^{K} \sum_{i=1}^{n} x_{jk} \right]^2}{N_K} = \frac{(3991)^2}{40} = 398,202.025$$

$$III = \sum_{k=1}^{K} \frac{\left[\sum_{i=1}^{n} x_{jk} \right]^2}{n_K} = \frac{(999.0)^2}{10} + \ldots \frac{(1000)^2}{10} = 398,203.462$$

$$SSB = III - II = 398,203.462 - 398,202.025 = 1.437$$

$$SSW = I - III = 398,207.04 - 398,203.462 = 3.578$$

$$SST = I - II = 398,207.04 - 398,202.025 = 5.015$$

ANOVA Table

Source	DF	SS	MS	F
Between	3	1.437	0.479	4.84
Within	36	3.578	0.099	
Total	39	5.015		

Decision: With $F > 2.87$, reject H_0, conclude that
$\mu_A = \mu_B = \mu_C = \mu_D$ is not true

3. Comparison of a raw material at three different production sites.
   Independent variable: production site (discrete, 3 levels)
   Dependent variable: oil viscosity (continuous)
   Statistical test: ANOVA (example of the computational formula)

Hypotheses: H_0: $\mu_A = \mu_B = \mu_C$
             H_1: H_0 is false

Decision rule: With $\alpha = .05$, reject H_0 if $F > F_{2,12}(.95) \approx 3.70$.

Viscosity Batch A	Viscosity Batch B	Viscosity Batch C	
10.23	10.24	10.25	
10.33	10.28	10.20	
10.28	10.20	10.21	
10.27	10.21	10.18	
10.30	10.26	10.22	
$\Sigma =$ 51.41	51.19	51.06	$\Sigma\Sigma = 153.66$

Calculations:

$$I = \sum_{k=1}^{K} \sum_{i=1}^{n} x_{jk}^2 = (10.23)^2 + (10.33)^2 + \ldots (10.22)^2 = 1574.1182$$

$$II = \frac{\left[\sum_{k=1}^{K} \sum_{i=1}^{n} x_{jk}\right]^2}{N_k} = \frac{(153.66)^2}{15} = 1574.0930$$

$$III = \sum_{k=1}^{K} \frac{\left[\sum_{i=1}^{n} x_{jk}\right]^2}{n_K} = \frac{(51.41)^2}{5} + \frac{(51.19)^2}{5} + \frac{(51.06)^2}{5} = 1574.1056$$

$$SS_B = III - II = 1574.1056 - 1574.0930 = 0.0126$$

$$SS_W = I - III = 1574.1182 - 1574.1056 = 0.0126$$

$$SS_T = I - II = 1574.1182 - 1574.0930 = 0.0252$$

ANOVA table:

Source	DF	SS	MS	F
Between	2	0.0126	0.0063	6.3
Within	12	0.0126	0.0010	
Total	14	0.0252		

Decision: With F > 2.83, reject H_0, conclude that $\mu_A = \mu_B = \mu_C$ is not true

4. Use of benzodiazepines and responses to a computerized simulated driving test.

Independent variable: drug or placebo (discrete, 4 levels)
Dependent variable: driving score (continuous)
Statistical test: ANOVA (example of the definitional formula)

Hypotheses: H_0: $\mu_A = \mu_B = \mu_C = \mu_{Placebo}$
 H_1: H_0 is false

Decision rule: With $\alpha = .05$, reject H_0 if $F > F_{3,44}(.95) \approx 3.85$.

	Benzo(A)	Benzo(B)	Benzo(C)	Placebo
Mean =	55.25	60.08	52.33	50.58
S.D. =	5.24	7.46	5.66	6.40
n =	12	12	12	12

Calculations:

$$MS_W = \frac{(n_1-1)S_1^2 + (n_2-1)S_2^2 + (n_3-1)S_3^2 + ...(n_k-1)S_k^2}{N-K}$$

$$MS_W = \frac{11(5.24)^2 + 11(7.46)^2 + 11(5.66)^2 + 11(6.40)^2}{44} = 39.02$$

$$\overline{X_G} = \frac{(n_1\overline{X_1}) + (n_2\overline{X_2}) + (n_3\overline{X_3}) + ...(n_k\overline{X_k})}{N}$$

$$\overline{X_G} = \frac{12(55.25) + 12(60.08) + 12(52.33) + 12(50.58)}{48} = 54.56$$

$$MS_B = \frac{n_1(\overline{X_1} - \overline{X_G})^2 + n_2(\overline{X_2} - \overline{X_G})^2 + n_3(\overline{X_3} - \overline{X_G})^2 + \dots n_k(\overline{X_k} - \overline{X_G})^2}{K-1}$$

$$MS_B = \frac{12(55.25 - 54.56)^2 + 12(60.08 - 54.56)^2 + \dots 12(50.58 - 54.56)^2}{3} = 207.04$$

$$F = \frac{MS_B}{MS_W} = \frac{207.04}{39.02} = 5.31$$

Decision: With F > 2.85, reject H_0, conclude that

$\mu_A = \mu_B = \mu_C = \mu_{Placebo}$ is not true

5. Evaluation of two formulations compared to the reference standard.
    Independent variable: formulations (discrete, 3 levels)
                               subjects (blocks)
    Dependent variable: plasma elimination half-life (continuous)
    Statistical design: complete randomized block design

Plasma Elimination Half-life (in minutes)

Blocks (Subjects)	Form. A	Form. B	Reference Standard	Σ	Mean
001	206	207	208	621	207.0
002	212	218	217	647	215.7
003	203	199	204	606	202.0
004	211	210	213	634	211.3
005	205	209	209	623	207.7
006	209	205	209	623	207.7
007	217	213	225	655	218.3
008	197	203	196	596	198.7
009	208	207	212	627	209.0
010	199	195	202	596	198.7
011	208	208	210	626	208.7
012	214	222	219	655	218.3
Σ	2,489	2,496	2,524	7509	
Mean	207.4	208.0	210.3		

Hypotheses: H_0: $\mu_A = \mu_B = \mu_{RS}$
             H_1: H_0 is false

Decision rule: With $\alpha = 0.05$, reject H_0 if F > $F_{2,11} \approx 3.98$

Calculations:

$$I = \sum_{k=1}^{K} \sum_{j=1}^{J} x_{kj}^2$$

$$I = (206\,)^2 + (212\,)^2 + (203\,)^2 + ...(219\,)^2 = 1567969$$

$$II = \frac{\left[\sum\limits_{k=1}^{K} \sum\limits_{j=1}^{J} x_{kj}\right]^2}{KJ}$$

$$II = \frac{(7509\,)^2}{36} = 1566252.25$$

$$III_R = \frac{\sum\limits_{k=1}^{K}\left[\sum\limits_{j=1}^{J} x_{kj}\right]^2}{K}$$

$$III_R = \frac{(621\,)^2 + (647\,)^2 + ...(655\,)^2}{3} = 1567729$$

$$III_C = \frac{\sum\limits_{j=1}^{J}\left[\sum\limits_{k=1}^{K} x_{kj}\right]^2}{J}$$

$$III_C = \frac{(2489\,)^2 + (2496\,)^2 + (2524\,)^2}{12} = 1566309.417$$

$$SS_{Total} = SS_T = I - II$$

$$SS_{Total} = 1567969 - 1566252.25 = 1716.75$$

$$SS_{Blocks} = SS_B = III_R - II$$

$$SS_{Blocks} = 1567729 - 1566252.25 = 1476.75$$

$$SS_{Treatment} = SS_{Rx} = III_C - II$$

$$SS_{Treatment} = 1566309.417 - 1566252.25 = 57.167$$

$$SS_{Error} = SS_{Residual} = SS_T - SS_B - SS_{Rx}$$

$$SS_{Residual} = 1716.75 - 1476.75 - 57.167 = 182.833$$

ANOVA Table

Source	df	SS	MS.	F
Treatment	2	57.167	28.58	3.44
Blocks	11	1476.75	134.25	
Residual	22	182.833	8.31	
Total	35	1716.75		

Decision: With $F < 3.98$, fail to reject H_0 and conclude that there is no significant difference among the three products.

6. Evaluation of replicate assays
   Independent variable: replicates, first vs. second (discrete, 2 levels)
                              batches (blocks)
   Dependent variable: percent recovered (continuous)
   Statistical design: complete randomized block

   Hypotheses: H_0: $\mu_1 = \mu_2$
                     H_1: $\mu_1 \neq \mu_2$

Decision rule: With $\alpha = 0.05$, reject H_0 if $F > F_{1,5} = 6.61$

Blocks	Treatment (% recovered)			
	Replicate 1	Replicate 2	Σ	Mean
Batch A	93.502	92.319	185.821	92.911
Batch C	91.177	92.230	183.407	91.704
Batch D	87.304	87.496	174.800	87.400
Batch D2	81.275	80.564	161.839	80.920
Batch G	79.865	79.259	159.124	79.562
Batch G2	81.722	80.931	162.653	81.327
Σ	514.845	512.799	1027.644	
Mean	85.808	85.467		

Calculations:

$$I = \sum_{k=1}^{K} \sum_{j=1}^{J} x_{kj}^2$$

$$I = (93.502)^2 + (92.319)^2 + ... (80.931)^2 = 88347.4815$$

$$II = \frac{\left[\sum_{k=1}^{K} \sum_{j=1}^{J} x_{kj}\right]^2}{KJ}$$

$$II = \frac{(1027.644)^2}{12} = 88004.3492$$

$$III_R = \frac{\sum_{k=1}^{K} \left[\sum_{j=1}^{J} x_{kj}\right]^2}{K}$$

$$III_R = \frac{(185.821)^2 + (183.407)^2 + ... (162.653)^2}{2} = 88345.4597$$

$$III_C = \frac{\sum_{j=1}^{J} \left[\sum_{k=1}^{K} x_{kj}\right]^2}{J}$$

$$III_C = \frac{(514.845)^2 + (512.799)^2}{6} = 88004.6980$$

$$SS_{Total} = SS_T = I - II$$

$$SS_{Total} = 88347.4815 - 88004.3492 = 343.1323$$

$$SS_{Blocks} = SS_B = III_R - II$$

$$SS_{Blocks} = 88345.4597 - 88004.3492 = 341.1105$$

$$SS_{Treatment} = SS_{Rx} = III_C - II$$

$$SS_{Treatment} = 88004.6980 - 88004.3492 = 0.3488$$

$$SS_{Error} = SS_{Residual} = SS_T - SS_B - SS_{Rx}$$

$$SS_{Residual} = 343.1323 - 341.1105 - 0.3488 = 1.673$$

ANOVA Table:

Source	df	SS	MS	F
Treatment	1	0.3488	0.3488	1.0424
Blocks	5	341.1105	68.2221	
Residual	5	1.6730	0.3346	
Total	11	343.1323		

Decision: With $F < 6.61$, fail to reject H_0, and conclude that there is no significant difference between the first and second replicates and that the second measurement is not influenced by the first measurement.

10

Post Hoc Procedures

As discussed in the previous chapter, rejection of the null hypothesis in the one-way analysis of variance simply proves that some significant difference exists between at least two levels of the discrete independent variable. Unfortunately the ANOVA does not identify the exact location of the difference(s). *Post hoc* procedure can be used to reevaluate the data for a *significant* ANOVA and identify where the difference(s) exist while maintaining an overall Type I error rate (α) at a level similar to that used to test the original null hypothesis for the one-way ANOVA. Assuming an analysis of variance was conducted with $\alpha = 0.05$ and the H_0 was rejected, then the *post hoc* comparisons should keep the error rate constant at 0.05.

Although the title "post hoc" would imply an after-the-fact process, these procedures should be considered an integral part of any one-way ANOVA when there are more than two levels associated with the discrete independent variable. The researcher should always be mindful that if the null hypothesis is rejected with an one-way ANOVA the one of the post hoc procedures described in this chapter serves as a logical extension of that analysis.

Sometimes researchers error in performing multiple t-tests between the various two levels of the independent variable (pair-wise combinations). By using **multiple t-tests** the researcher actually compounds the Type I error rate. This compounding of the error is referred to as **the experimentwise error rate**. For example, if there are three levels to the independent variable, there are three possible comparisons:

$$\binom{3}{2} = \frac{3!}{2!1!} = 3$$

such as A vs. B, B vs. C and A vs. C. A simple way of thinking about this compounding error rate would be that if each t-test were conducted with $\alpha = 0.05$, then the error rate would be three comparisons times 0.05, or a 0.15 error rate. As can be seen in Tables 10.1 and 10.2, as the number of levels of the independent variable increases, the number of inter-sample comparisons (i.e., pair-wise comparisons) increases at a rapid rate, thus greatly increasing the level of α. The actual calculation for compounding the error or experimentwise error rate is:

$$\alpha_{ew} = 1 - (1 - \alpha)^C \qquad \text{Equ. 10.1}$$

where C is the total possible independent t-tests comparing only two levels of the discrete independent variable. Table 10.1 lists the experimental error rate for various pair-wise combinations. The third column is for the 95% confidence level and the fourth for the 99% confidence level.

One method of controlling this experimental error rate is to use the **Bonferroni adjustment**. This relatively simple procedure involves dividing the level of significance (i.e., 0.05 or 0.01) by the number of possible pair-wise comparisons (C) and determine a new critical t-value. Table 10.2 lists various adjustments for an infinite number of observations. These were calculated under the assumption that the t-value is at infinity and uses the standardized normal distribution and z-values for the various adjusted p-values (α). Notice

Table 10.1 Experiment-wise Error Rates for Multiple Paired t-tests After a Significant ANOVA

Number of Groups (Discrete levels)	(c) Number of Possible Paired Comparisons	Level of Significance Used in each t-test (α_{ew})	
		0.05	0.01
2	1	0.05	0.01
3	3	0.143	0.030
4	6	0.265	0.059
5	10	0.401	0.096
6	15	0.536	0.140
7	21	0.659	0.190
8	28	0.762	0.245

Table 10.2 Bonferroni Adjustment for Maintaining an Experimental
Error Rate of 0.05

Number of Discrete Levels	Number of (c) Possible Paired Comparisons	(α/c) Bonferroni Adjustment	Estimate Critical (z) Value for Infinite Degrees of Freedom
2	1	0.05	1.96
3	3	0.0167	2.39
4	6	0.008	2.65
5	10	0.005	2.81
6	15	0.003	2.96
7	15 ²¹	0.002	3.08
8	21 ₂₈	0.0017	3.15
9	36	0.0013	3.23
10	45	0.0011	3.30

how the critical value increases as the number of levels of the discrete independent variable increases, thus controlling increased experimentwise error rate.

What if there are less than an infinite number of observations? Other tables are available in various textbooks for smaller sample sizes and smaller α values than those in the third column of Table 10.2. As seen in Table B3 (Appendix B), for larger samples sizes the critical t-value is very close to the t-value at infinity (1.96). For example, at 80 degrees of freedom the critical t-value = 2.00. Therefore, Table 10.2 can be used as a rough approximation for the required critical value.

To illustrate both multiple t-tests and Bonferroni's adjustment, consider the second problem in Chapter 9 where a significant difference was found with a Type I error rate of 0.05, leading to the rejection of the following "global" null hypothesis associated with the original one-way analysis of variance:

$$H_0: \mu_A = \mu_B = \mu_C = \mu_D$$

The data used for these examples were:

Concentration in mcg/ml:	Mean	S.D.	n
Formulation A	123.2	12.8	20
Formulation B	105.6	11.6	20
Formulation C	116.4	14.6	19
Formulation D	113.5	10.0	18

Since there are four levels of the discrete independent variable, there are six possible pair-wise comparisons, the Bonferroni's adjustment of the α would be 0.008 and a *very rough approximation* for the critical t-value would be 2.65 from Table 10.2. Confidence intervals can be created using the following formula (Eq. 8.4):

$$\mu_1 - \mu_2 = (\overline{X}_1 - \overline{X}_2) \pm 2.65 \sqrt{\frac{S_P^2}{n_1} + \frac{S_P^2}{n_2}}$$

If we compare the results for both six pair-wise t-tests and six tests with Bonferroni's adjustment, there are more significant findings with the multiple t-test due to the experimentwise error (Table 10.3).

Performing unadjusted multiple t-tests is one of the major errors found in the literature (Glantz, 1980). When the independent variable has more than two discrete levels, an ANOVA followed by an appropriate post hoc procedure is the correct test, not multiple t-tests; because as seen in Table 10.1, when multiple independent t-tests are applied to one set of data, it becomes increasingly likely that a significant outcome will result by chance alone.

Following the rejection of the global null hypothesis for the one-way ANOVA, a post hoc procedure should be used to identify specific significant differences. Three of these methods are described below and results will be expressed as confidence intervals similar to the previous example.

Dunn's Multiple Comparisons

Dunn's procedure (also called a **Bonferroni t statistic**) calculates mean differences for all pair-wise comparisons and compares these differences to a

Table 10.3 Comparison of Results with Multiple t-tests and the Bonferroni Adjustment

Pairing	Multiple t-tests Confidence Interval	Bonferroni Adjustments Confidence Interval
$\overline{X}_A - \overline{X}_B$	$+9.79 < \mu_A - \mu_B < +25.41$ *	$+7.38 < \mu_A - \mu_B < +27.82$ *
$\overline{X}_A - \overline{X}_C$	$-2.07 < \mu_A - \mu_C < +15.674$	$-0.24 < \mu_A - \mu_C < +13.84$
$\overline{X}_A - \overline{X}_D$	$+2.11 < \mu_A - \mu_D < +17.29$ *	$+3.29 < \mu_A - \mu_D < +16.11$ *
$\overline{X}_B - \overline{X}_C$	$-19.31 < \mu_B - \mu_C < -2.29$ *	$-21.95 < \mu_B - \mu_C < +0.35$
$\overline{X}_B - \overline{X}_D$	$-15.04 < \mu_B - \mu_D < -0.76$ *	$-17.26 < \mu_B - \mu_D < +1.46$
$\overline{X}_C - \overline{X}_D$	$-5.46 < \mu_C - \mu_D < 11.26$	$-8.06 < \mu_C - \mu_D < 13.86$

* Significant at $p < 0.05$

critical value extracted from a table. As an extension of the Bonferroni adjustment it involves the splitting of the level of significance (α) between all possible comparisons (C). For all the *post hoc* procedures we will continue using the second example from the previous chapter, where it was found that a significant difference existed somewhere between the following means:

Concentration in mcg/ml:	Mean	n	
Formulation A	123.2	20	$MS_W = MS_E = 153.51$
Formulation B	105.6	20	
Formulation C	116.4	19	$v_2 = N-K = 73$
Formulation D	113.5	18	

As seen previously, the total number of possible pair-wise comparisons is:

$$C = \binom{4}{2} = \frac{4!}{2!2!} = 6$$

The absolute difference for each pair-wise comparison is computed:

$$|\overline{X}_A - \overline{X}_B| = 17.6 \qquad |\overline{X}_B - \overline{X}_C| = -10.8$$
$$|\overline{X}_A - \overline{X}_C| = 6.8 \qquad |\overline{X}_B - \overline{X}_D| = -7.9$$
$$|\overline{X}_A - \overline{X}_D| = 9.7 \qquad |\overline{X}_C - \overline{X}_D| = 2.9$$

A value is extracted from the table of Dunn's percentage points (Table B8, Appendix B). This value takes into consideration: 1) the total number of possible pair-wise comparisons (C); 2) the original denominator degrees of freedom (N-K) for the ANOVA; and 3) the Type I error rate used in the original ANOVA (i.e., $\alpha = 0.05$), As seen in Table B8, the first column is the number of possible combinations, the Type I error rate is in the second column, and the remaining columns relate to the N-K degrees of freedom. In this particular example the table value is

$$t'D_{\alpha;C;N-K} = t'D_{.05;6;73} \approx 2.72$$

This number is then inserted into the calculation of a critical Dunn's value:

$$d = t'D_{\alpha/2;C;N-K} \sqrt{MS_E \cdot (\frac{1}{n_1} + \frac{1}{n_2})} \qquad \text{Eq. 10.2}$$

If the mean difference is greater than the critical d value there is a significant difference between the two means. The calculation of the critical d-value for the first pair-wise comparison is:

$$d = (2.72) \sqrt{153.51 \cdot (\frac{1}{20} + \frac{1}{20})} = (2.72)(3.92) = 10.66$$

Our decision, with $|\overline{X}_A - \overline{X}_B|$ greater than the critical d-value of 10.66, is to reject $\mu_A = \mu_B$ and conclude that there is a significant difference between these two population means.

An alternative method would be to create a confidence interval similar to the t-test:

$$\mu_1 - \mu_2 = (\overline{X}_1 - \overline{X}_2) \pm t' D_{\alpha/2;C;N-K} \sqrt{MS_E \cdot (\frac{1}{n_1} + \frac{1}{n_2})} \qquad \text{Eq. 10.3}$$

For the first pair-wise comparison:

$$\mu_A - \mu_B = (123.2 - 105.6) \pm 2.72 \sqrt{153.51 (\frac{1}{20} + \frac{1}{20})}$$

$$\mu_A - \mu_B = (17.6) \pm 10.66$$

$$6.94 < \mu_A - \mu_B < 28.26$$

Since zero does not fall within the interval, there is a significant difference between Formulations A and B. Note the same results occurred with the Bonferroni adjustment. However, two important features appear with Dunn's procedure: 1) the table of critical values allows for better corrections for smaller sample sizes and 2) by using the MS_E the entire variance from the original ANOVA is considered rather than only the pooled variance for the pair-wise comparison.

Using the original method for the calculation of the critical d-value, the d-value for this second pair-wise comparison is:

$$d = (2.72) \sqrt{153.51 (\frac{1}{20} + \frac{1}{19})} = (2.72)(3.97) = 10.80$$

Here the decision, with $|\overline{X}_A - \overline{X}_C| < 10.66$, is that we fail to reject $\mu_A - \mu_C$, thus we fail to find that there is a significant difference between these two levels. Similarly the confidence interval is:

$$\mu_A - \mu_C = (123.2 - 116.4) \pm 2.72 \sqrt{153.51 \cdot (\frac{1}{20} + \frac{1}{19})}$$

$$-4.00 < \mu_A - \mu_B < 17.60$$

With zero within the confidence interval, the same results are obtained and we cannot conclude that there is a difference. Table 10.4 presents a summary of all pair-wise comparisons.

Thus, we can conclude that Formulation B has a significantly lower maximum concentration than either Formulation A or C, and that there appears to be no other significant pair-wise comparisons.

Student Newman-Keuls Test

The **Student-Newman-Keuls (SNK) test** is a slight modification on Dunn's procedure, where a q-statistic is calculated and compared to a table of critical values. The q-statistic is calculated by the following:

$$q = \frac{\overline{X_1} - \overline{X_2}}{\sqrt{\frac{MS_E}{2} \left(\frac{1}{n_1} + \frac{1}{n_2} \right)}} \qquad \text{Eq. 10.4}$$

In this ratio, the numerator is identical to that of a t-test and the denominator resembles the formula employed in Dunn's procedure.

The calculated q-statistic is compared to the critical values listed in Table

Table 10.4	Results of Dunn's Multiple Comparisons	
Pairing	Confidence Interval	Results
$\overline{X}_A - \overline{X}_B$	$+6.94 < \mu_A-\mu_B < +28.26$	Significant
$\overline{X}_A - \overline{X}_C$	$-4.00 < \mu_A-\mu_C < +17.60$	
$\overline{X}_A - \overline{X}_D$	$-1.25 < \mu_A-\mu_D < +20.65$	
$\overline{X}_B - \overline{X}_C$	$-21.64 < \mu_B-\mu_C < +0.04$	
$\overline{X}_B - \overline{X}_D$	$-18.85 < \mu_B-\mu_D < +3.05$	
$\overline{X}_C - \overline{X}_D$	$-8.18 < \mu_C-\mu_D < +13.98$	

B9 of Appendix B. The denominator degrees of freedom used, like Dunn's procedure, is the same as the original denominator degrees of freedom for the F-test (N-K). One additional piece of information is required to read the critical value, namely the distance between the means if they are ranked in descending order. This distance is expressed as "steps" and is counted as the inclusive number of means. For example, listed below are means used previously, but reordered from the highest to the lowest mean:

Formulation A	123.2
Formulation C	116.4
Formulation D	113.5
Formulation B	105.6

The step difference between Formulation A and Formulation C is two and the number of steps between Formulation A and Formulation B is four. This difference is used to select the appropriate column from Table B9. As seen in Table B9, the first column is the denominator degrees of freedom (N-K), the Type I error rate is in the second column, and the remaining columns relate to the number of "mean steps." In the above example if we were to select the critical value for a comparison between Formulations A and D the step difference would be 3 and the N-K degrees of freedom is 73, giving a critical value for $\alpha = 0.05$ of approximately 3.39. The decision rule is with $\alpha = 0.05$, reject the H_0: $\mu_A = \mu_D$ if $q > q_{3,73}(0.05) \approx 3.39$ and the computation is:

$$q = \frac{123.2 - 113.5}{\sqrt{\dfrac{153.51}{2}\left(\dfrac{1}{20} + \dfrac{1}{18}\right)}} = \frac{9.7}{2.85} = 3.40$$

In this case, q is greater than the critical q-value; therefore, we would reject the H_0 that they are equal.

As with the Dunn's multiple comparisons the formula can be slightly modified to create a confidence interval:

$$\mu_1 - \mu_2 = (\overline{X_1} - \overline{X_2}) \pm q \cdot \sqrt{\frac{MS_E}{2}\left(\frac{1}{n_1} + \frac{1}{n_2}\right)} \qquad \text{Eq. 10.5}$$

Using this formula to calculate a confidence interval for Formulation A versus Formulation D is as follows:

$$\mu_A - \mu_D = (123.2 - 113.5) \pm 3.39 \cdot \sqrt{\frac{153.51}{2}\left(\frac{1}{20} + \frac{1}{18}\right)}$$

$$\mu_A - \mu_D = (9.7) \pm 9.66$$

$$0.04 < \mu_A - \mu_D < 19.36$$

again, since zero does not fall within the interval, the decision is that there is a significant difference between Formulations A and D.

Similarly, the comparison between Formulations B and D would involve only two means in the "step difference"; therefore, the decision rule for this comparison is, with $\alpha = 0.05$, reject H_0: $\mu_B = \mu_D$ if $q > q_{2,73}(0.05) \approx 2.82$ and the computation is:

$$q = \frac{113.5 - 105.6}{\sqrt{\frac{153.51}{2}\left(\frac{1}{20} + \frac{1}{18}\right)}} = \frac{7.9}{2.85} = 2.77$$

Here the calculated q-value is less than the critical q-value, therefore we cannot reject the hypothesis that Formulations are equal. The same results are found creating a confidence interval.

$$\mu_B - \mu_D = (105.6 - 113.5) \pm 2.82 \sqrt{\frac{153.51}{2}\left(\frac{1}{20} + \frac{1}{18}\right)}$$

$$-15.94 < \mu_B - \mu_D < +0.14$$

A summary of all possible pair-wise comparisons using the Newman-Keuls test is presented in Table 10.5.

Scheffé Procedure

Scheffé's procedure for multiple comparisons offers several advantages over the previous methods: 1) this procedure allows not only pair-wise, but also complex comparisons; 2) Scheffé's procedure guarantees finding a significant comparison if there was a significant F-value in the original ANOVA, this significant *post hoc* comparison however may not be expressible in logical terms; and 3) the Type I error rate remains constant with the error rate used in

Table 10.5   Results of Newman-Keuls' Comparisons

Pairing	Confidence Interval	Results
$\overline{X}_A - \overline{X}_B$	$+7.27 < \mu_A\text{-}\mu_B < +27.93$	Significant
$\overline{X}_A - \overline{X}_C$	$-1.12 < \mu_A\text{-}\mu_C < +14.72$	
$\overline{X}_A - \overline{X}_D$	$+0.04 < \mu_A\text{-}\mu_D < +19.36$	Significant
$\overline{X}_B - \overline{X}_C$	$-20.33 < \mu_B\text{-}\mu_C < -1.27$	Significant
$\overline{X}_B - \overline{X}_D$	$-15.94 < \mu_B\text{-}\mu_D < +0.14$	
$\overline{X}_C - \overline{X}_D$	$-5.22 < \mu_C\text{-}\mu_D < +11.02$	

the original ANOVA for both pair-wise and complex comparisons. Regarding the second point, results which might not be logical or interpretable, a hypothetical example may be useful for illustrative purposes. Assume that pharmacists are administered a cognitive test to assess there knowledge of some therapeutic class of medication. The findings below result in a significant one-way ANOVA for the four levels of a discrete independent variable (note that the levels are mutually exclusive and exhaustive).

Level	Years of Experience	Mean Score
A	10 or less	94.8
B	11-20	85.1
C	21-30	91.3
D	More than 30	87.9

However, no significant pair-wise comparisons could be found and when each experience level was compared to all the other three levels there were no significant differences. The only statistically significant difference was between levels A and C combined and levels B and D combined. With levels B and D significantly lower. How can these results be logically explained? Do pharmacists have a mental dormancy during their second decade of practice, but awaken during the third decade? What about the old adage, that parents appear to become smarter as a child pass into adulthood? Could it be that during the second decade that many of the pharmacists had teenage sons or daughters and really weren't very bright, but the pharmacists become smarter as their children enter adulthood and the real world? Whatever the reason, a logical assessment of the finding is difficult, if not impossible, to makes interpretation difficult.

The first step is to establish a Scheffé value, which is expressed as follows:

$$(Scheffe\ value\ )^2 = S^2 = (K - 1)(\,F_{K-1,N-K}\,(1 - \alpha\,))\qquad \text{Eq. 10.6}$$

This procedure does not require any additional tables. The Scheffé value is nothing more than the F_c value used in the original ANOVA multiplied by the numerator degrees of freedom (K-1). The Scheffé value is used in the following to create a confidence interval:

$$\psi_i < \hat{\psi}_i \pm \sqrt{S^2 \cdot Var(\hat{\psi}_i)} \qquad \text{Eq. 10.7}$$

where ψ_i (psi) is the estimated population difference and $\hat{\psi}_i$ (psi hat) is the sample difference. This $\hat{\psi}_i$ can represent either a pair-wise or complex comparison:

$$\hat{\psi}_i = \overline{X}_1 - \overline{X}_2 \ (pair\text{-}wise\ comparison)$$

$$\hat{\psi}_i = \overline{X}_1 - 1/2(\overline{X}_2 + \overline{X}_3) \ (complex\ comparison)$$

The measure of the standard error term for this equation is slightly more complex than the previous two methods:

$$Var(\hat{\psi}_i) = MS_E \cdot \Sigma \frac{a_k^2}{n_k} \qquad \text{Eq. 10.8}$$

In this formula, a_k represents the prefix to each of the mean values.

$$\hat{\psi}_i = (a_1)\overline{X}_1 + (a_2)\overline{X}_2 + ... (a_n)\overline{X}_n$$

For example, consider the following simple pair-wise example:

$$\hat{\psi}_i = \overline{X}_1 - \overline{X}_2$$

It can also be written as:

$$\hat{\psi}_i = (+1)\overline{X}_1 + (-1)\overline{X}$$

where the two a_ks equal +1 and -1. A second example, involving a complex comparison is:

$$\hat{\psi}_i = \overline{X}_1 - 1/2(\overline{X}_2 + \overline{X}_3)$$

Once again the formula can be rewritten as:

$$\hat{\psi}_i = (+1)\overline{X}_1 + (-1/2)\overline{X}_2 + (-1/2)\overline{X}_3$$

where the three a_ks equal $+1$, $-1/2$ and $-1/2$. As a quick check, for all comparisons the sum of the absolute a_ks ($\sum |a_k|$) must equal 2. In each example the a_k is squared and divided by the number of observations associated with the sample mean and the sum of these ratios is multiplied by MS_E, or MS_W, taken from the ANOVA table in the original analysis of variance (Eq. 10.8).

$$Var(\hat{\psi}_i) = MS_E \cdot \sum \frac{a_k^2}{n_k}$$

If zero does not fall within the confidence interval produced by the formula (Eq. 10.7), then it is assumed that there is a significant difference in the comparison being made. Conversely, if zero falls in the interval no significant difference is found.

Using the same example for the previous two *post hoc* procedures, where do the significant pair-wise differences exist between the various formulations?

$$(Scheffe\ value)^2 = S^2 = (3)(F_{3,73}(.95)) = 3(2.74) = 8.22$$

The first pair-wise comparison is between Formulations A and B, where:

$$\psi_1 = Formulation\ A\ vs.\ B \qquad \hat{\psi}_1 = 17.6$$

The computation is as follows:

$$var(\hat{\psi}_1) = 153.51 \left[\frac{(+1)^2}{20} + \frac{(-1)^2}{20} \right] = 15.35$$

$$\psi_1 = +17.6 \pm \sqrt{(8.22)(15.35)}$$

$$+6.37 < \psi_1 < +28.83$$

Because zero does not fall in the confidence interval, the decision is to reject H_0, that Formulation A and Formulation B have the same C_{max}, and conclude that a difference exists. The second pair-wise comparison is between Formulation A and C, with:

$$\psi_2 = Formulation\ A\ vs.\ C \qquad \hat{\psi}_2 = 6.8$$

The calculation of the confidence interval is:

$$var(\hat{\psi}_2) = 153.51 \left[\frac{(+1)^2}{20} + \frac{(-1)^2}{19} \right] = 15.75$$

$$\psi_2 = +6.8 \pm \sqrt{(8.22)(15.75)}$$

$$-4.58 < \psi_2 < +18.18$$

In this case, with zero inside the confidence interval, the decision is that the null hypothesis that Formulation A has the same C_{max} as Formulation C cannot be rejected.

A summary of all possible pair-wise comparisons using Scheffé's procedure appears in Table 10.6.

Interestingly each of the three methods give slightly different results. From this one example, the Scheffé and Dunn procedures appear to be the most conservative tests and the Newman-Keuls test more liberal (Table 10.7). All three procedures found significant difference between the two extreme means (Formulations A and B); however, results varied for the other pair-wise

Table 10.6 Results of Scheffé's Pair-wise Comparisons

Pairing	Confidence Interval	Results
$\overline{X}_A - \overline{X}_B$	$+6.37 < \mu_A-\mu_B < +28.83$	Significant
$\overline{X}_A - \overline{X}_C$	$-4.58 < \mu_A-\mu_C < +18.18$	
$\overline{X}_A - \overline{X}_D$	$-1.84 < \mu_A-\mu_D < +21.24$	
$\overline{X}_B - \overline{X}_C$	$-22.18 < \mu_B-\mu_C < +0.58$	
$\overline{X}_B - \overline{X}_D$	$-19.44 < \mu_B-\mu_D < +3.64$	
$\overline{X}_C - \overline{X}_D$	$-8.78 < \mu_C-\mu_D < +14.58$	

Table 10.7   Comparison of Results for Various *Post hoc* Procedures

Pairing	Mean Δ	Bonferroni Adjustment	Dunn's	Newman-Keuls	Scheffé
A vs. B	17.6	Significant	Significant	Significant	Significant
B vs. C	10.8	Significant		Significant	
A vs. D	9.5			Significant	
B vs. D	7.9				
A vs. C	6.8				
C vs. D	2.9				

comparisons. Comparison of various significant ANOVA results[1] find that the likelihood of rejecting the hypothesis of no difference is greatest with Newman-Keuls and least with Scheffé.

$$\text{Newman-Keuls} > \text{Dunn} > \text{Scheffé}$$

Scheffé Procedure for Complex Comparisons

In the above example it was possible, by all four methods used, to identify significant pair-wise differences comparing the means of sample groups and extrapolating those differences to the populations which they represent. But what if all possible pair-wise comparisons were made and no significant differences were found? For example, suppose we actually found slightly different data among the four formulations:

Concentration in mcg/ml::	Mean	S.D.	n
Formulation A	119.7	11.2	20
Formulation B	110.9	9.9	20
Formulation C	117.7	9.5	19
Formulation D	112.6	8.9	18

In this case the calculated F-value (3.48) exceeds the critical F-value of (2.74). Therefore, the null hypothesis that all formulations are equal is rejected.

---

[1] Such results can be seen in problems one and three at the end of this chapter or problem 7.2.4 in Daniel, W.W. (1978). Biostatistics: A Foundation for Analysis in the Health Sciences, Second Edition, John Wiley and Sons, New York, p. 222.

Unfortunately, none of the Scheffé pair-wise comparisons are significant.

As mentioned previously, the Scheffé test can also be used for complex comparisons. This process begins by comparing individual levels (one formulation), to the average of the other combined levels (average of remaining three formulations) and determining if one is significantly larger or smaller than the rest. For example, the formulation with the smallest C_{max} can be compared to the remaining three groups:

$$\hat{\psi}_7 = 110.9 - 1/3(119.7 + 117.7 + 112.6)$$

with the appropriate a_k being:

$$\hat{\psi}_7 = (+1)\ 110.9 + (-1/3)\ 119.7 + (-1/3)\ 117.7 + (-1/3)\ 112.6 = -5.77$$

The computations for the confidence interval, with the calculated MS_E of 98.86 from the original ANOVA, are:

$$var(\hat{\psi}_7) = 98.86\left[\frac{(+1)^2}{20} + \frac{(-.33)^2}{20} + \frac{(-.33)^2}{19} + \frac{(-.33)^2}{18}\right] = 6.64$$

$$\psi_7 = -5.77 \pm \sqrt{(8.22)(6.64)} = -5.77 \pm 7.39$$

$$-13.16 < \psi_7 < +1.62$$

Unfortunately, in this particular example all of the single group comparisons were found to be not significant.

Compared to All Others	Confidence Interval
Formulation A	$-1.45 < \psi_8 < +13.39$
Formulation B	$-13.16 < \psi_8 < +1.62$
Formulation C	$-4.25 < \psi_8 < +10.85$
Formulation D	$-11.19 < \psi_8 < +4.19$

With such results, the next logical step is to compare the two larger results with the two smallest. In this case the complex comparison would look as follows:

$$\frac{\mu_A + \mu_C}{2} - \frac{\mu_D + \mu_B}{2} = 0$$

this could also be written as follows:

$$+\frac{1}{2}(\mu_A) + \frac{1}{2}(\mu_C) - \frac{1}{2}(\mu_D) - \frac{1}{2}(\mu_B) = 0$$

The +1/2s and -1/2s before each population mean become the a_k in the equation for calculating the variance term:

$$Var(\hat{\psi}_i) = MS_E \cdot \Sigma \frac{a_k^2}{n_k}$$

Notice that in both this and the previous example, the $\Sigma |a_k|$ equals 2. The calculations for the confidence interval are as follows:

$$\psi_{11} = Formulations\ A\ and\ C\ vs.\ Formulations\ D\ and\ B$$

$$\hat{\psi}_{11} = 1/2(119.7 + 117.7) - 1/2(110.9 + 112.6) = 6.95$$

$$var(\hat{\psi}_{11}) = 98.86\left[\frac{(+.5)^2}{20} + \frac{(+.5)^2}{19} + \frac{(-.5)^2}{20} + \frac{(-.5)^2}{18}\right] = 5.15$$

$$\psi_{11} = 6.95 \pm \sqrt{(8.22)(5.15)} = 6.95 \pm 6.51$$

$$0.44 < \psi_7 < +13.46$$

Here we find a significant difference if we compare the two formulations with the highest means to those with the smallest means.

If a significant pair-wise comparison is found, then more complex comparisons do not need to be computed unless the researcher wished to analyze specific combinations. Once again it is assumed that the original analysis of variance was found to be significant, and rejection of the hypothesis that all the means are equal. In all the tests performed in this section the Type I error (α) remained constant with the original error rate used to test the analysis of variance for k levels of the independent variable.

Other Procedures

Several other *post hoc* procedures are also available for identifying the exact location or locations of significant differences when an analysis of variance results in rejection of the null hypothesis. These include: 1) the **Duncan new multiple range test** (Mason, 1989, p. 347), the **LSD test** (Least Significant Difference test) (Mason, 1989, pp. 341-342), and the **Tukey's HSD test** (Honestly Significant Difference test) all of which are similar to Newman-Keuls (Daniel, 1991); and 2) the **Dunnett test** can be used when the researcher is only interested in comparing each of the experimental groups to the control group (Zar, 1984).

References

Daniel, W.W. (1991). Biostatistics: A Foundation for Analysis in the Health Sciences, Second Edition, John Wiley and Sons, New York, p.292-294.

Glantz, S.A. (1980). "Biostatistics: How to detect correct and prevent errors in the medical literature," Circulation 61(1):1-7.

Mason, R.L. et al. (1989). Statistical Design and Analysis of Experiments, John Wiley and Sons, New York.

Zar, J.H. (1984). Biostatistical Analysis, Prentice Hall, Englewood Cliffs, NJ, pp. 194-195.

Suggested Supplemental Readings

Fisher, L.D. and van Belle, G. (1993). Biostatistics: A Methodology for the Health Sciences, John Wiley and Sons, New York, pp. 596-61.

Kirk, R.E. (1968). Experimental Design: Procedures for the Behavioral Sciences, Brooks/Cole, Belmont, CA, pp. 69-98.

Zar, J.H. (1984). Biostatistical Analysis, Prentice Hall, Englewood Cliffs, NJ, pp. 185-205.

Example Problems

Based on the information presented, identify where the significant differences exist using the various *post hoc* procedures for the following problems.

1. Problem 4 in Chapter 9, which compares the use of benzodiazepines and

responses to a computerized simulated driving test.

Hypotheses: H_0: $\mu_A = \mu_B = \mu_C = \mu_{Placebo}$
            H_1: H_0 is false

Decision rule: With $\alpha = .05$, reject H_0 if $F > F_{3,44}(.95) \approx 3.85$.

Data:	Benzo(A)	Benzo(B)	Benzo(C)	Placebo
Mean =	55.25	60.08	52.33	50.58
S.D. =	5.24	7.46	5.66	6.40
n =	12	12	12	12

Results:

$$F = \frac{MS_B}{MS_W} = \frac{207.04}{39.02} = 5.31$$

Decision: With F>3.85, reject H_0, conclude that $\mu_A=\mu_B=\mu_C=\mu_{Placebo}$ is not true.

2.   Problem 3 in Chapter 9, which compares the viscosity of a raw material delivered to three different sites.

Hypotheses: H_0: $\mu_A = \mu_B = \mu_C$
            H_1: H_0 is false

Decision rule: With $\alpha = .05$, reject H_0 if $F > F_{2,12}(.95) \approx 3.70$.

Data:	Batch A	Batch B	Batch C
Mean =	10.28	10.24	10.21
S.D. =	0.037	0.033	0.026
n =	5	5	5

Results:

$$F = \frac{MS_B}{MS_W} = \frac{0.0063}{0.0010} = 6.3$$

Decision: With F>3.70, reject H_0, conclude that $\mu_A=\mu_B=\mu_C$ is not true.

3. Problem 2 in Chapter 9, which compares four laboratories involving samples from a reservoir during a collaborative trial.

Hypotheses: H_0: $\mu_A = \mu_B = \mu_C = \mu_D$
 H_1: H_0 is false

Decision rule: With $\alpha = .05$, reject H_0 if $F > F_{3,36}(.95) \approx 2.90$.

Data:

	Lab(A)	Lab(B)	Lab(C)	Lab(D)
Mean =	99.90	99.69	99.51	100.00
S.D. =	0.25	0.41	0.22	0.34

Results: ANOVA Table

Source	df	SS	MS	F
Between	3	1.437	0.479	4.84
Within	36	3.578	0.099	
Total	39	5.015		

Decision: With $F > 2.90$, reject H_0, conclude that $\mu_A = \mu_B = \mu_C = \mu_D$ is not true

Answers to Problems

1. *Post hoc* tests for data comparing the use of benzodiazepines and responses to a computerized simulated driving test.

Sample Differences: $\overline{X}_A - \overline{X}_B = -4.83$
 $\overline{X}_A - \overline{X}_C = +2.92$ $MS_W = MS_E = 39.02$
 $\overline{X}_A - \overline{X}_P = +4.67$
 $\overline{X}_B - \overline{X}_C = +7.75$
 $\overline{X}_B - \overline{X}_P = +9.5$
 $\overline{X}_C - \overline{X}_P = +1.75$

a. Dunn's Multiple Comparisons

Dunn's percentage point: $t'D_{\alpha;C;N-K} = t'D_{.05;6;44} \approx 2.77$

Computation for $\overline{X}_A - \overline{X}_B$:

$$\mu_A - \mu_B = (\overline{X}_A - \overline{X}_B) \pm t' D_{\alpha/2;C;N-K} \sqrt{MS_E \left(\frac{1}{n_A} + \frac{1}{n_B}\right)}$$

$$\mu_A - \mu_B = (55.25 - 60.08) \pm 2.77 \sqrt{39.02 \left(\frac{1}{12} + \frac{1}{12}\right)}$$

$$\mu_A - \mu_B = (-4.83) \pm 7.06$$

$$-11.89 < \mu_A - \mu_B < +2.23$$

Results:

Pairing	Confidence Interval	Results
$\overline{X}_A - \overline{X}_B$	$-11.89 < \mu_A-\mu_B < +2.23$	
$\overline{X}_A - \overline{X}_C$	$-4.14 < \mu_A-\mu_C < +9.98$	
$\overline{X}_A - \overline{X}_P$	$-2.39 < \mu_A-\mu_P < +11.73$	
$\overline{X}_B - \overline{X}_C$	$+0.69 < \mu_B-\mu_C < +14.81$	Significant
$\overline{X}_B - \overline{X}_P$	$+2.44 < \mu_B-\mu_P < +16.56$	Significant
$\overline{X}_C - \overline{X}_P$	$-5.31 < \mu_C-\mu_P < +8.81$	

b. Newman-Keuls Test

q-statistic - two step: $q_{2,N-K}(\alpha) = q_{2,44} \approx 2.85$
three step: $q_{3,N-K}(\alpha) = q_{3,44} \approx 3.43$
four step: $q_{4,N-K}(\alpha) = q_{4,44} \approx 3.78$

Computation for $\overline{X}_A - \overline{X}_P$:

$$\mu_A - \mu_P = (\overline{X}_A - \overline{X}_P) \pm q \sqrt{\frac{MS_E}{2}\left(\frac{1}{n_A} + \frac{1}{n_B}\right)}$$

$$\mu_A - \mu_P = (55.25 - 50.58) \pm 3.43 \sqrt{\frac{39.19}{2}\left(\frac{1}{20} + \frac{1}{18}\right)}$$

$$\mu_A - \mu_P = (4.67) \pm 4.93$$

$$-0.26 < \mu_A - \mu_P < +9.60$$

Results:

Pairing	Confidence Interval	Results
$\overline{X}_A - \overline{X}_B$	$-9.97 < \mu_A\text{-}\mu_B < +0.31$	
$\overline{X}_A - \overline{X}_C$	$-2.22 < \mu_A\text{-}\mu_C < +8.06$	
$\overline{X}_A - \overline{X}_P$	$-1.52 < \mu_A\text{-}\mu_P < +10.86$	
$\overline{X}_B - \overline{X}_C$	$+1.56 < \mu_B\text{-}\mu_C < +13.94$	Significant
$\overline{X}_B - \overline{X}_P$	$+2.68 < \mu_B\text{-}\mu_P < +16.32$	Significant
$\overline{X}_C - \overline{X}_P$	$-3.39 < \mu_C\text{-}\mu_P < +6.89$	

c. Scheffé procedure

Scheffé value

$$(Scheffe\ value)^2 = S^2 = (K-1)(F_{K-1,N-K}(1-\alpha)) = 3(3.85) = 11.55$$

Computation for $\overline{X}_B - \overline{X}_P$:

$$\hat{\psi}_5 = 60.08 - 50.58 = 9.50$$

$$var(\hat{\psi}_5) = 39.02\left[\frac{(+1)^2}{12} + \frac{(-1)^2}{12}\right] = 6.50$$

$$\psi_5 = +9.50 \pm \sqrt{(11.55)(6.50)} = 9.50 \pm 8.66$$

$$+0.84 < \psi_5 < +18.16$$

Results:

Pairing	Confidence Interval	Results
$\overline{X}_A - \overline{X}_B$	$-13.49 < \mu_A - \mu_B < +3.83$	
$\overline{X}_A - \overline{X}_C$	$-5.74 < \mu_A - \mu_C < +11.58$	
$\overline{X}_A - \overline{X}_P$	$-3.99 < \mu_A - \mu_P < +13.33$	
$\overline{X}_B - \overline{X}_C$	$-0.91 < \mu_B - \mu_C < +16.41$	
$\overline{X}_B - \overline{X}_P$	$+0.84 < \mu_B - \mu_P < +18.16$	Significant
$\overline{X}_C - \overline{X}_P$	$-6.91 < \mu_C - \mu_P < +10.41$	

2. *Post hoc* tests for data comparing the site of raw materials and viscosity.

Sample Differences: $\overline{X}_A - \overline{X}_B = +0.04$

$\overline{X}_A - \overline{X}_C = +0.07$ $MS_W = MS_E = 0.001$

$\overline{X}_B - \overline{X}_C = +0.03$

a. Dunn's Multiple Comparisons

Dunn's percentage point: $t'D_{\alpha;C;N-K} = t'D_{.05;3,12} \approx 2.80$

Computation for $\overline{X}_A - \overline{X}_B$:

$$\mu_A - \mu_B = (\overline{X}_A - \overline{X}_B) \pm t' D_{\alpha/2;C;N-K} \sqrt{MS_E \left(\frac{1}{n_A} + \frac{1}{n_B}\right)}$$

$$\mu_A - \mu_B = (10.28 - 10.24) \pm 2.80 \sqrt{0.001 \left(\frac{1}{5} + \frac{1}{5}\right)}$$

$$\mu_A - \mu_B = +0.04 \pm 0.056$$

$$-0.016 < \mu_A - \mu_B < +0.096$$

Results:

Pairing	Confidence Interval	Results
$\overline{X}_A - \overline{X}_B$	$-0.016 < \mu_A\text{-}\mu_B < +0.096$	
$\overline{X}_A - \overline{X}_C$	$+0.014 < \mu_A\text{-}\mu_C < +0.126$	Significant
$\overline{X}_B - \overline{X}_C$	$-0.026 < \mu_B\text{-}\mu_C < +0.086$	

b. Newman-Keuls Test

q-statistic   two step: $q_{2,N\text{-}K}(\alpha) = q_{2,12} = 3.08$
               three step: $q_{3,N\text{-}K}(\alpha) = q_{3,12} = 3.77$

Computation for $\overline{X}_A - \overline{X}_C$:

$$\mu_A - \mu_P = (\overline{X}_A - \overline{X}_C) \pm q \sqrt{\frac{MS_E}{2}\left(\frac{1}{n_A} + \frac{1}{n_C}\right)}$$

$$\mu_A - \mu_C = (10.28 - 10.21) \pm 3.77 \sqrt{\frac{0.001}{2}\left(\frac{1}{5} + \frac{1}{5}\right)}$$

$$\mu_A - \mu_c = (0.07) \pm 0.053$$

$$+0.017 < \mu_A - \mu_C < +0.123$$

Results:

Pairing	Confidence Interval	Results
$\overline{X}_A - \overline{X}_B$	$-0.004 < \mu_A\text{-}\mu_B < +0.084$	
$\overline{X}_A - \overline{X}_C$	$+0.017 < \mu_A\text{-}\mu_C < +0.123$	Significant
$\overline{X}_B - \overline{X}_C$	$-0.014 < \mu_B\text{-}\mu_C < 0.074$	

c. Scheffé procedure

Scheffé value

$$(Scheffe\ value\ )^2 = S^2 = (K - 1)(F_{K-1,N-K}(1-\alpha)) = 2(3.70) = 7.40$$

Computation for $\overline{X}_B - \overline{X}_C$:

$$var(\hat{\psi}_3) = 0.001\left[\frac{(+1)^2}{5} + \frac{(-1)^2}{5}\right] = 0.0004$$

$$\psi_3 = +0.03 \pm \sqrt{(7.40)(0.0004)} = 0.03 \pm 0.054$$

$$-0.024 < \psi_3 < +0.084$$

Results:

Pairing	Confidence Interval	Results
$\overline{X}_A - \overline{X}_B$	$-0.014 < \mu_A - \mu_B < +0.094$	
$\overline{X}_A - \overline{X}_C$	$+0.016 < \mu_A - \mu_C < +0.124$	Significant
$\overline{X}_B - \overline{X}_C$	$-0.024 < \mu_B - \mu_C < +0.084$	

3. *Post hoc* tests for data comparing four laboratories in a collaborative study.

Sample Differences:

$\overline{X}_A - \overline{X}_B = +0.21$

$\overline{X}_A - \overline{X}_C = +0.39$ $MS_W = MS_E = 0.099$

$\overline{X}_A - \overline{X}_D = -0.10$

$\overline{X}_B - \overline{X}_C = +0.18$

$\overline{X}_B - \overline{X}_D = -0.31$

$\overline{X}_C - \overline{X}_D = -0.49$

a. Dunn's Multiple Comparisons

Dunn's percentage point: $t'D_{\alpha;C;N-K} = t'D_{.05;6;36} \approx 2.80$

Computation for $\overline{X}_A - \overline{X}_B$:

$$\mu_A - \mu_B = (\overline{X}_A - \overline{X}_B) \pm t'D_{\alpha/2;C;N-K}\sqrt{MS_E\left(\frac{1}{n_A} + \frac{1}{n_B}\right)}$$

$$\mu_A - \mu_B = (99.90 - 99.69) \pm 2.80 \sqrt{0.099 \left(\frac{1}{10} + \frac{1}{10}\right)}$$

$$\mu_A - \mu_B = 0.21 \pm 0.39$$

$$-0.18 < \mu_A - \mu_B < +0.60$$

Results:

Pairing	Confidence Interval	Results
$\overline{X}_A - \overline{X}_B$	$-0.18 < \mu_A\text{-}\mu_B < +0.60$	
$\overline{X}_A - \overline{X}_C$	$0 < \mu_A\text{-}\mu_C < +0.78$	
$\overline{X}_A - \overline{X}_D$	$-0.29 < \mu_A\text{-}\mu_D < +0.49$	
$\overline{X}_B - \overline{X}_C$	$-0.21 < \mu_B\text{-}\mu_C < +0.57$	
$\overline{X}_B - \overline{X}_D$	$-0.08 < \mu_B\text{-}\mu_D < +0.70$	
$\overline{X}_C - \overline{X}_D$	$+0.10 < \mu_C\text{-}\mu_D < +0.88$	Significant

b. Newman-Keuls Test

q-statistic   two step: $q_{2,N\text{-}K}(\alpha) = q_{2,36} \approx 2.87$
                   three step: $q_{3,N\text{-}K}(\alpha) = q_{3,36} \approx 3.46$
                   four step: $q_{4,N\text{-}K}(\alpha) = q_{4,36} \approx 3.81$

Computation for $\overline{X}_A - \overline{X}_B$:

$$\mu_A - \mu_B = (\overline{X}_A - \overline{X}_B) \pm q \sqrt{\frac{MS_E}{2}\left(\frac{1}{n_A} + \frac{1}{n_B}\right)}$$

$$\mu_A - \mu_B = (99.90 - 99.69) \pm 2.87 \cdot \sqrt{\frac{0.099}{2}\left(\frac{1}{10} + \frac{1}{10}\right)}$$

$$-0.08 < \mu_A - \mu_B < +0.50$$

Results:

Pairing	Confidence Interval	Results
$\overline{X}_A - \overline{X}_B$	$-0.08 < \mu_A{-}\mu_B < +0.50$	
$\overline{X}_A - \overline{X}_C$	$+0.05 < \mu_A{-}\mu_C < +0.73$	Significant
$\overline{X}_A - \overline{X}_D$	$-0.19 < \mu_A{-}\mu_D < +0.39$	
$\overline{X}_B - \overline{X}_C$	$-0.11 < \mu_B{-}\mu_C < +0.47$	
$\overline{X}_B - \overline{X}_D$	$+0.03 < \mu_B{-}\mu_D < +0.65$	
$\overline{X}_C - \overline{X}_D$	$+0.12 < \mu_C{-}\mu_D < +0.86$	Significant

c. Scheffé procedure

Scheffé value

$$(Scheffe\ value\ )^2 = S^2 = (K - 1)(F_{K-1,N-K}(1 - \alpha)) = 3(3.85) = 11.55$$

Computation for $\overline{X}_B - \overline{X}_D$:

$$\hat{\psi}_5 = 60.08 - 50.58 = 9.50$$

$$var(\hat{\psi}_5) = 39.19\left[\frac{(+1)^2}{20} + \frac{(-1)^2}{18}\right] = 4.13$$

$$\psi_5 = +9.50 \pm \sqrt{(11.55)(4.13)} = 9.50 \pm 6.91$$

$$+2.59 < \psi_5 < +16.41$$

Results:

Pairing	Confidence Interval	Results
$\overline{X}_A - \overline{X}_B$	$-0.21 < \mu_A{-}\mu_B < +0.63$	
$\overline{X}_A - \overline{X}_C$	$-0.03 < \mu_A{-}\mu_C < +0.81$	
$\overline{X}_A - \overline{X}_D$	$-0.52 < \mu_A{-}\mu_D < +0.32$	
$\overline{X}_B - \overline{X}_C$	$-0.24 < \mu_B{-}\mu_C < +0.60$	
$\overline{X}_B - \overline{X}_D$	$-0.73 < \mu_B{-}\mu_D < +0.11$	
$\overline{X}_C - \overline{X}_D$	$-0.91 < \mu_C{-}\mu_D < +0.07$	Significant

11

Factorial Designs:
An Introduction

As presented in Chapter 9, the simple, one-way analysis of variance is used to test the effect of one independent discrete variable. When using factorial designs it is possible to control for multiple independent variables and determine their effect on a single dependent continuous variable.

Through random sampling and an appropriate definition of the population, in an ideal world, the researcher should be able to control all variables not of interest to the particular research design. For example in a laboratory, the researcher should be able to control the temperature of the experiment, the quality of the ingredients used (the same batch, the same bottle), the accuracy of the measurements, and numerous other factors which might produce bias in the statistical analyses performed. However, in many research situations, several different factors must be considered at the same time as well as the relationship of these variables to each other. Therefore, the study must be designed to consider two or more independent variables at one time and their influence on the outcome of the dependent variable.

Factorial Designs

The ANOVA model discussed in Chapter 9 is referred to as a "simple" or "one-way" analysis of variance because only a single independent variable or **factor** is being assessed. The term factor is synonymous with the terms **independent variable, treatment variable, predictor variable** or **experimental variable.** Throughout this chapter the terms factor and independent variable will be used interchangeably.

Instead of repeating our experiment for each independent variable or factor, we can design a more efficient experiment that evaluates the effects of two or more factors at the same time. These types of designs are referred to as **factorial designs** because each level of one factor is combined with each level of the other factor, or independent variable. The primary advantage of a factorial design is that it allows us to evaluate the effects of more than one independent variable, both separately and in combination with each other. As will be seen, these factorial designs can be used to increase the control we have over our experiment by reducing the within-group variance. The factorial designs also offer economical advantages by reducing the total number of subjects or observations which would be needed if the two main effects were evaluated separately.

To illustrate this situation, consider the following example. A school of pharmacy is working on developing a new method of delivering their recently developed Pharm.D. curriculum to B.S. pharmacists desiring to obtain this new degree, but unable to take a one- or two-year sabbatical to return to school. Therefore, the school is working with different delivery systems to provide distance learning for the didactic portion of the course work. The primary investigator has developed a ten-point satisfaction index for the pharmacist, to evaluate the convenience, flexibility and usefulness of the course materials, as well as the user friendliness of the course work. It is assumed that the better the response (maximum score of 10), the more likely that pharmacists beginning the course work will continue to the end of the didactic portion of the program. A pilot study was conducted on a random sample of pharmacists. Two different delivery methods were considered: written monographs (M_1) and computer based training (M_2). However, early in the development of course work there was concern that institutional (primarily hospital) and ambulatory (mostly retail) pharmacists may possess different learning signs and may react differently with respect to their evaluation of the course materials. Therefore, the pilot study was designed to evaluate two independent variables, the delivery system used and the pharmacist's practice setting, either institutional (S_1) or ambulatory (S_2). This can be illustrated in the simplest possible experimental design, a 2 x 2 factorial design:

		S_1	S_2
Methods	M_1	A	B
	M_2	C	D

Settings

where A,B,C, and D represent the mean results for the continuous dependent variable (satisfaction index), and rows and columns represent the main factors tested. For example A represents the responses for pharmacist practicing in institutional settings who receive the written monongraphs; whereas D represents ambulatory pharmacists exposed to computer based training.

In this design we are interested in evaluating the main effects of both the factors used and the interaction of these two factors. In this case we are dealing with three different hypotheses:

H_{01}: $\mu_{M1} = \mu_{M2}$ (Main effect of the delivery method)
H_{02}: $\mu_{S1} = \mu_{S2}$ (Main effect of the practice setting)
H_{03}: $(\mu_{M1,S1} - \mu_{M1,S2}) = (\mu_{M2,S1} - \mu_{M2,S2})$
(Interaction of method and setting)

The first hypotheses (H_{01}) evaluates the main factor for the two methods used for distance leaning (M_1, M_2). Are they approximately the same or are they statistically different? The second hypothesis (H_{02}) assesses the influence of the pharmacists' practice setting (S_1, S_2) and what influence they might have on evaluations of the course materials. These first two hypotheses are called **tests of main effects** and are similar to separate tests using one-way analysis of variance. The third hypothesis (H03) evaluates the possibility of relationships between the row and column variables. As discussed below, two independent variables are considered to interact if differences in an outcome for specific levels of one factor are different at two or more levels of the second factor.

Whenever we evaluate the effect of two or more independent variables on a dependent variable, we must be cautious of a possible **interaction** between these independent variables. An interaction measures the joint effects of the factors being tested. If the factors are independent of each other, or have no relationship, there will be no interaction. We are interested in detecting interactions because the overall tests of main effects, without considering interactions, may cause us to make statements about our data that are incorrect or misleading. The validity of most multi-factorial designs are contingent on an assumption of no interaction effects among the independent variables. One might argue that a more appropriate procedure is to test for any interaction first and if no interaction is detected (i.e., the test is not significant), then perform separate tests for the main effects. However, if interaction exists, it is meaningless to test the main effects or to try to interpret main effects. The approach used in this book is to evaluate the main effect and interactions in concert as a more efficient and time-saving method. Granted, if the interaction is found to be significant, the results of the evaluation of main effects are without value, because the factors are not independent of each other.

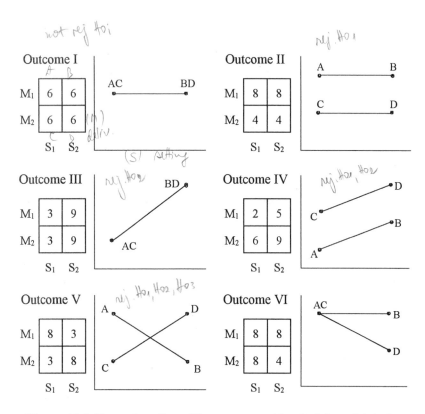

Figure 11.1 Examples of possible outcomes with a 2x2 factorial design.

To illustrate the various outcomes, consider the possible outcomes in Figure 11.1 for our experiment with the factors of delivery system and practice setting. Here results are plotted for one main factor (setting) on the x-axis and the second main factor (delivery system) on the y-axis. In Outcome I the results are the same for all four observations, therefore the investigator would fail to reject any of the three hypotheses and conclude that there was no significant effect for either of the main effects and no interaction between the two factors. For Outcome II, there is a significant difference between the two delivery methods used ($M_1 > M_2$) and the investigator could reject H_{01}, but would fail to reject the other two hypotheses. The opposite results are seen in Outcome III, where the investigator would find there is a significant difference between the two practice settings ($S_2 > S_1$) and reject H_{02}, but would fail to reject the other two hypotheses. Outcome IV represents a rejection of both H_{01} and H_{02} where $M_1 > M_2$ and $S_2 > S_1$, but there is no significant interaction and H_{03}

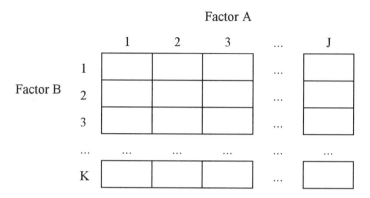

Figure 11.2 Layout for a two-way analysis of variance.

cannot be rejected.

Outcomes V and VI illustrate two possible interactions. In Outcome V there are significant differences in the main effects and a significant interaction between the two main factors. We can see that the two lines cross and there is a significant interaction between methods and settings. It appears that institutional pharmacists prefer monographs and ambulatory pharmacists favor the computer based training. Because of the interaction, it becomes meaningless to evaluate the results of the main effects, because if there was a significant difference between methods of delivery, it may be influenced by the practice setting of the pharmacists. In Outcome VI there is no difference in M_1 based on the practice setting, but there is a difference for M_2. Is this significant? Is there an interaction between the two main effects (factors)? A two-way analysis of variance can determine, with a certain degree of confidence, which hypotheses should be rejected as false.

Two-way Analysis of Variance

In the one-way ANOVA, we were only concerned with one major treatment effect or factor:

$$H_0: \mu_1 = \mu_2 = \mu_3 = \dots \mu_k$$
$$H_1: H_0 \text{ is false}$$

However, in a two-way ANOVA, we are concerned about the major effects of two variables and their potential interaction.

The number of factors and levels within each factor determine the dimensions of a factorial design. For example, if Factor A consists of three levels and Factor B only two, it would be presented as a 3 x 2 (read three by two) factorial design. Areas within the factorial design where dependent variable outcomes are reported are called **cells**. In the case of a 4 x 5 factorial design, there are 20 cells (4 x 5 = 20). In factorial designs there must be more than one observation per cell. If there were only one observation per cell, there would be no variance within the cells and therefore no sum of squares error available. Each of the two major factors are discrete independent variables and their significance is measured based on a single continuous dependent variable. The design for a two-way analysis of variance is presented in Figure 11.2. As seen in the previous illustration there are three hypotheses which are being tested simultaneously: two testing for the main effects and one for the interaction:

H_{01}: $\mu_{A1} = \mu_{A2} = \mu_{A3} = \dots \mu_{AJ}$ (Main effect of Factor A)

H_{02}: $\mu_{B1} = \mu_{B2} = \mu_{B3} = \dots \mu_{BK}$ (Main effect of Factor B)

H_{03}: $(\mu_{A1,B1}-\mu_{A1,B2}) = (\mu_{A2,B1}-\mu_{A2,B2}) = $ etc.   (Interaction of A and B)

Similarly, there are three alternative hypotheses to complement each of the null hypotheses:

H_{11}: H_{01} is false

H_{12}: H_{02} is false

H_{13}: H_{03} is false

With the one-way analysis of variance, the degrees of freedom for the critical F-value were associated with the number of levels of the independent variable (K-1) and the total number of observations (N-K). Because the two-way analysis of variance deals with two independent variables, we have a different F_c associated with each null hypotheses tested and these are directly associated with the number of rows and columns presented in the data matrix. The symbols used are: J for the number of levels of the column variable; K for the number of levels of the row variable; N is the total number of observations; and n is the number of observations per cell in the case of equal cell sizes.

There are three separate decision rules, one for each of the two main variables and one for the interaction between the two independent variables. Each hypothesis is tested with a different F-value, but each should be tested at the same α.

$$\text{Reject } H_0 \text{ if } F > F_{v1 v2}(1-\alpha).$$

Where the ν_2 degrees of freedom is always $J \cdot K \cdot (n-1)$ and ν_1 will vary depending upon which null hypothesis is being tested, then:

H_{01}: $\nu_1 = J-1$
H_{02}: $\nu_1 = K-1$
H_{03}: $\nu_1 = (J-1)(K-1)$

For equal cell sizes (the number of observations in each cell of the matrix are equal), the formulas are similar to those of the one-way ANOVA computational formulas. For intermediate value I, each observation (x_i) is squared, and then summed.

$$I = \sum_{k=1}^{K} \sum_{j=1}^{J} \sum_{i=1}^{I} x_i^2 \qquad \text{Eq. 11.1}$$

In the case of equal cell sizes the number observations in each cell for i=1 to I for be equal to n then Eq. 11.1 could be written as follows:

$$I = \sum_{k=1}^{K} \sum_{j=1}^{J} \sum_{i=1}^{n} x_i^2$$

However, in a later section of this chapter, equations will be presented for unequal cell sizes and the "i"-summation notation will be used for continuity.

In intermediate value II the total sum of all observations is squared and divided by the total number of observations in the data set.

$$II = \frac{\left[\sum_{k=1}^{K} \sum_{j=1}^{J} \sum_{i=1}^{I} x_i \right]^2}{N} \qquad \text{Eq. 11.2}$$

To compute the intermediate value IV, the sum of values for each cell of the matrix is squared and then all these values are summed and finally divided by the number of observations in each cell:

$$IV = \frac{\sum_{k=1}^{K} \sum_{j=1}^{J} \left[\sum_{i=1}^{I} x_i \right]^2}{n} \qquad \text{Eq. 11.3}$$

There are two intermediate III values, one for the main effect of Factor A (columns) and one for the main effect of Factor B (rows). In the former case the sum of all values for each column is totaled and squared. These squared values are then summed and divided by the product of the number columns multiplied by the number of observations per cell:

$$III_C = \frac{\sum\limits_{j=1}^{J}\left[\sum\limits_{k=1}^{K}\sum\limits_{i=1}^{I} x_i\right]^2}{K \cdot n}$$

Eq. 11.4

A similar procedure is used for the rows intermediate III, where the sum of all values for each row is totaled and squared. These squared values are then summed and divided by the product of the number of rows multiplied by the number of observations per cell:

$$III_R = \frac{\sum\limits_{k=1}^{K}\left[\sum\limits_{j=1}^{J}\sum\limits_{i=1}^{I} x_i\right]^2}{J \cdot n}$$

Eq. 11.5

The SS_{total} and SS_{error} are calculated in a similar way to the one-way ANOVA. Note that the former error term SS_W is now referred to as SS_E or SS_{error}.

$$SS_{Error} = SS_E = I - IV$$

Eq. 11.6

$$SS_{Total} = SS_T = I - II$$

Eq. 11.7

In the two-way ANOVA, SS_{rows}, $SS_{columns}$ and $SS_{interactions}$ are calculated from the sum of squares formulas III_R and III_C.

$$SS_{(Rows)} = SS_R = III_R - II$$

Eq. 11.8

$$SS_{Columns} = SS_C = III_C - II$$

Eq. 11.9

$$SS_{Interaction} = SS_{RC} = IV - III_R - III_C + II$$

Eq. 11.10

The key difference with this design is that the between group variance is further divided into the different sources of variation (row variable, column variable and interaction). A certain amount of variation can be attributed to the row variable and some to the column variable. The remaining left-over or **residual** variation is attributable to the "interaction" between these two factors.

The sum of squares information is inserted into an ANOVA table (Table 11.1) in which there are three levels of the between mean variability, the main effect of the rows variable, the main effect of the columns variable, and the effect of their interactions. The first column indicates the source of the variance. The second column is the degrees of freedom associated with each source. Note that the total number of degrees of freedom is one less than the total number of observations, again to correct for bias. The third column is the sum of squares calculated by Equations 11.6 through 11.10. The fourth column contains the mean square terms that are calculated by dividing the sum of squares by the corresponding degrees of freedom for each row. Finally, the F-values are calculated by dividing each of the mean square between values by the mean square error. Table 11.2 represents other symbols that can be used to represent an analysis of variance table. Computer programs, such as SPSS or SAS, present results of factorial design calculations in formats similar to those in Tables 11.1 or 11.2.

The within or error line in the ANOVA table represents the error factor or residual variance which cannot be accounted for by the variability among the

Table 11.1. Computations for the ANOVA Table for a Two-way Design

Source	Degrees of Freedom	Sum of Squares	Mean Squares (MS)	$\underline{F}$
Between:				
Rows	K-1	SS_R	$\dfrac{SS_R}{K-1}$	$\dfrac{MS_R}{MS_E}$
Columns	J-1	SS_C	$\dfrac{SS_C}{J-1}$	$\dfrac{MS_C}{MS_E}$
Interaction	(K-1)(J-1)	SS_{RC}	$\dfrac{SS_{RC}}{(K-1)(J-1)}$	$\dfrac{MS_{RC}}{MS_E}$
Within:				
Error	K·J·(n-1)	SS_E	$\dfrac{SS_E}{K \cdot J \cdot (n-1)}$	
Total	N-1	SS_T		

Table 11.2 ANOVA Table for a Two-way Design

Source	df	SS	MS	F
Between:				
Rows	K-1	SS_R	MS_R	F_R
Columns	J-1	SS_C	MS_C	F_C
Interaction	(K-1)(J-1)	SS_{RC}	MS_{RC}	F_{RC}
Within:				
Error	K·J·(n-1)	SS_E	MS_E	
Total	N-1	SS_T		

row means, column means, or cell means. As will be discussed later, the mean square error serves as the error term in the fixed-effects ANOVA. As seen in Table 11.1, the denominator of each ratio in the last column, is the variance estimate based on the pooled within groups sum of squared deviations. Once again this within groups variance (MS_E) is a measure of random "error" or chance differences among the variables.

If one or more of the F values calculated in the ANOVA table exceed their parallel critical F value defined in the decision rule, the hypothesis or hypotheses will be rejected in favor of the alternative hypothesis. It could be possible for all three null hypotheses to be rejected, meaning that both column and row variables were significantly different and that there was a significant interaction between the two variables. If a significant outcome is not identified for the interaction portion of the ANOVA table then the outcome of the F tests for the two main effects can be interpreted the same way as F-ratios in a one-way ANOVA. This measure of interaction is based upon the variability of the cell means. Therefore, when significant interaction occurs, caution must be used in interpreting the significance of the main effects. As mentioned previously, the validity of most factorial designs assume that there is no significant interaction between the independent variables. When interpreting the outcome of the two-way ANOVA, especially if there is a significant interaction, a plotting of the means (similar to Figure 11.1) can be extremely helpful to visualize the outcomes and identify the interaction.

As an example of a two-way ANOVA we will use a previous example associated with a two-sample t-test, where the investigator compared two formulations of the same drug and was interested in determining the maximum concentration (Table 8.2). However, in this case the study involved a two-period crossover study and the researcher wanted to make certain that the order in which the subjects received the formulation did not influence the C_{max} for the formulation received during the second period. The three hypotheses under test were:

H_{01}: $\mu_{\text{Formula A}}$ = $\mu_{\text{Formula B}}$

H_{02}: $\mu_{\text{Order 1}}$ = $\mu_{\text{Order 2}}$

H_{03}: $(\mu_{\text{Formula A,First}} - \mu_{\text{Formula B,First}})$ = $(\mu_{\text{Formula A,Second}} - \mu_{\text{Formula B,Second}})$

and the decision rules were: 1) with α = .05 and n = 12, reject H_{01} if F > $F_{1,44}(.95) \approx 4.06$; 2) with α = .05 and n = 12, reject H_{02} if F > $F_{1,44}(.95) \approx 4.06$; and 3) with α = .05 and n = 12, reject H_{03} if F > $F_{1,44}(.95) \approx 4.06$. The data observed by the investigator is presented in Table 11.3. Also

Table 11.3 Sample Data for a Two-way Crossover Clinical Trial (C_{max})

	Formulation A			Formulation B			$\sum_{j=1}^{J}\sum_{i=1}^{I}$	$\sum_{k=1}^{K}\sum_{j=1}^{J}\sum_{i=1}^{I}$
Formula	125	130	135	149	151	130		
A	128	121	123	132	141	129		
Received	131	129	120	142	130	122		
First	119	133	125	136	138	140		
$\sum_{i=1}^{I}$	= 1,519			1,640			3,159	
Formula	126	140	135	130	128	127		
B	126	121	133	141	145	132		
Received	117	126	127	133	136	138		
First	120	136	122	129	150	148		
$\sum_{i=1}^{I}$ =	= 1,529			1,637			3,166	
$\sum_{k=1}^{K}\sum_{i=1}^{I}$	= 3,048			3,277				6,325

included are: 1) the sum of observations for each cell (2x2 design); 2) the sum for each column (formulations A and B); 3) the sum for each row (order in which formulations were received); and 4) the total sum of all the observations. The initial computations of the intermediate values are:

$$I = \sum_{k=1}^{K} \sum_{j=1}^{J} \sum_{i=1}^{I} x_i^2 = (125)^2 + (130)^2 + \dots (148)^2 = 836,917$$

$$III_R = \frac{\sum_{k=1}^{K} \left[\sum_{j=1}^{J} \sum_{i=1}^{I} x_i \right]^2}{J \cdot n} = \frac{(3,159)^2 + (3,166)^2}{24} = 833,451.54$$

$$III_C = \frac{\sum_{j=1}^{J} \left[\sum_{k=1}^{K} \sum_{i=1}^{I} x_i \right]^2}{K \cdot n} = \frac{(3,048)^2 + (3,277)^2}{24} = 834,543.04$$

$$IV = \frac{\sum_{k=1}^{K} \sum_{j=1}^{J} \left[\sum_{i=1}^{I} x_i \right]^2}{n} = \frac{(1,519)^2 + \dots (1,637)^2}{12} = 834,547.58$$

The sum of squares required for the ANOVA table are:

$$SS_R = III_R - II = 833,451.54 - 833,450.52 = 1.02$$

$$SS_C = III_C - II = 834,543.04 - 833,450.52 = 1,092.52$$

$$SS_{RC} = IV - III_R - III_C + II$$

$$SS_{RC} = 834,547.58 - 833,451.54 - 834,543.04 + 833,450.52 = 3.52$$

$$SS_E = I - IV = 836,917 - 834,547.58 = 2,369.42$$

$$SS_T = I - II = 836,917 - 833,450.52 = 3,466.48$$

The resultant ANOVA table is as follows:

Source	df	SS	MS	F
Between				
Rows (order)	1	1.02	1.02	0.02
Column (formula)	1	1,092.52	1,092.52	20.29*
Interaction	1	3.52	3.52	0.07
Within (error):	44	2,369.42	53.85	
Total	47	3,466.48		

In this example, with $\alpha = .05$, the decision is to reject H_{02} and conclude that there is a significant difference between the two formulations. Note that this is a valid decision since there as not a significant interaction between the two factors. Also, there is no significant difference based on the order in which the drugs were administered. If the data is visually represented similar to the examples in Table 11.1, it is possible to see the significance in formulation, the closeness and insignificance of the order in which the drugs were administered, and the lack of any interaction (Figure 11.3).

A second example involving more levels of the independent variable involves a pharmaceutical manufacturer wishing to evaluate two automated systems for dissolution testing. Four separate batches of a particular agent were tested using each of the two automated systems and a technician-operated traditional dissolution system. Presented in Table 11.4 are the results of the experiment. Is there a significant difference between the batches or procedure used, or is there a significant interaction between the two factors?

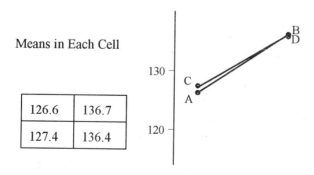

Means in Each Cell

126.6	136.7
127.4	136.4

Figure 11.3 Visual representation of clinical trial data.

Table 11.4 Comparison of Methods of Dissolution Testing

Batch	Statistic	Traditional Method	Automated System I	Automated System II	$\sum\sum x$
A	$\sum x =$	391	378	310	1079
	$\sum x^2 =$	25,627	23,968	16,189	
	Mean =	65.17	63.00	51.67	
	SD =	5.41	5.55	5.72	
B	$\sum x =$	369	360	358	1087
	$\sum x^2 =$	22,831	21,734	21,510	
	Mean =	61.50	60.00	59.67	
	SD =	5.24	5.18	5.46	
C	$\sum x =$	406	362	330	1098
	$\sum x^2 =$	27,612	21,982	18,284	
	Mean =	67.67	60.33	55.00	
	SD =	5.27	5.32	5.18	
D	$\sum x =$	401	383	345	1129
	$\sum x^2 =$	26,945	24,579	19,993	
	Mean =	66.83	63.83	57.50	
	SD =	5.38	5.11	5.09	
	$\sum\sum x =$	1567	1483	1343	4393

The header "Dissolution Results at 10 Minutes (%) n=6" spans the table.

Once again three hypotheses are being tested simultaneously (H_{01} for differences in the method used, H_{02} for differences in the batches tested, and H_{03} for possible interaction between the two factors):

H_{01}: $\mu_{Traditional} = \mu_{Automated\ I} = \mu_{Automated\ II}$

H_{02}: $\mu_{Batch\ A} = \mu_{Batch\ B} = \mu_{Batch\ C} = \mu_{Batch\ D}$

H_{03}: $(\mu_{Traditional,Batch\ A} - \mu_{Traditional,Batch\ B}) \ldots =$

$\qquad (\mu_{Automated\ II,Batch\ C} - \mu_{Automated\ II,Batch\ D})$

and the decision rules are, with $\alpha = .05$ and n = 6: 1) reject H_{01} if $F > F_{2,60}(.95) = 3.15$; 2) reject H_{02} if $F > F_{3,60}(.95) = 2.76$; and 3) reject H_{03} if $F > F_{6,60}(.95) = 2.25$. The computations are:

$$60 = 3.4 \cdot (6-1)$$

$$I = \sum_{k=1}^{K} \sum_{j=1}^{J} \sum_{i=1}^{I} x_i^2$$

$$I = (57)^2 + (62)^2 + (65)^2 + ...(44)^2 = 271,245$$

$$II = \frac{\left[\sum_{k=1}^{K} \sum_{j=1}^{J} \sum_{i=1}^{I} x_i \right]^2}{N}$$

$$II = \frac{(4393)^2}{72} = 268,034.0139$$

$$III_R = \frac{\sum_{k=1}^{K} \left[\sum_{j=1}^{J} \sum_{i=1}^{I} x_i \right]^2}{J \cdot n}$$

$$III_R = \frac{(1079)^2 + (1087) + ...(1129)^2}{18} = 268,114.1667$$

$$III_C = \frac{\sum_{j=1}^{J} \left[\sum_{k=1}^{K} \sum_{i=1}^{I} x_i \right]^2}{K \cdot n}$$

$$III_C = \frac{(1567)^2 + (1483)^2 + (1343)^2}{24} = 269,101.1250$$

$$IV = \frac{\sum_{k=1}^{K} \sum_{j=1}^{J} \left[\sum_{i=1}^{I} x_i \right]^2}{n}$$

$$IV = \frac{(391)^2 + (378)^2 + (345)^2 + ...(310)^2}{6} = 269,514.1667$$

$$SS_R = III_R - II = 268,114.1667 - 268,034.0139 = 80.1528$$

$$SS_C = III_C - II = 269,101.1250 - 268,034.0139 = 1067.1111$$

$$SS_{RC} = IV - III_R - III_C + II$$

$$SS_{RC} = 269,514.1667 - 268,114.1667 - 269,101.1250 + 268,034.0139$$

$$SS_{RC} = 332.8889$$

$$SS_E = I - IV = 271,245 - 269,514.1667 = 1730.8333$$

$$SS_T = I - II = 271,245 - 268,034.0139 = 3210.9861$$

The results of the statistical analysis are presented in an ANOVA table:

Source	df	SS	MS	F
Between				
Rows (batch)	3	80.1528	26.72	0.93
Column (method)	2	1067.1111	533.56	18.49*
Interaction	6	332.8889	55.48	1.92
Within (error):	60	1730.8333	28.85	
Total	71	3210.9861		

There was no significant interaction between the two factors; therefore, our decision is to reject the null hypothesis H_{02} for the main effect of methods used and assume that all three methods of dissolution testing are not all equal. There was no significant difference based on the batches tested.

Computational Formula with Unequal Cell Size

When data are used which do not contain equal cell sizes, the exact same procedure is used except that slightly modified formulas are substituted for Eq. 11.3 through 11.5. For intermediate value IV, each cell is summed, that value is squared and divided by the number of observations within the cell, and these values for all individual cells are summed:

$$IV = \sum_{k=1}^{K} \sum_{j=1}^{J} \frac{\left[\sum_{i=1}^{I} x_i \right]^2}{n_i}$$ Eq. 11.11

For the intermediate step involving the rows factor, all values within a row are summed, squared, and then divided by the number of observations within that row (N_R). Finally, all the calculated squared sums for each row are added together:

$$III_R = \sum_{k=1}^{K} \frac{\left[\sum_{j=1}^{J} \sum_{i=1}^{I} x_i \right]^2}{N_R}$$ Eq. 11.12

The intermediate step for the column is calculated in a similar manner as the III_R except the values in each column and the total number of observations per column (N_C) are used:

$$III_C = \sum_{j=1}^{J} \frac{\left[\sum_{k=1}^{K} \sum_{i=1}^{I} x_i \right]^2}{N_C}$$ Eq. 11.13

These modified intermediate steps, along with values I and II are then used to calculate the sum of squares value using the same formulas (Eq. 11.6 through 11.10) used for data with equal cell sizes.

As an example of this application, consider the previous clinical trials example. However in this case, due to dropouts in the study, there were three fewer subjects on the second leg of the clinical trial (Table 11.5). In this case the decision rules remain the same, except the denominator degrees of freedom decreases. With $\alpha = .05$ and $n = 12$: 1) reject H_{01} if $F > F_{1,41}(.95) \approx 4.08$; 2) reject H_{02} if $F > F_{1,41}(.95) \approx 4.08$; and 3) reject H_{03} if $F > F_{1,41}(.95) \approx 4.08$.

The initial computational steps are:

$$I = \sum_{k=1}^{K} \sum_{j=1}^{J} \sum_{i=1}^{I} x_i^2$$

$$I = (125)^2 + (130)^2 + (135)^2 + \dots (150)^2 + (148)^2 = 785,392$$

Table 11.5   Sample Data of a Clinical Trial with Unequal Cells (C_{max})

	Formulation A			Formulation B			$\Sigma\Sigma$	$\Sigma\Sigma\Sigma$
Formula	125	130	135	149	151	...		
A	128	121	123	132	141	129		
Received	131	129	120	142	130	122		
First	119	133	125	...	138	140		
Σ	= 1,519			1,374			2,893	
Formula	126	140	135	130	128	127		
B	126	121	133	141	145	132		
Received	117	126	...	133	136	138		
First	120	136	122	129	150	148		
Σ	= 1,402			1,637			3,039	
$\Sigma\Sigma$ =	2,921			3,011				5,932

$$II = \frac{\left[\sum_{k=1}^{K}\sum_{j=1}^{J}\sum_{i=1}^{I} x_i\right]^2}{N}$$

$$II = \frac{(5,932)^2}{45} = 781,969.42$$

$$III_R = \sum_{k=1}^{K} \frac{\left[\sum_{j=1}^{J}\sum_{i=1}^{I} x_i\right]^2}{N_R}$$

$$III_R = \frac{(2,893)^2}{22} + \frac{(3,039)^2}{23} = 781,973.89$$

$$III_C = \sum_{j=1}^{J} \frac{\left[\sum_{k=1}^{K}\sum_{i=1}^{I} x_i\right]^2}{N_C}$$

$$III_C = \frac{(2,921)^2}{23} + \frac{(3,011)^2}{22} = 783,063.41$$

$$IV = \frac{\sum\limits_{k=1}^{K}\sum\limits_{j=1}^{J}\left[\sum\limits_{i=1}^{I} x_i\right]^2}{n}$$

$$IV = \frac{(1,519)^2}{12} + \frac{(1.374)^2}{10} + \frac{(1,402)^2}{11} + \frac{(1,637)^2}{12} = 783,073.03$$

Calculation of the sum of squares:

$$SS_R = 781,973.89 - 781,969.42 = 4.47$$

$$SS_C = 783,063.41 - 781,969.42 = 1,093.99$$

$$SS_{RC} = 783,073.03 - 781,973.89 - 783,063.41 + 781,969.42 = 5.15$$

$$SS_E = 785,392 - 783,073.03 = 2,318.97$$

$$SS_T = 785,392 - 781,969.42 = 3,422.58$$

The ANOVA table from the sum of squares data and appropriate degrees of freedom appears as follows:

Source	df	SS	MS	F
Between				
Rows (order)	1	4.47	4.47	0.08
Column (formula)	1	1,093.99	1,093.99	19.34*
Interaction	1	5.15	5.15	0.09
Within (error):	41	2,318.97	56.56	
Total	44	3,422.58		

There is no significant interaction and the results, with $\alpha = .05$, is to reject H_{02} and conclude that there is a significant difference between the two formulations, but there is no significant difference based on the order that the drugs were administered. These results are identical to the ones found when all of the cell sizes were equal.

Fixed, Random and Mixed Effect Models

As seen with the previous examples of the two-way analysis of variance, the levels of the independent variable were purposefully set by the investigator as part of the research design. Such a design is termed a **fixed effects model** because the levels of the independent variables have been "fixed" by the researcher. The result of a fixed effect model cannot be generalized to values of the independent variables beyond those selected for the study. Any factor can be considered fixed if the researcher uses the same levels of the independent variable on replications of a study. The fixed-effects design is normally used for cost considerations and because studies usually involve only a specific number of levels for the independent variables of interest.

If the levels under investigation are chosen at random from a population then the model used would be called a **random effects model** and results can be generalized to the population from which the samples were selected. Usually, the researcher will randomly select the number of levels which he/she feels represents that independent variable. It is assumed that the selected levels represent all possible levels of that variable.

Lastly, there can be **mixed effects models** that contain both fixed effect variable(s) and random effects variable(s).

The computational formulas for all three models are identical except for the numerator used to calculate the F-value in the ANOVA table. In certain situations the mean square interaction is substituted for the traditional mean squares error (MS$_E$) term. The fixed-effect model would be calculated as presented in Table 11.1. Using the symbols presented in Table 11.2 the following modifications are required. For the random effects model modifications are made in the calculations for both the F$_C$ and F$_R$ values:

$$F_R = \frac{MS_R}{MS_{RC}}$$
Eq. 11.14

$$F_C = \frac{MS_C}{MS_{RC}}$$
Eq. 11.15

With the mixed effect model and fixed rows, the only modification involves the F$_R$ equation:

$$F_R = \frac{MS_R}{MS_{RC}}$$ Eq. 11.16

With the mixed effect model where the columns are fixed, the only modification involves the F_C equation:

$$F_C = \frac{MS_C}{MS_{RC}}$$ Eq. 11.17

Post Hoc Procedures

Similar to the one-way ANOVA, if there are significant findings to the tests of main effect in the two-way analysis, *post hoc* procedures must be used to determine where the differences occur. If there are no significant interactions, then *post hoc* procedures described in Chapter 10 can be performed on significant main effect factors. For example, consider the results of the analysis of the three methods for dissolution testing presented above. The findings were as follows, with the method providing the only significant difference:

Source	df	SS	MS	F
Between				
Column (method)	2	1067.1111	533.56	18.49*

Since there were no effects from the batch factor nor a significant interaction, the data can be combined for each method tested.

Dissolution Results at 10 Minutes (%) n=6

	Traditional Method	Automated System I	Automated System II
$\sum x =$	1567	1483	1343
$\sum x^2 =$	103,015	92,263	75,976
Mean =	65.29	61.79	55.96
SD =	5.52	5.21	5.99

One-way analysis of this data would produce an F = 17.11 with a MS_E = 31.165. Using Scheffé's procedure, the following results were observed:

Pairing	Confidence Interval	Results
$\overline{X}_T - \overline{X}_I$	$-0.54 < \mu_T-\mu_I < +7.54$	
$\overline{X}_T - \overline{X}_{II}$	$+5.28 < \mu_T-\mu_{II} < +13.37$	Significant
$\overline{X}_I - \overline{X}_{II}$	$+5.28 < \mu_I-\mu_{II} < +9.87$	Significant

Thus, based on the post hoc analysis there was no significant difference between the traditional dissolution testing method and the first automated process. However, both of these methods were significantly different than the second automated process.

Other Designs

As discussed in Chapter 9, the randomized block design allows the researcher to minimize experimental error by creating relatively homogeneous subgroups. This "blocking" of information reduces the variability. An extension of the randomized block design to include two extraneous factors in the same study is called **Latin-square design**. In the Latin square design one possible source of extraneous variation is assigned to the columns of the two-way matrix and a second source of extraneous variation is assigned to the rows. Like the randomized block design the outcome is measured once and only once in each row and each column. Therefore, the number of columns, rows, and treatments are all equal.

The **Graeco-Latin square design** is an extension of the Latin Square design and allows for the identification and isolation of three extraneous sources of variation. Greek letters are superimposed on the Latin letters in such a way that each Greek letter occurs once in each column, once in each row and once with each Latin letter.

In many cases a complete randomized block design will require a large number of treatments which may not be economically or practically feasible. The **balanced incomplete block design** includes only a part of the treatments in a block. There will be missing pieces of information but the design must be balanced; balanced by the fact that each level of each factor has the same number of observations. Because some of the information is missing at other levels for each factor, the method involves incomplete blocks.

Other types of designs include **fractional factorial designs**, **split plot designs** and **orthogonal array designs**. Each of these types of designs require stringent assumptions about the absence of interaction effects. We will not discuss formulas and calculations involved in these multi-factor designs because they are tedious and best run on a computer. Details can be found in advanced texts (Kirk, 1968; Mason, 1989).

Beyond a Two-way Factorial Design

Figure 11.4 represents a three-dimensional schematic comparing three independent variables. Each of the three independent variables (A, B, and C) are represented by a dimension of the drawing. The shaded cube represents the combined effect of the third level of Factor A, the first level of Factor B, and the second level of Factor C.

The advantage of these multi-factor designs is the increased efficiency for comparing different levels of several independent variables or factors at one time instead of conducting several separate single-factor experiments. However, as the number of independent variables increases the number of possible outcomes increases and designs get extremely complicated to interpret, especially the interactions between two or possibly more variables.

For example, with a two-way ANOVA there are two tests of the main effect and one interaction to interpret. With the three-way ANOVA these are increased to three tests of the main effect, three two-way interactions, and one three-way interaction. Lastly, with a four-way ANOVA the complexity of the outcomes includes four tests of main effects, six two-way interactions, four three-way interactions, and one four-way interaction (Table 11.7).

Because of this increased complexity, factorial designs involving more than three factors pose difficulties in the interpretation of the interaction effects. Therefore, most factorial designs are usually limited to three factors.

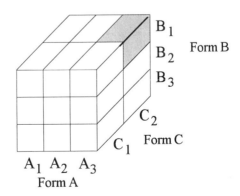

Figure 11.4 Example of a three-way ANOVA.

Table 11.7 Possible Significant Outcomes in Factorial Designs

	Main Effects	Interactions	
One Factor	A		
Two Factors	A	AxB	
	B		
Three Factors	A	AxB	AxBxC
	B	AxC	
	C	BxC	
Four Factors	A	AxB	AxBxC
	B	AxC	BxCxD
	C	AxD	AxCxD
	D	BxC	
		BxD	AxBxCxD
		CxD	
Five Factors	A	AxB	AxBxC
	B	AxC	AxCxD
	C	AxD	AxDxE
	D	AxE	BxCxD
	E	BxC	BxDxE
		BxD	CxDxE
		BxE	
		CxD	AxBxCxD
		CxE	AxBxCxE
		DxE	BxCxDxE
			AxBxCxDxE

References

Kirk, R.E. (1968). Experimental Design: Procedures for the Behavioral Sciences, Brooks/Cole Publishing, Belmont, CA.

Mason, R.L., Gunst, R.F. and Hess, J.L (1989). Statistical Design and Analysis of Experiments, John Wiley and Sons, New York, 1989.

Suggested Supplemental Readings

Havilcek, L.L. and Crain, R.D. (1988). Practical Statistics for the Physical Sciences, American Chemical Society, Washington, pp. 255-333.

Kachigan, S.K. (1991). Multivariate Statistical Analysis, Radius Press, New York, pp. 203-215.

Zar, J.H. (1984). Biostatistical Analysis, Prentice Hall, Englewood Cliffs, NJ, pp. 206-234, 244-252.

Example Problems

1. A preformulation department is experimenting with different fillers and various speeds on a tableting machine. Are there any significant differences in hardness based on the following samples?

Hardness (kP)
Speed of Tableting Machine (1000 units/hour)

Filler	80		100		120		180	
	7	8	6	7	5	7	6	7
Lactose	5	7	8	8	8	9	8	9
	8	9	6	7	7	7	7	7
	7	7	8	10	9	10	8	9
	7	7	8	9	5	7	7	6
Microcrystalline	7	9	6	7	8	8	6	6
Cellulose	5	7	8	7	5	7	8	7
	8	9	6	7	8	8	9	9
	7	5	4	6	6	7	4	6
Dicalcium	5	7	6	7	4	5	9	7
Phosphate	7	7	5	6	7	7	5	6
	5	8	7	8	5	6	7	6

2. An investigator compares three different indexes for measuring the quality of life of patients with a specific disease state. She randomly selects four hospitals and identifies twelve individuals with approximately the same state of disease. These patients are randomly assigned to each of the indexes and evaluated (note one patient's information was lost due to incomplete information). Are there any differences based on indexes or hospital used?

Quality of Life Index (Scores 0-100)

	Index 1		Index 2		Index 3	
Hospital A	67	73	85	91	94	95
	61	69	81	87	99	92
Hospital B	81	83	83	...	86	85
	85	80	81	84	89	80
Hospital C	82	77	79	74	81	85
	80	86	80	84	82	77

Answers to Problems

1. Experiment with different fillers and various speeds on a tableting machine.

Hypotheses: H_{01}: $\mu_{Speed\,1} = \mu_{Speed\,2} = \mu_{Speed\,3} = \mu_{Speed\,4}$
$\qquad\qquad$ H_{02}: $\mu_{Filler\,1} = \mu_{Filler\,2} = \mu_{Filler\,3}$
$\qquad\qquad$ H_{03}: No interaction between speed and filler

Hardness (kP)

Speed of Tableting Machine

Filler		80	100	120	180	
Lactose	$\Sigma =$	56	60	62	61	$\Sigma\Sigma = 239$
Microcrystalline Cellulose	$\Sigma =$	59	58	56	58	$\Sigma\Sigma = 231$
Dicalcium Phosphate	$\Sigma =$	51	49	47	50	$\Sigma\Sigma = 197$
$\Sigma\Sigma =$		166	167	165	169	$\Sigma\Sigma\Sigma = 667$

Decision Rules: With $\alpha = .05$ and $n = 8$: reject H_{01} if $F > F_{3,84}(.95) \approx$ 2.72; reject H_{02} if $F > F_{2,84}(.95) \approx 3.11$; and reject H_{03} if $F > F_{6,84}(.95) \approx 2.21$.

Calculations:

$$I = \sum_{k=1}^{K} \sum_{j=1}^{J} \sum_{i=1}^{I} x_i^2$$

$$I = (7)^2 + (5)^2 + (8)^2 \ldots + (6)^2 + (6)^2 = 4809$$

$$II = \frac{\left[\sum_{k=1}^{K} \sum_{j=1}^{J} \sum_{i=1}^{I} x_i \right]^2}{N}$$

$$II = \frac{(667)^2}{96} = 4634.26$$

$$III_R = \frac{\sum_{k=1}^{K} \left[\sum_{j=1}^{J} \sum_{i=1}^{I} x_i \right]^2}{J \cdot n}$$

$$III_R = \frac{(239)^2 + (231)^2 + (197)^2}{(4)(8)} = \frac{149291}{32} = 4665.344$$

$$III_C = \frac{\sum_{j=1}^{J} \left[\sum_{k=1}^{K} \sum_{i=1}^{I} x_i \right]^2}{K \cdot n}$$

$$III_C = \frac{(166)^2 + (167)^2 + (165)^2 + (169)^2}{(3)(8)} = \frac{111231}{24} = 4634.625$$

$$IV = \frac{\sum_{k=1}^{K} \sum_{j=1}^{J} \left[\sum_{i=1}^{I} x_i \right]^2}{n}$$

$$IV = \frac{(56)^2 + (60)^2 \ldots + (47)^2 + (50)(2)}{8} = \frac{37357}{8} = 4669.625$$

$$SS_R = III_R - II = 4,665.344 - 4,634.26 = 31.084$$

$$SS_C = III_C - II = 4,634.625 - 4,634.26 = 0.365$$

$$SS_{RC} = IV - III_R - III_C + II$$

$$SS_{RC} = 4,669.625 - 4,665.344 - 4,634.625 = 3.916$$

$$SS_E = I - IV = 4,809 - 4,634.26 = 174.74$$

$$SS_T = 785,392 - 781,969.42 = 3,422.58$$

ANOVA Table:

Source	df	SS	MS	F
Between				
Rows (filler)	2	31.084	15.542	9.368*
Column (speed)	3	0.365	0.122	0.074
Interaction	6	3.916	0.653	0.394
Within (error):	84	139.375	1.659	
Total	95	174.740		

Decision: With $\alpha = .05$, reject H_{01} and conclude that there is a significant difference between the three fillers used in the experiment, but there is no significant difference based on the speed of the tableting machine and no significant interaction between these two factors.

2. Experiment with quality of life indexes and various hospitals.

Hypotheses: H_{01}: $\mu_{Index\ 1} = \mu_{Index\ 2} = \mu_{Index\ 3}$
H_{02}: $\mu_{Hospital\ A} = \mu_{Hospital\ B} = \mu_{Hospital\ C}$
H_{03}: No interaction between index and hospital

Decision Rules: With $\alpha = .05$: reject H_{01} if $F > F_{2,26}(.95) \approx 3.39$; reject H_{02} if $F > F_{2,26}(.95) \approx 3.39$; and reject H_{03} if $F > F_{4,26}(.95) \approx 3.00$.

		Index 1	Index 2	Index 3	
Hospital A	$\Sigma =$	270	344	380	$\Sigma\Sigma = 994$
Hospital B	$\Sigma =$	329	248	340	$\Sigma\Sigma = 917$
Hospital C	$\Sigma =$	325	317	325	$\Sigma\Sigma = 967$
	$\Sigma\Sigma =$	924	909	1045	$\Sigma\Sigma\Sigma = 2878$

Calculations:

$$I = \sum_{k=1}^{K} \sum_{j=1}^{J} \sum_{i=1}^{I} x_i^2$$

$$I = (67\ )^2 + (73\ )^2 + (61\ )^2 \ldots + (82\ )^2 + (77\ )^2 = 238{,}646$$

$$II = \frac{\left[\sum_{k=1}^{K} \sum_{j=1}^{J} \sum_{i=1}^{I} x_i \right]^2}{N}$$

$$II = \frac{(2{,}878\ )^2}{35} = 236{,}653.83$$

$$III_R = \sum_{k=1}^{K} \frac{\left[\sum_{j=1}^{J} \sum_{i=1}^{I} x_i \right]^2}{N_R}$$

$$III_R = \frac{(994\ )^2}{12} + \frac{(917\ )^2}{11} + \frac{(967\ )^2}{12} = 236{,}704.87$$

$$III_C = \sum_{j=1}^{J} \frac{\left[\sum_{k=1}^{K} \sum_{i=1}^{I} x_i \right]^2}{N_C}$$

$$III_C = \frac{(924\ )^2}{12} + \frac{(909\ )^2}{11} + \frac{(1045\ )^2}{12} = 237{,}266.54$$

$$IV = \sum_{k=1}^{K} \sum_{j=1}^{J} \frac{\left[\sum_{i=1}^{I} x_i\right]^2}{N_i}$$

$$IV = \frac{(270\,)^2}{4} + \frac{(344\,)^2}{4} + \frac{(380\,)^2}{4} + \dots \frac{(325\,)^2}{4} = 238,305.33$$

$$SS_R = III_R - II = 236,704.87 - 236,653.83 = 51.04$$

$$SS_C = III_C - II = 237,266.54 - 236,653.83 = 612.71$$

$$SS_{RC} = IV - III_R - III_C + II$$

$$SS_{RC} = 238,305.33 - 236,704.87 - 237,266.54 + 236,653.83 = 987.75$$

$$SS_E = I - IV = 238,646 - 238,305.33 = 340.67$$

$$SS_T = I - II = 238,646 - 236,653.83 = 1,992.17$$

ANOVA Table:

Source	df	SS	MS	F
Between				
Rows (hospital)	2	51.04	25.52	1.95
Column (index)	2	612.71	306.36	23.39*
Interaction	4	987.75	246.94	18.85*
Within (error):	26	340.67	13.10	
Total	34	1,992.17		

Decision: With α = .05, reject H_{02} and conclude that there is a significant difference between the indexes used in this study. Reject H_{03} and conclude that a significant interaction exists between the two main factors, but there is no significant difference based on the hospital tested.

12

Correlation

Both correlation and regression analysis are concerned with continuous variables. Correlation does not require an independent variable, which as we will see in the next chapter, is a requirement for the regression model. With correlation, two or more variables may be compared to determine if there is a relationship and to measure the strength of that relationship. Correlation describes the degree to which two or more variables show interrelationships within a given population. The correlation may be either positive or negative. Correlation results do not explain why the relation occurs, only that such a relationship exists. Correlation is closely related to linear regression which will be discussed in Chapter 13, where the researcher controls at least one independent variable.

Graphic Representation of Two Continuous Variables

Graphs offer an excellent way of showing relationships between continuous variables based on either an interval or ratio scales. The easiest way to visualize the relationship between two continuous variables is graphically, using a **bivariate scatter plot**. Correlation usually involves only dependent or response variables. If one or more variables are under the researcher's control (for example, varying concentrations of a solution or specific speeds for a particular instrument) then the linear regression model would be more appropriate. Traditionally, with either correlation or regression, if an independent variable exists it is labeled X and plotted on the horizontal x-axis of the graph or the **abscissa**. The second, dependent variable Y is plotted on the vertical y-axis or the **ordinate** (Figure 12.1). In the correlation model, both variables are evaluated with equal import, vary at random (both referred to as dependent variables), and may be assigned to either axis.

The first role of correlation is to determine the strength of the relationship between the two variables represented on the x-axis and the y-axis. The measure of this magnitude is called the correlation coefficient (discussed in the next section). The data required to compute this coefficient are two continuous measurements (x,y) obtained on the same entity (a person, object or data point) and is refered to as the **unit of association**. As will be seen, the **correlation coefficient** is a well-defined mathematical index that measures the strength of relationships. This index measures both the magnitude and the direction of the relationships.

+1.0 perfect positive correlation
0.0 no correlation
-1.0 perfect negative correlation

If there is a perfect relationship (correlation coefficient of +1.00 or -1.00), all of the data points would fall on a straight line. The greater the change in Y for a constant change in X, the steeper the slope of the line. In a less than perfect relationship between two variables, the closer the data points are located on a straight line, the stronger the relationship and greater the correlation coefficient. In contrast, a zero correlation would indicate absolutely no linear relationship between the two variables.

Graph A in Figure 12.1 represents a **positive correlation** where data points with larger x-values tend to have corresponding large y-values. As seen later, an example of a positive correlation is height and weight of individuals. As the heights of people increase their weights also tend to increase. Graph B is a **negative correlation**, where Y appears to decrease as values for X increase (approaching a perfect negative correlation of -1.00). An example of a negative or **inverse correlation** might be speed versus accuracy. The faster an individual completes a given task, the lower the accuracy; whereas, the slower the person's speed, the greater the accuracy of the task. Graph C in Figure 12.1 shows a scattering of points with no correlation or discernable pattern.

More visual information can be presented by drawing a circle or an ellipse to surround the points in the scatter plot (D in Figure 12.1). If the points fall within a circle there is no correlation. If the points fall within an ellipse, the flatter the ellipse the stronger the correlation until the ellipse produces a straight line or a perfect correlation. The orientation of the ellipse indicates the direction of the correlation. An orientation from the lower left to the upper right is positive and from the upper left to the lower right is a negative correlation. Dashed lines can be drawn on the x- and y-axis to represent the centers of each distribution. These lines divide the scatter plot into **quadrants**. In an absolute 0.00 correlation, each quadrant would have an equal number of data points. As the correlation increases (in the positive or negative direction) the data point will increasingly be found in only two diagonal quadrants. An additional assumption involved with the correlation coefficient is that the two continuous variables possess a **joint normal distribution**. In other words, for any given value on the x-axis variable, the y-variable is sampled from a population which is normally distributed around some central point. If the populations, from which the samples are selected are not normal, inferential procedures are invalid (Daniel, 1978). In such cases the strength of the relationship can be calculated using an alternative nonparameteric procedure such as Spearman rank correlation (Chapter 17).

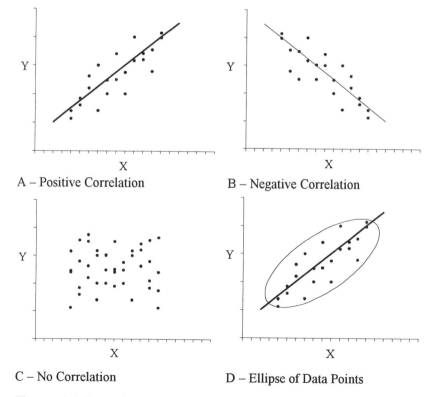

Figure 12.1 Examples of graphic representations of correlation data.

There are several different methods for calculating measures of correlation, the most widely used is the Pearson Product-Moment Correlation Coefficient (r).

Pearson Product Moment Correlation Coefficient

The simplest way to discuss correlation is to focus first on only two continuous variables. The **correlational relationship** can be thought of as an association which exists between the values representing two random variables. In this relationship we, as the investigators, have no control over the observed values for either variable.

The correlation coefficient assumes that the continuous variables are randomly selected from normally distributed populations. This coefficient is the average of the products of each x- and y-variable result measured as units in standardized normal distribution. Therefore r is the sum of the products divided by n - 1, or

$$r_{xy} = \frac{\sum z_x z_y}{n-1}$$
        Eq. 12.1

where z_x and z_y are standard scores for the variables at each data point and n is the number of pairs of data points, or the sample size. Ideally, we would know the population mean (μ) and standard deviation (σ) for each variable. This can be a very laborious process and involves computing the mean of each distribution, and then determining the deviation from the mean for each value in terms of a standard score.

$$z_x = \frac{x_i - \mu_x}{\sigma_x} \quad and \quad z_y = \frac{y_i - \mu_y}{\sigma_y}$$
        Eq. 12.2

Unfortunately, we usually do not know the parameters for the population and me must approximate the means and standard deviations using sample information.

A slightly more convenient formula for calculating the association of two variables is the Pearson product-moment correlation. This coefficient is the product of the **moments** ($x_i - \mu$) of the two variable observation. Where the moment deviation ($x_i - \overline{X}$) is the difference between the individual observations and the sample mean for that variable. The formula for this correlation coefficient is as following:

$$r = \frac{\sum(x-\overline{X})(y-\overline{Y})}{\sqrt{\sum(x-\overline{X})^2(y-\overline{Y})^2}}$$ Eq. 12.3

These calculations involve a determination of how values deviate from their respective means: how each x-value deviated from the mean for variable x ($\overline{X}$) and how each y-value varies from the mean for variable y ($\overline{Y}$). The convenience comes from not having to compute the individual z-values for each data point. Normally a table is set up for the terms required in the equation (Table 12.1). Using this method, the researcher must first calculate the sample mean for both the x- and y-variable. As seen in Table 12.1, values for the observed data are represented in the first two columns, where x is the value for each measurement associated with the x-axis and y is the corresponding measure on the y-axis for that same data point. The third and fourth columns reflect the deviations of the x- and y-scores about their respective means. The fifth column is the product of these deviations, the sum of which becomes the numerator in the Pearson product moment equation. The last two columns are the deviations squared for both the x- and y-variables and are used in the denominator.

As an example, consider the following data collected on six volunteer subjects during a Phase I clinical trial (Table 12.2). For whatever reason, the investigator is interested in determining if there is a correlation between the subjects' weight and height. First, both the volunteers' mean weight and mean height are calculated:

$$\overline{X}_x = \frac{\sum x}{n} = \frac{511.1}{6} = 85.18$$

Table 12.1 Data Layout for Computation of the Pearson Product Moment Correlation Coefficient - Definitional Formula

x	y	$x-\overline{X}$	$y-\overline{Y}$	$(x-\overline{X})(y-\overline{Y})$	$(x-\overline{X})^2$	$(y-\overline{Y})^2$
x_1	y_1	...	...	...	...	...
x_2	y_2	...	...	...	...	...
x_3	y_3	...	...	...	...	...
...	...	...	...	...	...	...
x_n	y_n	...	...	...	...	...
				$\sum(x-\overline{X})(y-\overline{Y})$	$\sum(x-\overline{X})^2$	$\sum(y-\overline{Y})^2$

Table 12.2 Clinical Trial Data for Six Volunteers

Subject	Weight (kg)	Height (m)
1	96.0	1.88
2	77.7	1.80
3	100.9	1.85
4	79.0	1.77
5	73.0	1.73
6	84.5	1.83
$\Sigma =$	511.1	10.86

$$\overline{X_y} = \frac{\Sigma y}{n} = \frac{10.86}{6} = 1.81$$

Table 12.3 shows the required sums for: 1) the deviations from the respective means; 2) the squares of those deviations; and 3) the products of deviations. Finally, each of the last three columns are summed and entered into the equation:

$$r = \frac{\Sigma(x - \overline{X})(y - \overline{Y})}{\sqrt{\Sigma(x - \overline{X})^2 (y - \overline{Y})^2}}$$

Table 12.3 Sample Data for Pearson's *r* Calculation - Definitional Formula

x	y	$x - \overline{X}$	$y - \overline{Y}$	$(x - \overline{X})(y - \overline{Y})$	$(x - \overline{X})^2$	$(y - \overline{Y})^2$
96.0	1.88	10.52	0.07	0.7574	117.07	0.0049
77.7	1.80	-7.48	-0.01	0.0748	55.96	0.0001
100.9	1.85	15.72	0.04	0.6288	247.12	0.0016
79.0	1.77	-6.18	- 0.04	0.2472	38.19	0.0016
73.0	1.73	-12.18	- 0.08	0.9744	148.35	0.0064
84.5	1.83	-0.68	0.02	-0.0136	0.46	0.0004
			$\Sigma =$	2.6690	607.15	0.0150

$$r = \frac{2.6690}{\sqrt{(607.15)(0.015)}} = \frac{2.6690}{3.0178} = +0.884$$

The results of the **product moment correlation coefficient** or simply the correlation coefficient shows a positive relationship and can be noted as a very strong relationship considering a perfect correlation is +1.00.

A third formula is available which further simplifies the mathematical process and is easier to compute, especially for hand-held calculators or computers. This computational formula is:

$$r = \frac{n \sum xy - \sum x \sum y}{\sqrt{n \sum x^2 - (\sum x)^2} \sqrt{n \sum y^2 - (\sum y)^2}} \qquad \text{Eq. 12.4}$$

Once again a table is developed based on the sample data (Table 12.4). In this case there are only five columns and the calculation of the sample means ($\overline{X}_x, \overline{X}_y$) are not required. Similar to the previous table, these first two columns represent the observed data, paired for both the x and y measurement scale. The third and fourth columns represent the individual x- and y-values squared and the last column is the product of x and y for each data point. Using this method to compute the correlation coefficient for the previous example of height and weight would produce the results seen in Table 12.5. The calculation of the correlation coefficient would be:

Table 12.4 Data Layout for Computation of the Pearson Product Moment Correlation Coefficient - Computational Formula

$\underline{X}$	$\underline{Y}$	$\underline{X^2}$	$\underline{Y^2}$	$\underline{XY}$
x_1	y_1	x_1^2	y_1^2	$x_1 y_1$
x_2	y_2	x_2^2	y_2^2	$x_2 y_2$
x_3	y_3	x_3^2	y_3^2	$x_3 y_3$
...	...	...	...	...
x_n	y_n	X_n^2	y_n^2	$x_n y_n$
$\sum x$	$\sum y$	$\sum x^2$	$\sum y^2$	$\sum xy$

Table 12.5. Sample Data for Pearson's r Calculation - Computational Formula

X	y	x^2	y^2	xy
96.0	1.88	9216.00	3.5344	180.480
77.7	1.80	6037.29	3.2400	139.860
100.9	1.85	10180.81	3.4225	186.665
79.0	1.77	6241.00	3.1329	139.830
73.0	1.73	5329.00	2.9929	126.290
84.5	1.83	7140.25	3.3489	154.635
511.1	10.86	44144.35	19.6716	927.760

$$r = \frac{n\sum xy - \sum x \sum y}{\sqrt{n\sum x^2 - (\sum x)^2}\sqrt{n\sum y^2 - (\sum y)^2}}$$

$$r = \frac{6(927.76) - (511.1)(10.86)}{\sqrt{6(44144.35) - (511.1)^2}\sqrt{6(19.6716) - (10.86)^2}}$$

$$r = \frac{5566.56 - 5550.546}{(60.356)(0.3)} = \frac{16.014}{18.107} = +0.884$$

The results from using either formula (Eq. 12.3 or 12.4) produce the identical answers since algebraically these formulas are equivalent.

Correlations can be measured on variables that have completely different scales with completely different units (i.e., a correlation between weight in kilograms and height in meters). Thus, the value of the correlation coefficient is completely independent of the values for the means and standard deviations of the two variables being compared.

Correlation Line

The correlation coefficient is an index which can be used to describe the linear relationship between two continuous variables and deals with paired relationships (each data point represents a value on the x-axis as well as a value on the y-axis). As will be seen in the next chapter, the best line to be fitted between the points on the bivariate scatter plot is very important for the regression model where predictive is required for y at any given value on the x-axis. However, it is also possible, and some times desirable to approximate a line which best fits between the data point in our correlation model. As will be discussed in greater detail in Chapter 13, a straight line between our data points can be define as follows:

$$y = a + bx \qquad \text{Eq. 12.5}$$

where (y) is a value on the vertical axis, (x) is a corresponding value on the horizontal axis, (a) indicates the point where the line crosses the vertical axis, and (b) represents the amount by which the line rises for each increase in x, (the slope of the line). We can define the line which fits best between our data points using the following formulas and data from Table 12.3 for our computational method of determining the correlation coefficient.

$$b = \frac{n \sum xy - (\sum x)(\sum y)}{n \sum x^2 - (\sum x)^2} \qquad \text{Eq. 12.6}$$

$$a = \frac{\sum y - b \sum x}{n} \qquad \text{Eq. 12.7}$$

Such lines are illustrated in Figure 12.1. The correlation coefficient provides an indication of how close the data points are to this line. As mentioned

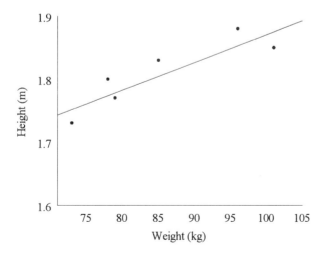

Figure 12.2   Correlation line representing data presented in Table 12.4.

previously, if we produce a correlation coefficient equal to +1.00 or −1.00, then all the data points will fall directly on the straight line. Any value other than a perfect correlation, positive or negative, indicated some deviation from the line. The closer the correlation coefficient to zero, the greater the deviation from this line.

In our previous example of weight and heights for our six subjects, the correlation line which fits based between these points is calculated as follows:

$$b = \frac{(6)(927.76) - (511.1)(10.86)}{(6)(44144.35) - (511.1)^2} = \frac{16.014}{3642.89} = +0.0044$$

$$a = \frac{(10.86) - (0.0044)(511.1)}{6} = 1.43$$

The data and resultant line with the slope of +0.044 and y-intercept 1.43 of are presented in Figure 12.2. As can be seen data are relatively close to the straight line, indicative of the high correlation value of $r = +0.884$.

Statistical Significance of a Correlation Coefficient

A positive or negative correlation between two variables shows that a relationship exists. Whether one considers it as a strong or weak correlation, important or unimportant, is a matter of interpretation. For example in the behavioral sciences a correlation of 0.80 would be considered a high correlation. However, for individuals in the pharmaceutical industry data involved with process validation may require a correlation >0.99.

Verbal descriptions of correlations are inconsistent. The simplest might be: less than 0.2 is a "weak" correlation; 0.2 to 0.39 represents a "fair" correlation; and 0.4 or more can be considered a "good" correlation. Another rough guide (Guilford, 1956) is as follows:

<0.20	slight; almost negligible relationship
0.20-0.40	low correlation; definite but small relationship
0.40-0.70	moderate correlation; substantial relationship
0.70-0.90	high correlation; marked relationship
>0.90	very high correlation; very dependable relationship

Similar levels, but slightly different terminology can be seen with yet another guide (Roundtree, 1981):

<0.20	very weak, negligible
0.20-0.40	weak, low
0.40-0.70	moderate
0.70-0.90	strong, high, marked
>0.90	very strong, very high

The sign (+ or -) would indicate a positive or negative correlation. In the previous example of weight vs. height the result of +0.884 would represent a "high," "strong," or "marked" positive correlation.

The values for correlation coefficients do not represent equal distances along a linear scale. For example, a correlation of 0.50 is not twice as large as $r = 0.25$. Instead, the coefficient is always relative to the conditions under which it was calculated. The larger the r, either in the positive or negative direction, the greater the consistency of the two measures.

In addition to identifying the strength and direction of a correlation coefficient, there are statistical methods for testing the significance of a given correlation. Two will be discussed here: 1) use of a Pearson product-moment table and 2) the conversion to a student t-statistic. In both cases, the symbol r_{xy} or ρ (rho) can be used to represent the correlation for the populations from which the samples were randomly selected. The hypotheses being tested are:

$$H_0: \quad r_{yx} = 0 \qquad \text{or} \qquad H_0: \quad \rho = 0$$
$$H_1: \quad r_{yx} \neq 0 \qquad \qquad\quad H_1: \quad \rho \neq 0$$

The null hypothesis indicates that a correlation does not exist between the two continuous variables, the population correlation coefficient is zero. Whereas, the alternative hypothesis states that a significant relationship exists between variables x and y. Pearson's correlation coefficient, symbolized by the letter r, symbolizes the sample value for the relationship; whereas ρ represents true population correlation.

Using the Table B10 in Appendix B, it is possible to identify a critical r-value and if the correlation coefficient exceeds the critical value, H_0 is rejected. The first column in the table represents the degrees of freedom and the remaining columns are the critical values at various allowable levels of Type I error (α). For correlation problems the number of degrees of freedom is the number of data points minus two (n-2). The decision rule is to reject H_0 (no correlation) if the calculated r-value is greater than $r_{n-2}(\alpha)$. In the previous example comparing weights and heights of volunteers in a clinical trial, the decision rule would be with $\alpha = 0.05$, reject H_0 if $r > r_4(.05) = 0.8114$. The result of the calculations was that the correlation coefficient was 0.884, which is greater than the critical r-value of 0.8114; therefore, we would reject H_0 and conclude that there is a significant correlation with 95% confidence. One might question how well we can trust a correlation coefficient from a sample size of only six to predict the relationship in the population from which the sample is drawn. Two factors will influence this decision: 1) the strength of the correlation (the r-value itself); and 2) the sample size. Looking at the table of critical values for the correlation coefficient (Table B10, Appendix B) it is possible to find significance for a relatively small r-value if it comes from a large sample.

The second method for calculating the level of significance for the sample r-value is to enter the results into a special formula for a t-test and compare the results to a critical value from a student t-distribution (Table B3, Appendix B). This converted t-value from an r-value is compared to the critical t-value with n-2 degrees of freedom. The decision rule is to reject H_0 (no correlation) if t > $t_{n-2}(1-\alpha/2)$ or t < $-t_{n-2}(1-\alpha/2)$. The statistical formula is:

$$t = \frac{r\sqrt{n-2}}{\sqrt{1-r^2}}$$
Eq. 12.8

The correlation coefficient (r) incorporates the concept of how scores vary within a given distribution. These potential deviations are considered as a standard error of the correlation coefficient and represents the standard deviation for the theoretical distribution of correlation coefficients for samples from the population with a given size. The closer the correlation coefficient to a perfect result (+1.00 or −1.00), the smaller this standard error. Approximately 95% of all possible correlation coefficients will be within two standard deviations of the population ρ. Therefore, we can use information used in Chapter 8 to create a t-statistic to calculate significance of the correlation coefficient.

Using our previous example (weight vs. height) to illustrate the correlation t-conversion, the decision rule is with $\alpha = 0.05$, reject H_0 if t > $t_4(.975)$ = 2.776. The computations are:

$$t = \frac{.884\sqrt{6-2}}{\sqrt{1-(.884)^2}} = \frac{1.768}{0.467} = 3.78$$

In this case the decision, with t > 2.776, is to reject H_0 and conclude that there is a significant correlation between the volunteers' weight and height. Based on the t-conversion, a significant result would indicate that the results could not have occurred by chance alone from a population with a true zero correlation.

Table 12.6 Comparison of Critical *r*-Values and *t*-Values

Table of Critical Values	Statistical Results	$\alpha = 0.05$		$\alpha = 0.01$	
		C.V.	Result	C.V.	Result
Table B11	r = 0.884	0.8114	Significant	0.9172	NS
Table B3	t = 3.78	2.776	Significant	4.604	NS

Note in Table 12.6 that both methods produce identical outcomes.

The *r*-value can be considered a ratio of the actual amount of deviation divided by the total possible deviation. Whereas the square of the *r*-value,^{2} is the amount of actual deviation which the two distributions have in common. The interpretation of the correlation between two variables is concerned with the degree to which they **covary**. In other words, how much of the variation in one of the continuous variables can be attributed to variation in the other. The square of the correlation coefficient, r^2, indicates the proportion of variance in one of the variables accounted for by the variance of the second variable. The r^2 term is sometimes referred to as the "**common variance**." In the case of $r^2 = 0.49$ (for $r = 0.7$), 49% of the variance in scores for one variable is associated with the variance in scores for the second variable.

Correlation and Causality

As a correlation approaches a +1.0 or -1.0 there is a tendency for numbers to concentrate closer to a straight line. However, one should not assume that just because correlations come closer to a perfect correlation that they form a straight line. The correlation coefficient says nothing about the percentage of the relationship, only its relative strength. It represents a convenient ratio, not an actual measurement scale. It serves primarily as a data reduction technique and as a descriptive method. Figure 12.2 illustrates this point where four different data sets can produce the same "high" correlation (r = 0.816). As discussed in the next chapter, if lines were drawn which best fit between the points in each data set, they would be identical with a slope of 0.5 and a y-intercept of 3.0. This table also shows the advantage of plotting the data on graph paper, or a computer generated visual, to actually observe the distribution of the data points.

The correlation coefficient does not suggest nor prove the reason for this relationship; only that it exists, and whether the two variables vary together either positively or negatively and the degree of this relationship. It does not indicate anything about the **causality** of this relationship. Did the x-variable cause the result in y? Did y effect variable x? Could a third variable have effected both x and y? There could be many reasons for this relationship.

With correlation the relationship identified between two dependent variables is purely descriptive and no conclusions about causality can be made. By contrast, with experimental or regression studies, where the predictor or independent variable is controlled by the researcher, there is a better likelihood that interpretations about causality can be stated. However, with correlation, this relationship may be due to external variables not controlled for by the experiment. These are called **confounding variables** and represent other unidentified variables that are entwined or confused with the variables being tested. Two factors must be established before the researcher can say that x, assumed to be the independent variable, caused the result in y. First, x must have preceded y in time. Second, the research design was such, that it controlled for other factors that might cause or influence y.

Even a significant result from a correlation coefficient does not necessarily imply a cause and effect relationship between the two variables. In the previous example, does the height of the person directly contribute to his/her weight? Does the weight of the person influence the person's height? The former assumption may be true, but probably not the latter. In this particular case, both variables were influenced by a third factor. The patients volunteering to take part in the study were screened using an inclusion criteria that they must fall within 10% of the ideal height/weight standards established by the Metropolitan Life Insurance Company. Thus, if we approximate ideal weight/height standards, taller volunteers will tend to weigh more and shorter volunteers will weight less because of the ratio established between these variables based on the standardized tables used by Metropolitan Life.

In some cases causality may not be as important as the strength of the relationship. For example if the researchers were comparing two methods (i.e., analytical assays, cognitive scales, physiological measures), the individual is not interested in whether one method produced a higher mean value than the other, rather they are interested in whether there is a significant correlation between the two methods.

Various types of relationships can exist between two continuous variables and still produce a correlation coefficient. Many are illustrated in Figures 12.1 and 12.3. A **monotonic relationship** is illustrated by Figure 12.1-A, -B and -D where the relationship is ever-increasing or ever-decreasing. The monotonic relationship could be linear (best represented by a straight line) or **nonlinear** or **curvilinear relationships** where a curved line best fits the data points. In

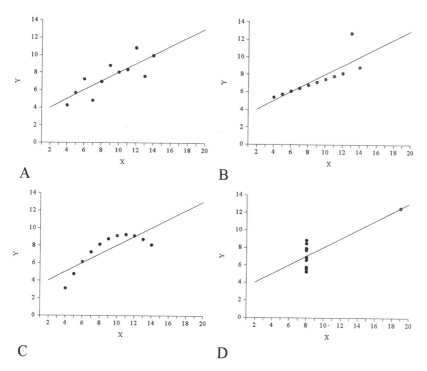

Figure 12.3 Graphs of four sets of data with identical correlations (r = 0.816). From: Anscombe, F.J. (1973). "Graphs in statistical analysis" <u>American Statistician</u> <u>27</u>:17-27.

contrast, the Figure 12.3-C is an example of a **non-monotonic relationship**. In this case the relationship is not ever-increasing or ever-decreasing, the points begin as a positive correlation but change near 10 on the x-axis and become a negative correlation. This figure represents a non-monotonic, concave downward relationship. One last type of relationship is a **cyclical relationship** where waves are formed as the correlation continues to change from a positive to a negative to a positive relationship.

In vivo – In vitro Correlation

One example of the use of the correlation coefficient is to establish a relationship between an *in vitro* measure for a pharmaceutical product and an *in vivo* response in living systems. This relationship is referred to as an *in vivo–in vitro* **correlation**, or an **IV/IV correlation**.

In 1977, the Food and Drug Administration issued regulations on bioequivalency and bioavailability and included a list of drugs described as having "known or potential bioequivalency or bioavailability problems" (Fed.Reg.,1977). In these regulations, it was pointed out that bioequivalence requirement for the majority of products could be the form of an *in vitro* test in which the product is compared to a reference standard. This point will be discussed in greater detail in Chapter 18. Preferably, these *in vitro* tests should be correlated with human *in vivo* data. In most cases the *in vitro* tests are dissolution tests.

Dissolution is a measure of the percent of drug entering a dissolved state over varying periods of time. Tests of dissolution are used to determine if drug products are in compliance with compendia standards in the United States Pharmacopeia (USP) or new drug application (NDA). In USP XXIII there are 532 dissolution tests. Dissolution testing can be performed on a variety of dosage forms including immediate release and extended release solids, transdermal patches and topical preparations. For immediate release solid dosage forms, one of the most commonly used comparisons for IV/IV correlation are between an *in vivo* parameter (i.e., AUC) and the mean *in vitro* dissolution time (Skelly and Shiu, 1993). If we can establish a strong relationship between this internal response and an equivalent external laboratory measurement we may be able to avoid the risks inherent with human clinical trials. In addition *in vivo* studies can be very expensive and equivalent laboratory results offer a considerable economic advantage.

In an ideal world we would see a correlation of +1.00 or a straight line relationship between the two parameters. This represents a comparison between single point measures of outcome and rate (Figure 12.4). Using this model it is possible to perform *in vitro* laboratory exercises and predict the response on *in vivo* systems. Unfortunately we do not live in an ideal world and both of these continuous variables will contain some error or variability resulting in an $r <$ 1.00. The larger the r-value, the more meaningful the predictive abilities. As will be discussed in the next chapter, the strength of a correlation is commonly characterized by r^2, the square of the correlation coefficient. The r^2 is useful because it indicates the proportion of the variance explained by the line which best fits between the data points in the linear relationship.

In some cases *in vitro* dissolution testing can substitute for bioequivalency testing. This is particularly true for extended release dosage forms. To use dissolution data as a substitute for bioequivalency testing, one is required to have a very strong correlation. In other words, the IV/IV correlation must be highly predictive of *in vivo* performance. Thus, *in vitro* dissolution information

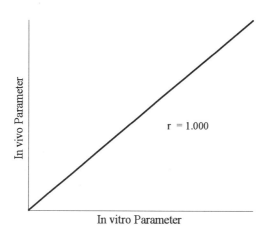

Figure 12.4   Hypothetical example of a perfect IV/IV correlation.

may be meaningful for predicting an *in vivo* response. However, there is no complete assurance that *in vitro* dissolution equals *in vivo* dissolution. One needs to be confident that for a given product tested that this IV/IV equality exists and that *in vivo* dissolution leads to absorption and absorption results in an in vivo response. The processes and potential problems associated with IV/IV correlation are beyond the scope of the book and readers interested in more information are referred to a series of papers in the book edited by Blume and Midha (1995) or the article by Amidon, et. al. (1995).

Pair-wise Correlations Involving More Than Two Variables

When there are more than just two continuous variables affecting each data point, it is possible to calculate pair-wise correlations. For example if we are evaluating three continuous variables (XYZ) on the same subjects, we can calculate the correlations (r_{xy}, r_{xz}, r_{yz}). The simplest way to evaluate the relationship between these variables is to create a table referred to as an **intercorrelation matrix**. Also called a **correlation matrix** it arranges the correlation coefficients in a systematic and orderly fashion represented by a square with an equal number of rows and columns (Table 12.7). The diagonal coefficients have a perfect relationship (r=1.00) between each variable correlated with itself. The number of cells above, or below the diagonal can be

Table 12.7 Example of an Intercorrelation Matrix

Variables	$\underline{X}$	$\underline{Y}$	$\underline{Z}$
X	r_{xx}	r_{xy}	r_{xz}
Y	r_{xy}	r_{yy}	r_{yz}
Z	r_{xz}	r_{yz}	r_{zz}

Table 12.8 Abbreviated Intercorrelation Matrix

Variables	$\underline{Y}$	$\underline{Z}$
X	r_{xy}	r_{xz}
Y	...	r_{yz}

calculated using either of the following determinants:

$$C = \frac{k(k-1)}{2}$$
Eq. 12.9

$$C = \binom{k}{2} = \frac{k!}{2!(k-2)!}$$
Eq. 12.10

where k equals the number of variables and Eq. 12.10 is simply the combination formula (discussed in Chapter 2) for paired comparisons.

The cells in the lower portion of the correlation matrix are a mirror image of the cells above the diagonal. We could simplify the matrix by discarding the diagonal cells and either the lower or upper portion of the cells and express the matrix as seen in Table 12.8.

To illustrate the use of an intercorrelation matrix, consider the data presented in Table 12.9. In this table more information is presented for the volunteer included in the earlier clinical trial. These additional data include: 1) entry laboratory values for blood urea nitrogen (BUN) and serum sodium; and study pharmacokinetic results are represented by the area under the curve (AUC).

Table 12.9 Leveled Variables from Six Subjects in a Clinical Trial

		Entry Lab Values		Results
Weight (kg)	Height (m)	BUN (mg/dl)	Sodium (mmol/l)	AUC (ng/ml)
96	1.88	22	144	806
77.7	1.80	11	141	794
100.9	1.85	17	139	815
79.0	1.77	14	143	775
73.0	1.73	15	137	782
84.5	1.83	21	140	786

Table 12.10 Layout of Correlation Matrix for Table 12.8

Variables	Weight	Height	BUN	Na	AUC
Weight(A)	1.00	r_{ab}	r_{ac}	r_{ad}	r_{ae}
Height (B)	r_{ab}	1.00	r_{bc}	r_{bd}	r_{be}
BUN (C)	r_{ac}	r_{bc}	1.00	r_{cd}	r_{ce}
Na (D)	r_{ad}	r_{bd}	r_{cd}	1.00	r_{de}
AUC (E)	r_{ae}	r_{be}	r_{ce}	r_{de}	1.00

Table 12.11 Correlation Matrix for Table 12.8

Variables	Height	BUN	Na	AUC
Weight(A)	.884	.598	.268	.873
Height(B)		.665	.495	.781
BUN (C)			.226	.334
Na (D)				.051

Using the data presented in Table 12.9, the intercorrelation matrix is shown in Table 12.10 and the actual pair-wise correlations in Table 12.11. Based on the correlation coefficients presented on this matrix and the descriptive terminology discussed earlier, the results of the multiple correlation would be: 1) a high correlation between weight and height, weight and AUC, and height and AUC; 2) a moderate correlation between weight and BUN, height and BUN, and height and sodium; 3) a low correlation exists between weight and sodium, BUN and sodium, and BUN and AUC; and 4) an almost negligible relationship between sodium and AUC.

This matrix can be extended to include the intercorrelations for any number of continuous variables. Using the correlation matrix it is possible to identify those variables which correlate most highly with each other. Unfortunately, just by inspection of the matrix its not possible to determine any joint effects of two or more variables on another variable.

Multiple Correlations

Many times in a multiple correlation we are interested in one key variable which has special importance to us and we are interested in determining how other variables influence this factor. This variable is labeled as our **criterion variable**. Other variables assist in the evaluation of this variable. These additional variables are referred to as **predictor variables** because they may have some common variance with the criterion variable; thus information about these latter variables can be used to predict information about our criterion variable. The terms **criterion variable** and **predictor variable** may be used interchangeably with dependent and independent variables respectively.

In the next chapter we will discuss regression, where the researchers are able to control at least one variable in "controlled experimental studies" and the criterion or dependent variable becomes synonymous with the **experimental variable**. In these experimental studies we will reserve the expression independent variable to variables independent of each other.

In **multiple correlation** we use techniques which allow us to evaluate how much of the variation in our criterion variable is associated with variances in a set of predictor variables. This procedure involves weighing the values associated with our respective predictor variables. The procedures are complex and tedious to computer. However, through the use of computer programs it is possible to derive these weights (usually the higher weights are associated with predictor variables with the higher common variance with our criterion variable).

In a multiple correlation we once again computer a line which fits best between our data points and compute the variability around that line. The formula for a straight line (y=a+bx) can be expanded to the following for multiple predictor variables.

$$y_i = \beta_o + \beta_1 x_{1i} + \beta_2 x_{2i} + ... + \beta_k x_{ki} + e_i \qquad \text{Eq. 12.11}$$

In this equation the e_i a common variance associated with the y-variable and β_o the point on the where a plane created by the other variables will intercept with the y-axis. The remaining βs in Eq. 12.12 are weights that are applied to each of the predictor variables, which result in composite scores that correlate most highly with the scores of our criterion variable, are referred to as **beta coefficients** or **beta weights**. These weights are a function of the correlation between the specific predictor variables and the criterion variables, as well as the correlations that exist among all the predictor variables.

The result of the mathematical manipulation, which is beyond the scope of this book, is a **multiple correlation coefficient** (R). It is the correlation resulting from the weighted predictor scores. Multiple correlations are closely related to multiple regression models. An excellent source for additional information on multiple correlation is presented by Kachigan (1991, pp.147-153). Others sources would include Zar (1984, pp.328-338) and Daniel (1978, pp.325-327).

Partial Correlations

An alternative method for the evaluation of multiple correlations is to calculate a **partial correlation** that shows the correlation between two continuous variables, while removing the effects of any other continuous variables. The simplest type of partial correlation is to extract the common effects of one variable from the relationship between two other variables of interest:

$$r_{yx,z} = \frac{r_{yx} - (r_{xz})(r_{yz})}{\sqrt{(1 - r_{xz}^2)(1 - r_{yz}^2)}}$$
                        Eq. 12.12

where $r_{xy,z}$ is the correlation between variables x and y, eliminating the effect of variable z. This formula can be slightly modified to evaluate the correlations for the other two combinations (XZ and YZ). In this formula all three paired correlations must be calculated first and then placed into Equation 12.12.

As an example of a partial correlation for three continuous variables, assume that only the first two columns and fifth column from Table 12.9 were of interest to the principle investigator involved in the clinical trial and that the researcher is interested in the correlation between the AUC and the weight, removing the effect that height might have on the results. The partial correlation would be as follows:

$$r_{ae,b} = \frac{r_{ae} - (r_{ab})(r_{be})}{\sqrt{(1 - r_{ab}^2)(1 - r_{be}^2)}}$$

$$r_{ae,b} = \frac{.873 - (.884)(.781)}{\sqrt{(1 - (.884)^2)(1 - (.781)^2)}} = \frac{.183}{.292} = .627$$

Therefore, we see a moderate correlation between AUC and weight when we control the influence of height. In other words, what we have accomplished is to determine the relationship (r = 0.63) between our two key variables (AUC and weight) while holding a third variable (height) constant. Is this a significant relationship? We can test the relationship by modifying of t-statistic which was used to compare only two dependent variables.

$$t_{yx.z} = \frac{r_{yx.z}\sqrt{n - k - 1}}{\sqrt{1 - (r_{yx.z})^2}}$$ Eq. 12.13

In this case, k represents the number of variables being evaluated which might influence the outcome in against the y-variable. In our example, k equal 2 for variables x and z. Decision rule is to reject the null hypotheses of no correlation if t is greater the critical t-value the n-k-1 degrees of freedom. In t-conversion to evaluate the significance of $r = 0.63$ the critical value would be $t_3(.975) = 2.78$ and the calculations would be as follows:

$$t_{yx.z} = \frac{(.627)\sqrt{6 - 2 - 1}}{\sqrt{1 - (.627)^2}} = \frac{1.086}{0.779} = 1.394$$

Would fail to reject the null hypothesis and conclude that there is no significant correlation between the AUC and weight excluding the influence of height.

The partial correlation can be expanded to control for more than one additional continuous variable.

Non-linear Correlations

For nonlinear correlations the best measure of a relationship is the **correlation ratio**. This **eta-statistic** (η) can be used when data tend to be curvilinear in their relationship. Based on visual inspection the test data is divided into categories, at least seven, but no more than 14 categories. These categories represent clusters of data with observable breaking points in the data. If there are fewer than seven categories the eta-statistic may not be sensitive to the curvilinear relationship. The statistic is based on a comparison of the differences, on the y-axis, between observed data points and their category mean and the total mean for all of the observations:

$$\eta = \sqrt{1 - \frac{\Sigma(y_i - \overline{Y_c})^2}{\Sigma(y_i - \overline{Y_t})^2}} \qquad \text{Eq. 12.14}$$

where y_i represents the data point, $\overline{Y}_c$ is the mean for the category and $\overline{Y}_t$ is the mean for all of the y-observations.

If there is a nonlinear relationship, the traditional correlation coefficient tends to underestimate the strength of this type of relationship. For example consider the relationship presented in Figure 12.5 where the data appears to curve. Calculation of a traditional correlation coefficient (Eq. 12.4) produces an $r = 0.883$. In this case the total mean for all the observations on the y-axis is $\overline{Y}_t = 20.25$. Calculation of the η is based on the data in Table 12.12.

$$\eta = \sqrt{1 - \frac{15.6167}{4140.50}} = \sqrt{0.9962} = 0.9981$$

Note that η is larger than r.

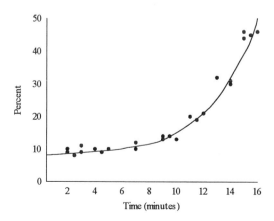

Figure 12.5 Graphic of a curvilinear relationship.

Table 12.12 Sample Data Comparing Time and Percent Response

x (time)	y (%)	$\overline{Y}_c$	$(y-\overline{Y}_c)$	$(y-\overline{Y}_c)^2$	$(y-\overline{Y}_t)$	$(y-\overline{Y}_t)^2$
2	9	9.40	-0.40	0.16	-11.25	126.5625
2	10		0.60	0.36	-10.25	105.0625
2.5	8		-1.40	1.96	-12.25	150.0625
3	9		-0.40	0.16	-11.25	126.5625
3	11		1.60	2.56	-9.25	85.5625
4	10	9.67	0.33	0.1089	-10.25	105.0625
4.5	9		-0.67	0.4489	-11.25	126.5625
5	10		0.33	0.1089	-10.25	105.0625
7	10	11.00	-1.00	1.00	-10.25	105.0625
7	12		1.00	1.00	-8.25	68.0625
9	13	13.50	-0.50	0.25	-7.25	52.5625
9	14		0.50	0.25	-6.25	39.0625
9.5	14		0.50	0.25	-6.25	39.0625
10	13		-0.50	0.25	-7.25	52.5625
11	20	20.00	0.00	0.00	-0.25	0.0625
11.5	19		-1.00	1.00	-1.25	1.5625
12	21		1.00	1.00	0.75	0.5625
13	32	31.00	1.00	1.00	11.75	138.0625
14	30		-1.00	1.00	9.75	95.0625
14	31		0.00	0.00	10.75	115.5625
15	44	45.25	-1.25	1.5625	23.75	564.0625
15	46		0.75	0.5625	25.75	663.0625
15.5	45		-0.25	0.0625	24.75	612.5625
16	46		0.75	0.5625	25.75	663.0625
		$\Sigma =$	0	15.6167	0	4140.5000

References

"Bioequivalency requirements and in vivo bioavailability procedures" Federal Register 42: 1621-1653 (1977).

Amidon, G.L., et al. (1995). "A theoretical basis for a biopharmaceutic drug classification: the correlation of in vitro drug product dissolution and in vivo bioavailability." Pharmaceutical Research 12:413-420.

Blume, H.H. and Midha, K.K. eds. (1995). Bio-International 2: Bioavailability, Bioequivalence and Pharmacokinetic Studies, Medpharm Scientific Publishers, Stuttgart, pp. 247-318.

Daniel, W.W. (1978). Biostatistics: A Foundation for Analysis in the Health Sciences, John Wiley and Sons, New York, pp.282, 325-327.

Guilford, J.P. (1956). Fundamental Statistics in Psychology and Education, McGraw-Hill, New York, p.145

Rowntree, D. (1981). Statistics Without Tears: A Primer for Non-Mathematicians, Charles Scribner's Sons, New York, p. 170.

Kachigan, S.K. (1991). Multivariate Statistical Analysis, Second Edition, Radius Press, New York, , pp.147-153.

Skelly, J.P. and Shiu, G.F. (1993). "In vitro/in vivo correlations in biopharmaceutics: scientific and regulatory implications" European Journal of Drug Metabolism and Pharmacokinetics 18:121-129.

Zar, J.H. (1984). Biostatistical Analysis, 2nd ed., Prentice Hall, Englewood Cliffs, NJ, pp.328-338.

Suggested Supplemental Readings

Bolton, S. (1997). Pharmaceutical Statistics: Practical and Clinical Applications, Marcel Dekker, New York, pp. 249-257.

Cutler, D.J. (1995). "In Vitro/In Vivo Correlation and Statistics" Bio-International 2: Bioavailability, Bioequivalence and Pharmacokinetic Studies, Blume, H.H. and Midha, K.K. eds., Medpharm Scientific Publishers, Stuttgart, pp. 281-289.

Havilcek, L.L. and Crain, R.D. (1988). <u>Practical Statistics for the Physical Sciences</u>, American Chemical Society, Washington, DC, pp. 83-93, 106-108.

Example Problems

1. Two different scales are used to measure patient anxiety levels upon admission to a hospital. Method A is an established test instrument, while Method B (which has been developed by the researchers) is a quicker and easier instrument to administer. Is there a correlation between the two measures?

Method A	Method B	Method A	Method B
55	90	52	97
66	117	36	78
46	94	44	84
77	124	55	112
57	105	53	102
59	115	67	112
70	125	72	130
57	97		

2. Two drugs (A and B) are commonly used together to stabilize patients after stokes and the dosing for each is individualized. Listed below are the dosages administered to eight patients randomly selected from admission records at a specific hospital over a six- month period. Did the dosage of either drug result in a stronger correlation with shortened length of stay (LOS) in the institution?

Patient	LOS (days)	Drug A (mg/Kg)	Drug B (mcg/Kg)
1	3	2.8	275
2	2	4.0	225
3	4	1.5	250
4	3	3.0	225
5	2	3.7	300
6	4	2.0	225
7	4	2.4	275
8	3	3.5	275

3. It is believed that two assay methods will produce identical results for analyzing a specific drug. Various dilutions are assayed using both the

currently accepted method (GS) and the proposed alternative (ALT). Based on the results listed below, does a high correlation exist?

Method GS	Method ALT	Method GS	Method ALT
90.1	89.8	60.2	61.0
85.2	85.1	35.5	34.8
79.7	80.2	24.9	24.8
74.3	75.0	19.6	21.1

4. A random sample of twelve students graduating from a School of Pharmacy were administered an examination to determine retention of information received during classes. The test contained four sections covering pharmacy law, pharmaceutical calculations (math), pharmacology (p'cology) and medicinal chemistry (medchem). Listed below are the results of the tests.

Student	Law	Math	P'cology	Medchem	Total
001	23	18	22	20	83
002	22	20	21	18	81
003	25	21	25	17	88
004	20	19	18	20	77
005	24	23	24	14	85
006	23	22	22	20	87
007	24	20	24	15	83
008	20	17	15	22	74
009	22	19	21	23	85
010	24	21	23	19	87
011	23	20	21	19	83
012	21	21	20	21	83

Create a correlation matrix to compare the results and relationships between the various sections and total test score. Which of the two sections most strongly correlated together? Which section has the greatest correlation with the total test score?

Answers to Problems

1. Comparison of two different scales to measure patient anxiety levels.
   Variables: continuous (two measurement scales)

a. Pearson Product Moment

Method A - variable x - mean = 57.7
Method B - variable y - mean = 105.5

x	y	x-$\overline{X}$	y-$\overline{Y}$	(x-$\overline{X}$)(y-$\overline{Y}$)	(x-$\overline{X}$)^2	(y-$\overline{Y}$)^2
55	90	-2.7	-15.5	41.85	7.29	240.25
66	117	8.3	11.5	95.45	68.89	132.25
46	94	-11.7	-11.5	134.55	136.89	132.25
77	124	19.3	18.5	357.05	372.49	342.25
57	105	-0.7	-0.5	0.35	0.49	0.25
59	115	1.3	9.5	12.35	1.69	90.25
70	125	12.3	19.5	239.85	151.29	380.25
57	97	-0.7	-8.5	5.95	0.49	72.25
52	97	-5.7	-8.5	48.45	32.49	72.25
36	78	-21.7	-27.5	596.75	470.89	756.25
44	84	-13.7	-21.5	294.55	187.69	462.25
55	112	-2.7	6.5	-17.55	7.29	42.25
53	102	-4.7	-3.5	16.45	22.09	12.25
67	112	+9.3	6.5	60.45	86.49	42.25
72	130	+14.3	24.5	350.35	204.49	600.25
				2236.85	1750.95	3377.75

Calculations:

$$r = \frac{\Sigma(x-\overline{X})(y-\overline{Y})}{\sqrt{\Sigma(x-\overline{X})^2(y-\overline{Y})^2}} = \frac{2236.85}{\sqrt{(1750.95)(3377.75)}} = 0.92$$

b. Computational formula (data in Table 12.13):

Calculations:

$$r = \frac{15(93571)-(866)(1582)}{\sqrt{15(51748)-(866)^2}\sqrt{15(170226)-(1582)^2}}$$

$$r = \frac{1403565-1370012}{(162.06)(225.09)} = \frac{33553}{36478.08} = 0.92$$

Table 12.13 Data for Problem 1, Computational Formula

x	y	x²	y²	xy
55	90	3025	8100	4950
66	117	4356	13689	7722
46	94	2116	8836	4324
77	124	5929	15376	9548
57	105	3249	11025	5985
59	115	3481	13225	6785
70	125	4900	15625	8750
57	97	3249	9409	5529
52	97	2704	9409	5044
36	78	1296	6084	2808
44	84	1936	7056	3696
55	112	3025	12544	6160
53	102	2809	10404	5406
67	112	4489	12544	7504
72	130	5184	16900	9360
$\sum=$ 866	1582	51748	170226	93571

c. Conversion to t-statistic:

Hypothesis: H_0: $r_{xy} = 0$

H_1: $r_{xy} \neq 0$

Decision Rule: With $\alpha = 0.05$, reject H_0 if $t > t_{13}(.975) = 2.16$.

Calculations:

$$t = \frac{r\sqrt{n-2}}{\sqrt{1-r^2}} = \frac{.92\sqrt{15-2}}{\sqrt{1-(.92)^2}} = \frac{3.32}{0.39} = 8.51$$

Decision: With $t > 2.16$, is to reject H_0 and conclude there is a significant relationship between Method A and Method B.

2. Comparison of two drugs and length of stay at a specific hospital.
Variables: continuous (two measurement scales)

Calculation of the three paired correlations produced the following intercorrelation matrix:

Variables	LOS	Drug A	Drug B
LOS	...	-0.923	-0.184
Drug A	...	...	+0.195
Drug B	...	...	...

The partial correlation for length of stay vs. Drug A is:

$$r_{la,b} = \frac{r_{la} - (r_{lb})(r_{ab})}{\sqrt{(1 - r_{lb}^2)(1 - r_{ab}^2)}} = \frac{-0.923 - (-0.184)(+0.195)}{\sqrt{(1 - (-0.184)^2)(1 - (0.195)^2)}} = 0.920$$

The partial correlation for length of stay vs. Drug B is:

$$r_{lb,a} = \frac{r_{lb} - (r_{la})(r_{ab})}{\sqrt{(1 - r_{la}^2)(1 - r_{ab}^2)}} = \frac{-0.184 - (-0.923)(+0.195)}{\sqrt{(1 - (-0.923)^2)(1 - (0.195)^2)}} = -0.011$$

Evaluation of the partial correlation for length of stay vs. Drug A:

Decision rule is with $\alpha = 0.05$, reject H_0 if $|t| > t_5(.975) = 2.57$.

$$t_{la.b} = \frac{r_{la.b}\sqrt{n - k - 1}}{\sqrt{1 - (r_{la.b})^2}}$$

$$t_{yx.z} = \frac{(-0.92)\sqrt{8 - 2 - 1}}{\sqrt{1 - (-0.92)^2}} = \frac{-2.057}{0.392} = -5.24$$

Decision: There is a strong correlation, statistically significant with 95% confidence, between the length of stay and administration of Drug A, but Drug B have very little influence on the length of stay.

3. Comparison of two analytical procedures on different concentrations of a drug.
Variables: continuous (two measurement scales)

Method GS	Method ALT			
x	y	x^2	y^2	xy
90.1	89.8	8,118.01	8,064.04	8,090.98
85.2	85.1	7,259.04	7,242.01	7,250.52
79.7	80.2	6,352.09	6,432.04	6,391.94
74.3	75.0	5,520.49	5,625.00	5,572.50
60.2	61.0	3,624.04	3,721.00	3,672.20
35.5	34.8	1,260.25	1,211.04	1,235.40
24.9	24.8	620.01	615.04	617.52
19.6	21.1	384.16	445.21	413.56
469.5	471.8	33,138.09	33,355.38	33,244.62

Calculations:

$$r = \frac{n\sum xy - \sum x \sum y}{\sqrt{n\sum x^2 - (\sum x)^2}\ \sqrt{n\sum y^2 - (\sum y)^2}}$$

$$r = \frac{8(33,244.62) - (469.5)(471.8)}{\sqrt{8(33,138.09) - (469.5)^2}\ \sqrt{8(33,355.38) - (471.8)^2}}$$

$$r = \frac{265,956.96 - 221,510.1}{(211.36)(210.35)} = \frac{44,446.86}{44,459.58} = +0.9997$$

Conclusion: A very strong correlation between methods GS and ALT.

4. Comparison of multiple test results:
   Variables: continuous (five measurement scales)

   Example of correlation coefficient for scores on law and pharmaceutical calculations sections (Table 12.14).

   Calculations:

$$r = \frac{n\sum xy - \sum x \sum y}{\sqrt{n\sum x^2 - (\sum x)^2}\ \sqrt{n\sum y^2 - (\sum y)^2}}$$

Table 12.14 Data for Problem 4, Computational Formula

Law (x)	Calculations (y)	x^2	y^2	xy
23	18	529	324	414
22	20	484	400	440
25	21	625	441	525
20	19	400	361	380
24	23	576	529	552
23	22	529	484	506
24	20	576	400	480
20	17	400	289	340
22	19	484	361	418
24	21	576	441	504
23	20	529	400	460
21	21	441	441	441
271	241	6149	4871	5460

$$r = \frac{12(5460) - (271)(241)}{\sqrt{12(6149) - (271)^2} \sqrt{12(4871) - (241)^2}} = \frac{209}{358.8} = +0.582$$

Conclusion: A moderate correlation between law and calculation scores.

Correlation Matrix:

	Law	Math	P'cology	Medchem	Total
Law	1.000	0.582	0.943	-0.674	0.832
Math	0.582	1.000	0.678	-0.591	0.712
P'cology	0.943	0.678	1.000	-0.689	0.877
Medchem	-0.674	-0.591	-0.689	1.000	-0.324
Total	0.832	0.712	0.877	-0.324	1.000

Results: Strongest correlation between two sections is +0.943 between law and pharmacology.

13

Linear Regression

Unlike the correlation coefficient, regression analysis requires at least one independent variable. Where correlation describes pair-wise relationships between continuous variables, linear regression is a statistical method to evaluate how one or more independent (predictor) variables influence outcomes for one continuous dependent (response) variable through a linear relationship. A regression line is computed that best fits between the data points. If a linear relationship is established, the independent variable can be used to predict the corresponding value on the dependent variable. For example a person's weight can be used to predict body surface area. The strength of the relationship between the two variables can be determined by calculating the amount of variance that is explained by the regression line.

Both linear regression and correlation are similar, in that both describe the strength of the relationship between two or more continuous variables. However, with linear regression, also termed **regression analysis**, a relationship is established between the two variables and a response for the dependent variable can be made based on a given value for the independent variable. For correlation, two dependent variables can be compared to determine if a relationship exists between them. Similarly, correlation is concerned with the strength of the relationship between two continuous variables. In regression analysis, or **experimental associations**, researchers control the values of at least one of the variables and assign objects at random to different levels of these variables. Where correlation simply described the strength and direction of the relationship, regression analysis provides a method for describing the nature of the relationship between two or more continuous variables.

The correlation coefficient can be very useful in exploratory research where the investigator is interested in the relationship between two or more continuous variables. One of the disadvantages of the correlation coefficient is that it is not very useful for predicting the value of y from a value of x, or vice versa. Because, as seen in the previous chapter, the correlation coefficient (r) is the extent of the linear relationship between x and y. However, there may be a close correlation between the two variables that are based on a relationship other than a straight line (for example, Figure 12.3). The processes of correlation and regression are closely related with similar calculations based upon the same sums and sums of squares. Therefore, if an independent variable is involved, calculating both is useful because the correlation coefficient can support the interpretation associated with regression. This chapter will focus primarily with simple linear regression, where these is only one independent or predictor variable.

There are several assumptions associated with the linear regression model. First, values the x-axis, which represent the independent variable are "fixed". This nonramdom variable is predetermined by the researcher so that responses on the y-axis are measured at only predetermined points on the x-axis. Because the researcher controls the x-axis it is assumed that these measures are without error. Second, for each value on the x-axis there is a subpopulation of values for the corresponding dependent variable on the y-axis. For any inferential statistics or hypothesis testing, as discussed later, it is assumed that these subpopulations are normally distributed. For data which may not be normally distributed, for example AUC or C_{max} measures in bioavailability studies, log transformations may be required to convert such positively skewed data to normal distributions. Coupled with the assumption of normality is homogeneity of variance, in that it is assumed that the variances for all the subpopulations are approximately equal. Third, it is assumed that these subpopulations have a linear relationship and that a straight line can be drawn between them. The formula for this line is:

$$\mu_{y/x} = \alpha + \beta x \qquad \text{Eq. 13.1}$$

where $\mu_{y/x}$ is mean for any given subpopulation for an x-value for the predictor independent variable. The terms α and β represent the true population y-intercept and slope for the regression line. Unfortunately, we do not know these population parameters and must estimate these by creating a line which is our best estimate based on our sample data.

The Regression Line

As seen above, linear regression is involved with the characteristics of a straight line or **linear function**. This line can be estimated from sample data. Similar to correlation, a graph offers an excellent method for visualizing the relationship between the continuous variables. In the simple regression design there are only two variables (x and y). As mentioned in the previous chapter, the x-axis, or abscissa, represents the independent variable and the y-axis, the ordinate, is the dependent outcome. The scatter plot presented in Figure 13.1 shows a typical representation of these variables with y on the vertical axis and x on the horizontal axis. In this case x is a specific amount of drug (mcg) administered to mice, with y representing some measurable physiological response.

The first step in a linear regression analysis is to draw a straight line which best fits between the points. The slope of the line and its intercept of the y axis are then used for the regression calculation as introduced in the previous chapter. The general equation (Eq. 12.5) for a straight line is:

$$y = a + bx$$

In this formula, y is a value on the vertical axis, x is a corresponding value on the horizontal axis, a indicates the point where the line crosses the vertical axis, and b represents the amount by which the line rises for each increase in x, (the slope of the line). A second method for defining these values is that a is the value on the y-axis where $x=0$ and b is the change in the y-value (the response value) for every unit increase in the x-value (the predictor variable).

Unfortunately, our estimate of the straight line is based on sample data and therefore subject to sampling error. Therefore we need to modify our definition of the regression line to the following, where e is an error term associated with our sampling.

$$y = \alpha + \beta x + e \qquad \text{Eq. 13.2}$$

Once again, it is assumed that the e's associated with each subpopulation are normally distributed with a variances approximately equal.

Our best estimate of the true population regression line, would be the straight line which we can draw through our sample data. However, if asked to draw this line using a straight edge, it is unlikely that any two people would draw exactly the same line to best fit these points. Thus, a variety of slopes and intercepts could be approximated. There are in fact an infinite number of possible lines, $y=a+bx$, which could be drawn between our data points. How

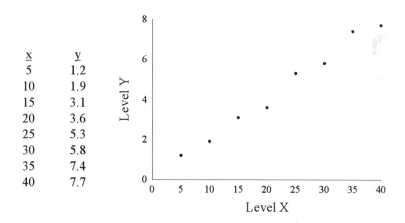

x	y
5	1.2
10	1.9
15	3.1
20	3.6
25	5.3
30	5.8
35	7.4
40	7.7

Figure 13.1 Simple example of data points for two continuous variables.

can we select the "best" line of all the possible lines that can pass through these data points?

The **least-squares line** is the line which best describes the linear relationship between the independent and dependent variables. The data points are usually scattered on either side of this straight line that fits best between the points on the scatter diagram. Also called the **regression line**, it represents a line from which the smallest sum of squared differences are observed between the observed (x,y) coordinates and the line (x,y) coordinates along the y axis (sum of the squared vertical deviations). In other words, this **'best fit'** line represents that line for which the sum of squares of the distances from the points in the scatter diagram to the regression line, in the direction of the y-variable is smallest. The calculation of the line which best fits between the data points, is presesented below. The slope of this line (Eq. 12.6) is:

$$b = \frac{n\sum xy - (\sum x)(\sum y)}{n\sum x^2 - (\sum x)^2}$$

Data to solve this equation can be generated in a table similar to that used for the correlation coefficient (Table 12.4).

The greater the change in y for a constant change in x, the steeper the slope of the line. With the calculated slope of the line which best fits the observed points in the scatter diagram, it is possible to calculate the y-intercept

Table 13.1 Data Manipulation of Regression Line for Figure 13.1

	x	y	x^2	y^2	xy
	5	1.2	25	1.44	6.00
	10	1.9	100	3.61	19.00
	15	3.1	225	9.61	46.50
n=8	20	3.6	400	12.96	72.00
	25	5.3	625	28.09	132.50
	30	5.8	900	33.64	174.00
	35	7.4	1225	54.76	259.00
	40	7.7	1600	59.29	308.00
$\Sigma =$	180	36.0	5100	203.40	1017.00

using Eq.12.7 (that point where the x-value is zero):

$$a = \frac{\Sigma y - b \Sigma x}{n}$$

An alternative approach to the scatter diagram is to display the information in a table. The regression line can be calculated for the data points in Figure 13.1 by arranging the data in tabular format as present in Table 13.1. Similar to the manipulation of data for the correlation coefficient, each x-value and y-value are squared, and the product is calculated for the x- and y-value at each data point. These five columns are then summed to produce a Σx, Σy, Σx^2, Σy^2, and Σxy. Note that Σy^2 is not required for determining the regression line, but will be used later in additional calculations required for the linear regression model. Using the results in Table 13.1, the computations for the slope and y-intercept would be as follows:

$$b = \frac{8(1017) - (180)(36)}{8(5100) - (180)^2} = \frac{8136 - 6480}{40800 - 32400} = \frac{1656}{8400} = 0.197$$

$$a = \frac{36 - 0.197(180)}{8} = \frac{36 - 35.46}{8} = \frac{0.54}{8} = 0.0675$$

Based on these data, the regression line is presented in Figure 13.2, where the slope is in a positive direction +0.197 (as values of x increase, values of y will

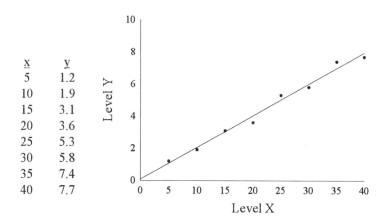

x	y
5	1.2
10	1.9
15	3.1
20	3.6
25	5.3
30	5.8
35	7.4
40	7.7

Figure 13.2 Regression line for two continuous variables.

also increase) and the intercept is slightly above zero (0.0675).

A quick check of the position of the regression line on the scatter diagram would be to calculate the means for both variables ($\overline{X}_x$, $\overline{X}_y$) and see if the line passes through this point. This can be checked by placing the slope, y-intercept, and $\overline{X}_x$ in the straight line equation and then determining if the y-value equals $\overline{X}_y$. In this example the mean for the abscissa is:

$$\overline{X}_x = \frac{\Sigma x}{n} = \frac{180}{8} = 22.5$$

the mean for the ordinate is:

$$\overline{X}_y = \frac{\Sigma y}{n} = \frac{36}{8} = 4.5$$

and the y-value for the mean of x is the same as the mean of y:

$$y = a + bx = 0.0675 + 0.197(22.5) = 0.0675 + 4.4325 = 4.5$$

If there is a linear relationship (a statistical procedure will be presented later to prove that the line is straight), then it is possible to determine any point on the y-axis for a given point on the x-axis using the formula for a straight line (Eq. 12.5). Mechanically we could draw a vertical line up from any point on the x-axis, where in intercepts our line we draw a horizontal line to the y-axis and read the value at that point. Mathematically we can accomplish the same result using the formula for a straight line. For example, based on the regression line calculated above, if x = 32 mcg the corresponding physiological response for the y-value would be:

$$y = a + bx = 0.0675 + (0.197)(32) = 0.0675 + 6.304 = 6.372$$

If instead the x-value is 8 mcg, the expected y-value physiological response would be:

$$y = a + bx = 0.0675 + (0.197)(8) = 0.0675 + 1.576 = 1.644$$

Note that both of these results are approximations. As will be discussed later, if we can establish a straight line relationship between the x- and y-variables, the slope of the line of best-fit will itself vary based on sampling error. Our estimate of the population slope (β) will be based on our best quest, b, plus or minus a certain deviation. This will in fact create a confidence interval around any point on our regression line and provide a range of y-values. However, for the present time the use of the straight line equation provides us with a quick estimate of the corresponding y-value for any given x-value. Conversely, for any given value on the y-axis it is possible to estimate a corresponding x-value using a modification of the previous formula for a straight line:

$$x = \frac{y-a}{b} \qquad \text{Eq. 13.3}$$

If one wishes to determine, the corresponding x-value for a physiological response of 5.0, the calculation for the appropriate dose of drug would be:

$$x = \frac{y-a}{b} = \frac{5.0 - 0.0675}{0.197} = \frac{4.9325}{0.197} = 25.04 \, mcg$$

A method for calculating whether or not a relationship between two variables is in fact linear will be discussed subsequently. Many of the relationships which are encountered in research are linear, and those that are not can often be made linear with appropriate data transformation techniques. For example, if a scatter diagram shows that a non-linear pattern is feasible, it is possible to produce a linear pattern by doing a transformation on one of the variables.

Coefficient of Determination

As the spread of the scatter dots along the vertical axis (y-axis) decreases, the precision of the estimated μ_y increases. A perfect (100%) estimate is possible only when all the dots lie on the straight regression line. The **coefficient of determination** offers one method to evaluate if the linear regression equation adequately describes the relationship. It compares the scatter of data points about the regression line with the scatter about the mean of the sample values for the dependent y-variable. Figure 13.3 shows a scattering of points about both the mean of the y-distribution ($\overline{X}_y$) and the regression line itself for part of the data presented in Figure 13.2. As discussed in Chapter 5, in normally distributed data we expect to see data vary around the mean, in this case $\overline{X}_y$. It is also possible to measure the deviation of each point (C). If the data is truly represented by the straight regression line, then a certain amount of this total variation can be explained by the deviation from the mean to the line (B). However, most data points will not fall exactly on the regression line and this deviation (A) must be caused by other sources (random error).

The coefficient of determination is calculated using the sum of the squared deviations which takes into consideration these deviations (A, B and C). In this case the total deviation equals the explained plus the unexplained deviations:

$$\Sigma(y_i - \overline{X}_y)^2 = \Sigma(y_c - \overline{X}_y)^2 + \Sigma(y_i - y_c)^2 \qquad \text{Eq. 13.4}$$

Where the total deviation is the vertical difference between the observed data point and the mean of y ($y_i - \overline{X}_y$). The explained deviation is the vertical difference between the point on the regression line and the mean of Y ($y_c - \overline{X}_y$). The unexplained deviation is the vertical difference between the observed data point and the corresponding point on the regression line ($y_i - y_c$). This vertical distances between the data points and the regression line are called **residuals**. The residuals for this example are presented in Table 13.2. With the line of best fit between the data points, the sum of the residuals should equal zero, an equal amount of deviation above and below the line. This can be a long and cumbersome calculation involving a calculation of the mean of the y-values ($\overline{X}_y$), the y-value on the regression line (y_c) for each level of the independent x-value, various differences between those values, and then summation of the various differences. A more manageable set of formulas use the sums computed in Table 13.1 to calculate the sum of squares due to linear regression:

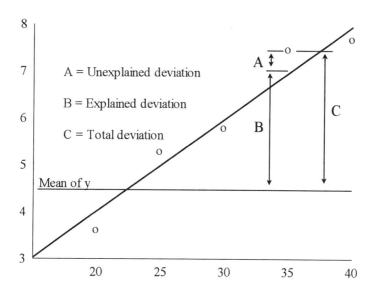

Figure 13.3 Variability of data points around the mean of the y-variable and the regression line.

$$SS_{Total} = SS_{Explained} + SS_{Un\,exp\,lained}$$ Eq. 13.5

These would produce the same results as the more time consuming formula in Equation 13.5. The sum of the total variation between the mean ($\overline{X}_y$) and each observed data point (y_i) would be the total sum of squares (SS_{total}):

$$SS_{total} = \Sigma(y_i - \overline{X}_y)^2 = \Sigma y^2 - \frac{(\Sigma y)^2}{n}$$ Eq. 13.6

The variability explained by the regression line of the deviations between the mean ($\overline{X}_y$) and the line (y_c) is the explained sum of squares ($SS_{explained}$):

$$SS_{explained} = \Sigma(y_c - \overline{X}_y)^2 = b^2 \cdot \left[\Sigma x^2 - \frac{(\Sigma x)^2}{n}\right]$$ Eq. 13.7

Table 13.2 Residuals for Data Points from the Regression Line

X	y	y_c	Residual
5	1.2	1.0525	- 0.1475
10	1.7	2.0375	+0.1375
15	3.1	3.0225	- 0.0775
20	3.6	4.0075	+0.4075
25	5.3	4.9925	- 0.3075
30	5.8	5.9925	+0.1775
35	7.4	6.9625	- 0.4327
40	7.7	7.9475	+0.2475
		$\Sigma =$	0

The remaining, unexplained deviation between the regression line (y_c) and the data points (y_i) is the unexplained sum of squares ($SS_{unexplained}$). This can be computed by subtracting the explained variability for the total dispersion:

$$SS_{unexplained} = SS_{total} - SS_{explained} \qquad \text{Eq. 13.8}$$

Calculation for these sums of squares for the previous example (Figure 13.2) would be:

$$SS_{total} = \Sigma y^2 - \frac{(\Sigma y)^2}{n} = 203.4 - \frac{(36)^2}{8} = 41.40$$

$$SS_{explained} = b^2 \cdot \left[\Sigma x^2 - \frac{(\Sigma x)^2}{n} \right] = (0.197)^2 \left[5100 - \frac{(180)^2}{8} \right] = 40.75$$

$$SS_{unexplained} = SS_{total} - SS_{explained} = 41.40 - 40.75 = 0.65$$

The sum of squares due to linear regression is synonymous with the explained sum of squares and measures the total variability of the observed values that are associated with the linear relationship. The coefficient of determination (r^2) is the proportion of variability accounted for by the sum of squares due to linear regression.

$$r^2 = \frac{SS_{explained}}{SS_{total}} = \frac{b^2 \cdot \left[\sum x^2 - \frac{(\sum x)^2}{n} \right]}{\sum y^2 - \frac{(\sum y)^2}{n}}$$

Eq. 13.9

In our previous example the coefficient of determination would be:

$$r^2 = \frac{(0.197)^2 \cdot \left[5100 - \frac{(180)^2}{8} \right]}{203.4 - \frac{(36)^2}{8}} = \frac{40.75}{41.40} = .984$$

The coefficient of determination measures the exactness of fit of the regression equation to the observed values of y. In other words, the coefficient of determination identifies how much variation in one variable can be explained by variations in the second. The rest of the variability $(1-r^2)$ is explained by other factors, most likely unidentifiable by the researcher. In our example the computed r^2 is .984, this indicates that approximately 98% of the total variation is explained by the linear regression model. If the r^2 is large, the regression equation accounts for a great proportion of the total variability in the observed values.

Similar to the correlation coefficient, the coefficient of determination is a measure of how closely the observations fall on a straight line. In fact, the square root of the coefficient of determination is the correlation coefficient:

$$r = \sqrt{r^2}$$

Eq. 13.10

In this example the correlation coefficient is the square root of 0.984 or 0.992. As proof of this relationship the correlation coefficient is calculated using Equation 12.4 and the data in Table 13.1:

$$r = \frac{8(1017) - (180)(36)}{\sqrt{8(5100) - (180)^2} \sqrt{8(203.4) - (36)^2}} = \frac{1656}{1668.94} = 0.992$$

This linear correlation (correlation coefficient) can be strongly influenced by a few extreme values. One rule of thumb is to first plot the data points on graph paper and examine the points visually before reporting the linear correlation.

An opposite approach would be to consider the correlation coefficient as a measure of the extent of linear correlation. If all the data points fall exactly on a straight line, the two variables would be considered to be perfectly correlated ($r = +1.00$ or -1.00). Remember that the correlation coefficient measures the extent to which the relationship between two continuous variables is explained by a straight line.

Also termed the **common variance**, r^2 represents that proportion of variance in the criterion (dependent) variable that is accounted for by variance in the predictor (independent) variable. As the coefficient of determination increases we are able to account for more of the variation in the dependent variable with values predicted from the regression equation. Obviously, the amount of error associated with the prediction of criterion variable from the predictor variable will decrease as the degree of correlation between the two variables increases. Therefore, the r^2 is a useful measure when predicting value for one variable from a second variable.

ANOVA Table

Once we have established that there is a strong positive or negative relationship between the two continuous variables, we can establish the type of relationship (linear, curvilinear, etc.). This final decision on the acceptability of the linear regression model is based on an objective ANOVA test where a statistical calculation will determine whether or not the data is best represented by a straight line:

$$H_0: \text{ X and Y are not linearly related}$$
$$H_1: \text{ X and Y are linearly related}$$

In this case the ANOVA statistic is:

$$F = \frac{Mean\ Square\ Linear\ Regression}{Mean\ Square\ Residual} \qquad \text{Eq. 13.11}$$

where the amount of variability explained by the regression line is placed in the numerator and the unexplained residual, or error, variability is the denominator. Obviously as the amount of explained variability increases the F-value will increase and it becomes more likely that the result will be a rejection of the null hypothesis in favor of the alternative that a straight line relationship exists. The decision rule is, with $\alpha = 0.05$, reject H_0 if $F > F_{1,n-2}(1-\alpha)$. The numerator degrees of freedom is *one* for the regression line and the denominator degrees of freedom is n-2, where n equals the number of data points. Table B11 in Appendix B is a expanded version of Table B5 from the same Appendix for one as the numerator degrees of freedom and a larger finite set of denominator degrees of freedom. Similar to the one-way ANOVA, the computed F is compared with the critical F-value in Table B11, and if it is greater than the critical value, the null hypothesis that no linear relationship exists between x and y is rejected. The ANOVA table is calculated as follows:

Source of Variation	SS	df	MS	F
Linear Regression	Explained	1	$\frac{SS_{Explained}}{1}$	$\frac{MS_{Explained}}{MS_{Unexplained}}$
Residual	Unexplained	n-2	$\frac{SS_{Unexplained}}{n-2}$	
Total	Total	n-1		

As an example for linear regression, assume that twelve healthy male volunteers received a single dose of various strengths of an experimental anticoagulant. As the primary investigators, we wished to determine if there is a significant relationship between the dosage and corresponding prothrombin times. In this case the independent variable is the dosage of the drug administered to the volunteers and the dependent variable is their response, measured by their prothrombin times. Results of the study are presented in Table 13.3. The hypotheses in this case are:

H_0:   Dose (x) and Pro-time (y) are not linearly related
H_1:   Dose and Pro-time are linearly related

and the decision rule with $\alpha = .05$, is to reject H_0 if $F > F_{1,10}(.95)$, which is 4.96. The tabular arrangement of the data needed to calculate an ANOVA table is presented in Table 13.4. First the slopes and y-intercept for the regression line would be:

$$b = \frac{n \sum xy - (\sum x)(\sum y)}{n \sum x^2 - (\sum x)^2}$$

$$b = \frac{12(46315) - (2430)(228)}{12(495650) - (2430)^2} = \frac{1740}{42900} = 0.0406$$

Table 13.3 Prothrombin Times for Volunteers Receiving Various Doses of an Anticoagulant

Subject	Dose (mg)	Prothrombin Time (seconds)	Subject	Dose (mg)	Prothrombin Time (seconds)
1	200	20	7	220	19
2	180	18	8	175	17
3	225	20	9	215	20
4	205	19	10	185	19
5	190	19	11	210	19
6	195	18	12	230	20

Table 13.4 Summations of Data Required for Linear Regression

Subject	Dose (mg)	Time (seconds)	x^2	y^2	xy
8	175	17	30625	289	2975
2	180	18	32400	324	3240
10	185	19	34225	361	3515
5	190	19	36100	361	3610
6	195	18	38025	324	3510
4	205	19	42025	361	3895
11	210	19	44100	361	3990
9	215	20	46225	400	4300
7	220	19	48400	361	4180
3	225	20	50625	400	4500
12	230	20	52900	400	4600
$\Sigma =$	2430	228	495650	4342	46315

$$a = \frac{\Sigma y - b \Sigma x}{n}$$

$$a = \frac{228 - (0.0406)(2430)}{12} = \frac{129.34}{12} = 10.79$$

In this case there would a gradual positive slope to the line (as dosage increases, the prothrombin time increases) and the predicted y-intercept would be 10.79 seconds. The total variability around the mean prothrombin time is:

$$SS_T = \sum y^2 - \frac{(\sum y)^2}{n}$$

$$SS_T = 4342 - \frac{(228)^2}{12} = 10.0$$

of which the regression line explains a certain amount of variation:

$$SS_E = b^2 \cdot \left[\sum x^2 - \frac{(\sum x)^2}{n} \right]$$

$$SS_E = (0.0406)^2 \left[495650 - \frac{(2430)^2}{12} \right] = 5.88$$

However, an additional amount of variation remains unexplained:

$$SS_U = SS_T - SS_E = 10.0 - 5.88 = 4.12$$

For this particular example the coefficient of determination is:

$$r^2 = \frac{SS_{explained}}{SS_{total}} = \frac{5.88}{10} = 0.588$$

meaning that approximately 59% of the total variability is explained by the straight line which we draw between the data points. The ANOVA table would be:

Source	SS	df	MS	F
Linear Regression	5.88	1	5.88	14.27
Residual	4.12	10	0.412	
Total	10.00	11		

The resultant F-value is greater than the critical value of 4.96, therefore we would reject H_0 and conclude that a linear relationship exists between the dosage of the new anticoagulant and the volunteers' prothrombin times.

Once the type of relationship is established, it is possible to predict values for the dependent variable (prothrombin time) based on the corresponding value for the independent variable (dose). Obviously, the accuracy of any prediction, based on a regression line, depends on the strength of the relationship between the two variables (the higher coefficient of determination the better our predictive abilities). Use of the regression analysis enables the researcher to determine the nature (i.e., linear) and strength of the relationship, and allows for predictions to be made.

It is important to realize that the linear regression line, which fit best between our data points, can not be extrapolated beyond the largest or smallest point for our observations. Using the ANOVA table we can reject the null hypothesis and conclude with 95% confidence that there is a linear relationship. However, be cannot extend these assumption beyond the extremes in the data. For example, in our previous example we identified a linear relationship between the dose of the experimental anticoagulant and volunteer prothrombin times. This linear relationship is illustrated by the solid line in Figure 13.4. What we don't know is what will happen beyond 230 mg, the highest dose. Could a linear relationship continue (A), might there be an acceleration in the anticoagulant effect (B), a leveling of response (C) or an actual decrease in prothromin time with increased doses (D)? Correspondingly, we do not know what the relationship is for responses at dosages less than 175 mg of the experimental anticoagulant. Thus, if more data were available beyond the last data point, it might be found that the regression line would level out or decrease sharply. Therefore, the regression line and the regression equation apply only within the range of the x-values actually observed in the data.

Confidence Intervals and Hypothesis Testing for the Population Slope (β)

The correlation coefficient (r) and slope of the line (b) are descriptive statistics that describe different aspects of the relationship between two continuous variables. When either r or b equal zero, there is no linear correlation and variables x and y can be considered independent of each other, and no mutual interdependence exists. An alternative test to our previously discussed ANOVA test for linearity, is a null hypothesis that no linear relationship exists between two variables. This is based on the population slope (β) of the regression line. In general, a positive ß indicates that y increases as x increases, and represents a direct linear relationship between the two variables. Conversely, a negative β indicates that values of y tend to increase as values of x decrease, and an inverse linear relationship between x and y exists.

The hypothesis under test assumes that there is no slope; therefore, a relationship between the variables does not exist:

$$H_0: \quad \beta = 0$$
$$H_1: \quad \beta \neq 0$$

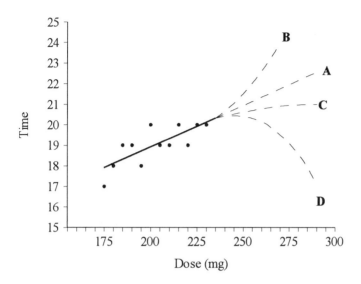

Figure 13.4 Example of the problems associated with extrapolation.

In this case we can either: 1) calculate a t-value and compare it to a critical value or 2) compute a confidence interval for the possible slopes for the population (β). The calculation of the t-value is similar to a paired t-test with an observed difference in the numerator and an error term in the denominator:

$$t = \frac{b - \beta_0}{S_b}$$ Eq. 13.12

Based on the null hypothesis, β_0 is an expected outcome of zero or no slope and S_b is an error term that is defined below.

Calculation of the error term involves variability about the regression line. The variation in the individual y_i values about the regression line can be estimated by measuring their variation from the regression line for the sample. The standard deviation for these observed y_i values is termed the **standard error of estimate** ($S_{y/x}$) and is calculated as follows:

$$S_{y/x} = \sqrt{\frac{\Sigma (y_i - y_c)^2}{n - 2}} = \sqrt{MS_{residual}}$$ Eq. 13.13

where the numerator is $SS_{unexplained}$ and denominator is the degree of freedom associated with the unexplained error. Thus, the standard error of estimate equals the square root of the mean square residual. If there is no relationship between the two continuous variables, the slope of the regression equation should be zero. To test the null hypothesis H_0: $\beta=0$, we need to calculate a standard error of the sample slope (b), which is our estimate of population slope (β):

$$S_b = \frac{S_{y/x}}{\sqrt{\Sigma(x_i - \overline{X})^2}}$$ Eq. 13.14

where:

$$\Sigma(x_i - \overline{X})^2 = \Sigma x^2 - \frac{(\Sigma x)^2}{n}$$ Eq. 13.15

from data collected in tables such as Table 13.3 and the mean square residual from the ANOVA table. The formula can be simplified to:

$$S_b = \sqrt{\frac{MS_{residual}}{\Sigma x^2 - \frac{(\Sigma x)^2}{n}}}$$ Eq. 13.16

The value $S_{y/x}$ is also referred to as the **residual standard deviation**.

The decision rule is to reject H_0 (no slope) if $t > |t_{n-2}(1-\alpha/2)|$. With regression, we are dealing with sample data which provides the information for the calculation for an intercept (a) and slope (b), which are estimates of the true population α and β. Because they are samples, they are subject to sampling error similar to previously discussed sample statistics. The number of degrees of freedom is n-2. The number two subtracted from the sample size represents the two approximations in our data: 1) the sample slope as an estimate of β and 2) the sample y-axis intercept as an estimate of α.

As noted, a second parallel approach would be to calculate a confidence interval for the possible slopes for the population:

$$\beta = b \pm t_{n-2}(1-\alpha/2) \cdot S_b$$ Eq. 13.17

In this case the sample slope (b) is the best estimate of the population slope (β) defined in Eq. 13.1:

$$\mu_{y/x} = \alpha + \beta x$$

By creating a confidence interval we can estimate, with 95% confidence, the true population slope (β). As with previous confidence intervals, if zero falls within the confidence interval the result of no slope is a possible outcome; therefore, one fails to reject the null hypothesis and must assume there is no slope in the true population and thus no relationship between the two continuous variables.

Using our example of the twelve healthy male volunteers who received a single dose of various strengths of an experimental anticoagulant (Tables 13.2 and 13.3), one could determine if there was a significant relationship between the dosage and the corresponding prothrombin time by determining if the regression line for the population, based on sample data, has a slope. Once again, the null hypothesis states that there is no slope in the population:

$$H_0: \quad \beta = 0$$
$$H_1: \quad \beta \neq 0$$

The decision rule is, with $\alpha = 0.05$, reject H_0 if $t > |t_{10}(1-\alpha/2)|$ which equals 2.228 (Table B3, Appendix B). The calculation of S_b is:

$$S_b = \sqrt{\frac{MS_{residual}}{\sum x^2 - \frac{(\sum x)^2}{n}}}$$

$$S_b = \sqrt{\frac{0.412}{495650 - \frac{(2430)^2}{12}}} = \sqrt{\frac{0.412}{3575}} = 0.0107$$

and the calculation of the t-statistics is:

$$t = \frac{b - 0}{S_b} = \frac{0.0406 - 0}{0.0107} = 3.79$$

The decision in this case is, with $t > 2.228$, to reject H_0 and conclude that there is a slope, thus a relationship exists between dosage and prothrombin times. Note that the results are identical to those seen the ANOVA test. In fact, the square of the t-statistic equals our previous F-value ($3.79^2 \approx 14.27$, with rounding errors).

A possibly more valuable piece of information would be obtained by calculating the 95% confidence interval for the population slope:

$$\beta = b \pm t_{n-2}(1 - \alpha/2) \cdot S_b$$

$$\beta = 0.04 \pm 2.23(0.011) = 0.04 \pm 0.02$$

$$0.02 < \beta < 0.06$$

Since zero does not fall within the confidence interval, $\beta=0$ is not a possible outcome, therefore H_0 is rejected again and one concludes that a relationship exists between the two variables. It is possible to predict, with 95% confidence, that the true population slope is somewhere between +0.02 and +0.06.

If the null hypothesis is rejected in favor of the alternate hypothesis, that $\beta \neq 0$ then higher values of x would correspond with higher predicted values of y. In this case, there would be a positive correlation.

The population slope (β) is sometimes referred to as the **population regression coefficient**. An alternative formula for calculating the slope is:

$$b = r \cdot \frac{S_y}{S_x} \qquad \text{Eq. 13.18}$$

where r is our correlation coefficient and the standard deviations for each variable is represented by S_x and S_y. In the above example of prothrombin times the standard deviation of the x-variable (dosage) is 18.0278, the standard deviation for the y-variable (protime) is 0.9535 and the correlation coefficient is 0.7675 (square root of $r^2 = 0.589$).

$$b = (0.7675)\frac{0.9535}{18.0278} = 0.0406$$

This result is identical to our previous calculation for the slope of the line.

By testing the significance associated with the slope of the regression line we can be certain that the observed linear equation did not represent simply a chance departure from a horizontal line, when there would be no relationship between the two continuous variables. However, using a t-test to determine the significance of the relationship, we make additional assumptions that the y-values at different levels of x have equal variances and that their distributions are normal in shape.

Confidence Intervals for the Regression Line

The differences between the observed value and predicted value on our regression line (y_i- $\overline{X}_y$) is our best estimate of the variation of the y population around the true regression line. The variance term $S_{y.x}^2$ or the mean square residual is an estimate of the variance of the $\overline{Y}$ population about the true population regression line. The **standard deviation about regression** is another term used to describe $S_{y/x}$ and is more meaningful than the variance term and signifies the standard deviation of y at a given x-value.

As discussed previously for a given value on the x-axis it is possible to estimate a corresponding y value using $y=a+bx$. A confidence interval for the expected y value can be computed using a modification of the formula for the hypothesis test of the slope.

$$y = y_c \pm t_{n-2}(1-\alpha/2) \cdot \sqrt{MS_{residual}} \cdot \sqrt{\frac{1}{n} + \frac{(x_i - \overline{X})^2}{\sum x^2 - \frac{(\sum x)^2}{n}}} \qquad \text{Eq. 13.19}$$

where the $MS_{residual}$ is the mean square residual from the ANOVA table in the original regression analysis. Assuming that each point on the regression line (y_c) gives the best representation (mean) of the distribution of scores, it is possible to estimate the mean of y for any point on the x-axis.

In calculating the 95% confidence interval around the regression line, it is assumed that data are distributed approximately normally in the direction of the y-variable. If we have a large sample size, we would expect that approximately 95% of our prediction errors fall within ± 1.96 $S_{y/x}$. The errors in predicting y for a given value of x are due to several factors. Obviously, there is random variation of y about the true regression line that is expressed as $S_{y/x}$. In addition there is error in estimating the y-axis intercept of the true regression line (α) and error in estimating the slope of the true regression line (β). Because of the error due to estimating the slope of the line, the error in the estimate of the slope will become more pronounced for values of the independent variable (x_i) as those values deviate more from the center (the mean x-value). This produces a bowing of the **confidence bands** as seen in Figure 13.5. The point at which the deviation is least, or where the confidence interval is the smallest, is at the mean for the observed x-values. This would seem logical since we expect less error as one moves to the middle of the distribution (x-values) and we expect a larger error as one approaches the extreme areas of the data.

Once again, we will use the previous anticoagulant example to illustrate the determination of confidence intervals. With 95% confidence, what is the

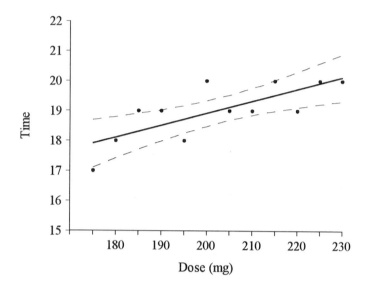

Figure 13.5   Graphic illustration of 95% confidence intervals.

expected mean prothrombin time at a dosage of 210 mg of the anticoagulant? Based on the previous data in Table 13.3 we know the following: $\sum x = 2,430$; $\sum x^2 = 495,650$ and n = 12. The mean for the independent variable is:

$$\overline{X} = \frac{\sum x}{n} = \frac{2430}{12} = 202.5$$

Based on previous calculations the slope (b) is 0.04 and the y-intercept (a) is 10.9. Lastly, from the analysis of variance table, the mean square residual $(S_{x/y}{}^2)$ is 0.41. Using this data the first step is to calculate the y_c value for each point on the regression line for known values of the independent variable (x_i). The y_c would be the best estimate of the center for the interval. For example, the expected value on the regression line at 210 mg would be:

$$y_c = a + bx_i = 10.9 + 0.04(210) = 19.3$$

The calculation of the confidence interval around the regression line at 210 mg of drug would be:

Table 13.5 95% Confidence Intervals at Selected Dosages

Dose (mg)	Time (seconds)	y_c	Lower Limit	Upper Limit	Range
175	17	17.9	17.10	18.70	1.60
180	18	18.1	17.40	18.80	1.40
190	19	18.5	17.98	19.02	1.04
200	20	18.9	18.47	19.33	0.86
210	19	19.3	18.85	19.75	0.90
220	19	19.7	19.10	20.30	1.20
230	20	20.1	19.31	20.89	1.58

$$\overline{y} = 19.3 \pm 2.23\sqrt{0.41}\sqrt{\frac{1}{12} + \frac{(210 - 202.5)^2}{495650 - \frac{(2430)^2}{12}}}$$

$$\overline{y} = 19.3 \pm 2.23(0.64)\sqrt{0.083 + \frac{56.25}{3575}} = 19.3 \pm 0.45$$

$$18.85 < \overline{y} < 19.75$$

Thus, based on sample data and the regression line that fits best between the data points, the researcher could conclude with 95% confidence that the true population mean for a dosage of 210 mg would be between 18.85 and 19.75 seconds. Results of the calculation of the confidence intervals at the various levels of drug used are presented in Table 13.5 and is graphically represented in Figure 13.5.

Multiple Linear Regression Models

Multiple regression is a logical extension of the concepts presented for a simple regression model involving only two continuous variables. With the simple regression analysis, we were concerned with identifying the line which best fits between our data points (Eq. 13.2):

$$y = a + \beta x + e$$

Rather than using values on one predictor or independent variable, as we did with the simple regression analysis (to estimate values on a criterion or dependent variable), we can control several independent variables. By using many predictor variables, we will hopefully reduce our error of prediction even further, by accounting for more of the variance. Multiple linear regression is a powerful multivariate statistical technique for controlling any number of confounding variables:

$$y_j = a + \beta_1 x_1 + \beta_2 x_2 + \beta_2 x_2 + ... + \beta_j x_j + e_j \qquad \text{Eq. 13.20}$$

where y is the value of the independent variable and k is the number of independent variables. The values of β_1, β_2 ... β_k in the equation are referred to as β **coefficients, beta weights** or **regression coefficients**.

The beta coefficients indicate the relative importance of the various independent predictor variables and are based on their standardized z score. The prediction equation can be written as:

$$z_y = \beta_1 z_1 + \beta_2 z_2 + \beta_3 z_3 + ... \beta_k z_k \qquad \text{Eq. 13.21}$$

These beta weights are estimates of their corresponding coefficients for the population equation in standardized z score form. These beta coefficients are also referred to as **partial regression coefficients**, because these regression coefficients are related to the partial correlation coefficients, which were discussed in Chapter 12.

As seen in the previous chapter, the multiple correlation coefficient (R) indicates the correlation for a weighted sum of the predictor variables and the criterion variable. The squared multiple correlation coefficient (R^2) will indicate the proportion of the variance for the dependent criterion variable, which is accounted for by combining the various predictor variables.

Unlike simple regression analysis, which was represented by a straight line, multiple regression represents "planes in multi-dimensional space, a concept admittedly difficult to conceive and virtually impossible to portray graphically" (Kachigan, 1991). Instead of thinking of a least squares line to fit our data, we must think of a least squares solution based on weighted values for each of the various predictor variables. Using computer software it is possible to calculate the appropriate beta weights to create the least squares solution, with those having the greatest correlation having the largest weight.

The calculations for multiple linear regression analysis are extensive and complex and fall beyond the scope of this book. Excellent references for additional information on this topic include Zar (1984), Snedecor and Cochran (1989), and the Sage University series (Berry and Feldman, 1985; Achen, 1982; Schroeder, 1986).

Regression analysis allows us to make **predictions**, and could be referred to as **prediction analysis**. In the simple linear regression model, discussed previously, we can predict a value on the criterion variable, given its corresponding value on a predictor variable. With multiple regression we are interested in predicting a value for the criterion variable given the value on each of several corresponding predictor variables. The primary objectives of a multiple regression analysis are to: 1) determine whether or not a relationship exists between two continuous variables; 2) if a relationship exists, describe the nature of the relationship; and 3) assess the relative importance of the various predictor variables to contribute variation in the criterion variable.

References

Achen, C.H. (1982). Interpreting and Using Regression (paper 29), Sage University Series on Quantitative Applications in the Social Sciences, Sage Publications, Newbury Park, CA.

Berry, W.D. and Feldman, S. (1985). Multiple Regression in Practice (paper 50), Sage University Series on Quantitative Applications in the Social Sciences, Sage Publications, Newbury Park, CA.

Kachigan, S.K. (1991). Multivariate Statistical Analysis, second edition, Radius Press, New York, p. 181.

Schroeder, L.D. et al. (1986). Understanding Regression Analysis: An Introductory Guide (paper 57), Sage University Series on Quantitative Applications in the Social Sciences, Sage Publications, Newbury Park, CA.

Snedecor, G.W. and Cochran, W.G. (1989). Statistical Methods, eighth edition, Iowa State University Press, Ames, IA, pp. 333-365.

Zar, J.H. (1984). Biostatistical Analysis, second edition, Prentice Hall, Englewood Cliffs, NJ, p. 328-359.

Suggested Supplemental Readings

Bolton, S. (1997). Pharmaceutical Statistics: Practical and Clinical Applications, Marcel Dekker, Inc., New York, pp. 216-241.

Daniel, W.W. (1978). Biostatistics: A Foundation for Analysis in the Health Sciences, John Wiley and Sons, New York, pp. 366-398, 439-462.

Fisher, L.D. and van Belle, G. (1993). Biostatistics: A Methodology for the Health Sciences, John Wiley and Sons, New York, pp. 630-638.

Example Problems

1. Samples of a drug product are stored in their original containers under normal conditions and sampled periodically to analyze the content of the medication.

time (months)	assay (mg)
6	995
12	984
18	973
24	960
36	952
48	948

Does a linear relationship exist between the two variables? If such a relation exists, what is the slope, y-intercept, and 95% confidence interval?

2. Acme Chemical is testing various concentrations of a test solution and the effect the concentration has on the optical density of each concentration.

Concentration (%)	Optical Density
1	0.24
2	0.66
4	1.15
8	2.34

Is there a significant linear relationship between the concentration and optical density. If there is a relationship, create a plot representing this relationship and 95% confidence intervals.

3. During early Phase I clinical trials of a new therapeutic agent the following AUCs (area under the curve) were observed at different dosages of the formulation.

Dosage	AUC (hr·μg/ml)
100	1.07
300	5.82
600	15.85
900	25.18
1200	33.12

Does a linear relationship exist between the dose and observed AUC? If such a relation exists, calculate the slope, y-intercept, and 95% confidence interval.

Answers to Problems

1. Comparison of content of a medication at different time periods.
    Variables: continuous independent variable (time in months)
                 continuous dependent variable (amount of drug in mg)

Hypothesis: H_0:   Time (x) and assay results (y) are not linearly related
            H_1:   Time and assay results are linearly related

Decision Rule: With $\alpha = .05$, reject H_0 if $F > F_{1,4}(.95) = 7.71$

x = time (months)   y = assay (mg)

x	y	x^2	y^2	xy
6	995	36	990025	5970
12	984	144	968256	11808
18	973	324	946729	17514
24	960	576	921600	23040
36	952	1296	906304	34272
48	948	2304	898704	45504
$\Sigma =$ 144	5812	4680	5631618	138108

n=6

Calculations:

Slope and intercept:

$$b = \frac{n\sum xy - (\sum x)(\sum y)}{n\sum x^2 - (\sum x)^2} = \frac{6(138108) - (144)(5812)}{6(4680) - (144)^2} = -1.13$$

$$a = \frac{\Sigma y - b \Sigma x}{n} = \frac{5812 - (-1.13)(144)}{6} = 995.78$$

Coefficient of determination:

$$SS_{explained} = b^2 \left[\Sigma x^2 - \frac{(\Sigma x)^2}{n} \right] = (1.13)^2 \left[4680 - \frac{(144)^2}{6} \right] = 1562.93$$

$$SS_{total} = \Sigma y^2 - \frac{(\Sigma y)^2}{n} = 5631618 - \frac{(5812)^2}{6} = 1727.33$$

$$SS_{unexplained} = SS_{total} - SS_{explained} = 1727.33 - 1562.93 = 164.40$$

$$r^2 = \frac{SS_{explained}}{SS_{total}} = \frac{1562.93}{1727.33} = 0.905$$

ANOVA Table:

Source	SS	df	MS	F
Linear Regression	1562.93	1	1562.93	38.03
Residual	164.40	4	41.10	
Total	1727.33	5		

Decision: With $F > 7.71$, reject H_0 and conclude that a linear relationship exists between the storage time and the assayed amount of drug.

Slope of the population:

Hypotheses: H_0: $\beta = 0$
                       H_1: $\beta \neq 0$

Decision Rule: With $\alpha = .05$, reject H_0 if $t > |t_4(1-\alpha/2)| = 2.776$

Calculations:

$$S_b = \sqrt{\frac{MS_{residual}}{\Sigma x^2 - \frac{(\Sigma x)^2}{n}}}$$

$$S_b = \sqrt{\frac{41.10}{4680 - \frac{(144)^2}{6}}} = 0.183$$

$$t = \frac{b - 0}{S_b} = \frac{-1.13 - 0}{0.183} = -6.17$$

Decision: With t > 2.776, reject H_0, conclude that there is a slope and thus a relationship between time and assay results.

95% C.I. for the slope:

$$\beta = b \pm t_{n-1}(1 - \alpha/2) \cdot S_b$$

$$\beta = -1.13 \pm 2.776(0.183) = -1.13 \pm 0.51$$

$$-1.64 < \beta < -0.62$$

Decision: Since zero does not fall within the confidence interval, reject H_0 and conclude a relationship exists. With 95% confidence the slope of the line (β) is between -1.64 and -0.62.

Confidence interval around the regression line:

Example at 48 months, where $\overline{X}$ = 24

$$\overline{y} = y_c \pm t_{n-2}(1 - \alpha/2) \cdot \sqrt{MS_{residual}} \cdot \sqrt{\frac{1}{n} + \frac{(x_i - \overline{X})^2}{\Sigma x^2 - \frac{(\Sigma x)^2}{n}}}$$

$$\bar{y} = 941.54 \pm 2.776\sqrt{41.102}\sqrt{\frac{1}{6} + \frac{(48-24)^2}{4680 - \frac{(144)^2}{6}}}$$

$$\bar{y} = 941.54 \pm (17.78)\sqrt{0.167 + \frac{576}{1224}}$$

$$\bar{y} = 941.54 \pm 14.20$$

$$927.34 < \bar{y} < 955.74$$

Results:

95% Confidence Intervals

Time (months)	Sample (mg)	y_c	Lower Limit	Upper Limit	Range
6	995	989.00	977.40	1000.60	23.20
12	984	982.22	972.84	991.60	18.76
18	973	975.44	967.69	983.19	15.50
24	960	968.66	961.54	975.78	14.24
36	952	955.10	945.72	964.48	18.75
48	948	941.54	927.34	955.74	28.40

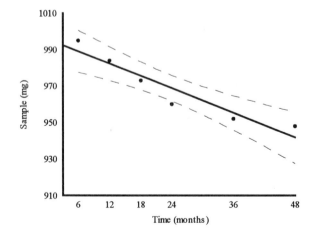

2. Comparison of various concentrations to effect on the optical density
    Variables: continuous independent variable (concentration)
                  continuous dependent variable (optical density)

    Hypotheses: H_0: Concentration and density are not linearly related
                 H_1: Concentration and density are linearly related

    Decision Rule: With $\alpha = 0.05$, reject H_0 if $F > F_{1,2}(1-\alpha) = 18.5$

	Concentration	Density			
	$\underline{x}$	$\underline{y}$	$\underline{x^2}$	$\underline{y^2}$	$\underline{xy}$
	1	0.24	1	0.058	0.24
	2	0.66	4	0.436	1.32
n=4	4	1.15	16	1.323	4.60
	$\underline{8}$	$\underline{2.34}$	$\underline{64}$	$\underline{5.476}$	$\underline{18.72}$
$\Sigma =$	15	4.39	85	7.293	24.88

Calculations:

Slope and y-intercept:

$$b = \frac{4(24.88) - (15)(4.39)}{4(85) - (15)^2} = 0.293$$

$$a = \frac{4.39 - 0.293(15)}{4} = -0.00125$$

Coefficient of determination:

$$SS_{total} = \Sigma y^2 - \frac{(\Sigma y)^2}{n} = 7.293 - \frac{(4.39)^2}{4} = 2.47498$$

$$SS_{explained} = b^2 \cdot \left[\Sigma x^2 - \frac{(\Sigma x)^2}{n} \right] = (.293)^2 \left[85 - \frac{(15)^2}{4} \right] = 2.46816$$

$$SS_{unexplained} = SS_{total} - SS_{explained} = 2.47498 - 2.46816 = 0.00682$$

$$r^2 = \frac{SS_{explained}}{SS_{total}} = \frac{2.46816}{2.47498} = .997$$

ANOVA table:

Source of Variation	SS	df	MS	F
Linear Regression	2.46816	1	2.46816	723.80
Residual	0.00682	2	0.00341	
Total	2.47498	3		

Decision: With F>18.5, reject H_0 and conclude that a linear relationship exists between the concentration and amount of optical density.

Slope of the population:

Hypotheses: H_0: $\beta = 0$
 H_1: $\beta \neq 0$

Decision Rule: With $\alpha = .05$, reject H_0 if t > $|t_2(1-\alpha/2)|$ = 4.302

Calculations:

$$S_b = \sqrt{\frac{MS_{residual}}{\Sigma x^2 - \frac{(\Sigma x)^2}{n}}}$$

$$S_b = \sqrt{\frac{0.00341}{85 - \frac{(15)^2}{4}}} = 0.0109$$

$$t = \frac{b - 0}{S_b} = \frac{0.293 - 0}{0.0109} = 26.88$$

Decision: With t > 4.302, reject H_0, conclude that there is a slope and thus a relationship between concentration and density.

95% C.I. for the slope:

$$\beta = b \pm t_{n-1}(1 - \alpha/2) \cdot S_b$$

$$\beta = 0.23 \pm 4.302(0.0109) = 0.293 \pm 0.047$$

$$0.246 < \beta < 0.340$$

Decision: Since zero does not fall within the confidence interval, reject H_0 and conclude a relationship exists. With 95% confidence the slope of the line (β) is between +0.246 and +0.340.

Confidence interval around the regression line:

Example at 4% concentration, where $\overline{X} = 3.75$

$$\overline{y} = y_c \pm t_{n-2}(1 - \alpha/2) \cdot \sqrt{MS_{residual}} \cdot \sqrt{\frac{1}{n} + \frac{(x_i - \overline{X})^2}{\Sigma x^2 - \frac{(\Sigma x)^2}{n}}}$$

$$\overline{y} = 1.17 \pm 4.302\sqrt{0.00341}\sqrt{\frac{1}{4} + \frac{(4 - 3.75)^2}{85 - \frac{(15)^2}{4}}}$$

$$\overline{y} = 1.17 \pm 0.13$$

$$1.04 < \overline{y} < 1.30$$

Results:

95% Confidence Intervals

Concentration	Density	y_c	Lower Limit	Upper Limit	Range
1	0.24	0.29	0.11	0.47	0.36
2	0.66	0.58	0.43	0.73	0.30
4	1.15	1.17	1.04	1.30	0.26
8	2.34	2.34	2.11	2.57	0.46

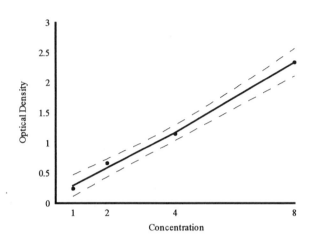

Concentration

3. Comparison of pharmacokinetic measurement and amount of active ingredient.

Variables: continuous independent variable (dosage in mg)
              continuous dependent variable (assay percent)

Hypotheses:
   H_0:   Dosage (x) and AUC results (y) are not linearly related
   H_1:   Dosage and AUC results are linearly related

Decision Rule: With $\alpha = .05$, reject H_0 if $F > F_{1,3}(.95) = 10.1$

Dosage (x)	AUC (y)	x^2	y^2	xy
100	1.07	10000	1.1449	107
300	5.82	90000	33.8724	1746
600	15.85	360000	251.2225	9510
900	25.18	810000	634.0324	22662
1200	33.12	1440000	1096.9344	39744
3100	81.04	2710000	2017.2066	73769

Calculations:

Slope and intercept:

$$b = \frac{n\sum xy - (\sum x)(\sum y)}{n\sum x^2 - (\sum x)^2}$$

$$b = \frac{5(73769) - (3100)(81.04)}{5(2710000) - (3100)^2} = \frac{117621}{3940000} = 0.0299$$

$$a = \frac{\Sigma y - b \Sigma x}{n}$$

$$a = \frac{81.04 - (0.0299)(3100)}{5} = \frac{-11.65}{5} = -2.33$$

Coefficient of determination:

$$SS_E = b^2 \cdot \left[\Sigma x^2 - \frac{(\Sigma x)^2}{n} \right]$$

$$SS_E = (0.0299)^2 \cdot \left[2710000 - \frac{(3100)^2}{5} \right] = 704.48$$

$$SS_T = \Sigma y^2 - \frac{(\Sigma y)^2}{n}$$

$$SS_T = 2017.2066 - \frac{(81.04)^2}{5} = 703.71$$

$$SS_U = SS_T - SS_E = 704.48 - 703.71 = 0.77$$

$$r^2 = \frac{SS_{explained}}{SS_{total}} = \frac{703.71}{704.48} = 0.9989$$

Correlation:

$$r = \sqrt{r^2} = \sqrt{.9989} = 0.9994$$

ANOVA Table:

Source	SS	df	MS	F
Linear Regression	703.71	1	703.71	2706.57
Residual	0.77	3	0.26	
Total	704.48	4		

Decision: With $F > 10.1$, reject H_0 and conclude that a linear relationship exists between the length and percent assay.

Slope of the population:

Hypothesis: H_0: $\beta = 0$
                     H_1: $\beta \neq 0$

Decision Rule: With $\alpha = .05$, reject H_0 if $t > \left| t_{n-2}(1-\alpha/2) \right| = 3.18$

Calculations:

$$S_b = \sqrt{\frac{MS_{residual}}{\Sigma x^2 - \frac{(\Sigma x)^2}{n}}}$$

$$S_b = \sqrt{\frac{0.26}{2710000 - \frac{(3100)^2}{5}}} = 0.0006$$

$$t = \frac{b - 0}{S_b} = \frac{0.0299 - 0}{0.0006} = 49.83$$

Decision: With $t > 3.18$, reject H_0, conclude that there is a slope and thus a relationship between dosage and AUC.

95% C.I. for the slope:

$$\beta = b \pm t_{n-1}(1 - \alpha/2) \cdot S_b$$

$$\beta = 0.0299 \pm 3.18(0.0006) = 0.0299 \pm 0.0019$$

$$0.0299 < \beta < 0.0318$$

Decision: Since zero does not fall within the confidence interval, reject H_0 and conclude a relationship exists. With 95% confidence the slope of the line (β) is between 0.960 and 1.196.

Confidence intervals around the regression line:

Example at 900, where $\overline{X} = 620$:

$$\overline{y} = y_c \pm t_{n-2}(1-\alpha/2) \cdot \sqrt{MS_{residual}} \cdot \sqrt{\frac{1}{n} + \frac{(x_i - \overline{X})^2}{\Sigma x^2 - \frac{(\Sigma x)^2}{n}}}$$

$$\overline{y} = 24.58 \pm 3.18\sqrt{0.26}\sqrt{\frac{1}{5} + \frac{(900 - 620)^2}{2710000 - \frac{(3100)^2}{5}}}$$

$$\overline{y} = 24.58 \pm 0.89$$

95% Confidence Intervals

Dose	AUC	y_c	Lower Limit	Upper Limit	Range
100	1.07	0.66	-0.53	1.85	2.38
300	5.82	6.64	5.71	7.57	1.86
600	15.85	15.61	14.88	16.34	1.46
900	25.18	24.58	23.69	25.47	1.78
1200	33.12	33.55	32.27	34.83	2.56

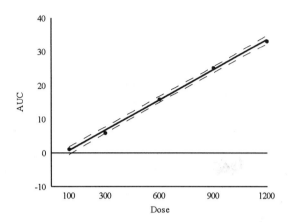

14

z-tests of Proportions

As an introduction to this new set of z-tests, consider the following two problems. First, we are presented with a coin and we wish to determine if the coin is "fair" (an equal likelihood of tossing a head or a tail). To test the assumption of fairness, we toss the coin 20 times and find that we have 13 heads and only 7 tails. Is the coin unfair, loaded in such a way that heads occur more often, or could the outcome be the result of chance error? In a second situation, 50 patients are randomly divided into two groups each receiving a different treatment for their condition. In one group 75% show improvement and in the second group only 52% improve. Do the results prove that the first therapy results in a significantly greater therapeutic response, or is this difference due to chance alone?

Z-tests of proportions can address each of these examples, when comparisons are made between proportions or percentages for one or two levels of a discrete independent variable. They are useful when comparing proportions of two discrete levels of an independent variable or when comparing a sample proportion to a known population proportion. The formula and procedures are similar to those used for the t-tests.

z-test of Proportions – One-sample Case

The z-tests of proportions involve a dependent variable that has only two discrete possible outcomes (i.e., pass or fail, live or die). These outcomes should be mutually exclusive and exhaustive. Similar to the statistics used for t- and F-tests, this z-statistic involves the following ratio:

$$z = \frac{\textit{difference between proportions}}{\begin{array}{c}\textit{standard error of the}\\\textit{difference of the proportions}\end{array}} \qquad \text{Eq. 14.1}$$

The simplest example would be the tossing of a fair coin. We would expect the proportion of heads to be equal to the proportion of tails. Therefore, we would expect a head to occur 50% of the time, or have a proportion of 0.50. Our null hypothesis is that we are presented with a fair coin:

$$H_0: \quad P_{heads} = 0.50$$

The only alternative is that the likelihood of tossing a head is something other than 50%.

$$H_1: \quad P_{heads} \neq 0.50$$

If we toss the coin 100 times and this results in 50 heads and 50 tails the numerator of the above ratio (Eq. 14.1) would be zero, resulting in a $z = 0$. As the discrepancy between what we observe and what we expect (50% heads) increases, the resultant z-value will increase until it eventually becomes large enough to be significant. Significance is determined using the critical z-values for a normalized distribution previously discussed in Chapter 6. For example, from Table B2 in Appendix B, +1.96 or -1.96 are the critical values in the case of a 95% level of confidence. For a 99% level of confidence the critical z-values would be +2.57 or −2.57.

In the one sample case the proportions found for a single sample are compared to a theoretical population to determine if the sample is selected from that same population.

$$H_0: \quad \hat{p} = P_0$$
$$H_1: \quad \hat{p} \neq P_0$$

The test statistic is as follows:

$$z = \frac{\hat{p} - P_0}{\sqrt{\dfrac{P_0(1 - P_0)}{n}}} \qquad \text{Eq. 14.2}$$

where P_0 is the expected proportion for the outcome, $1-P_0$ is the complement proportion for the "not" outcome, $\hat{p}$ is the observed proportion of outcomes in the sample, and n is the number of observations (sample size). The decision rule is, with a certain α, reject H_0 if $z > z_{(1-\alpha/2)}$ or $z < -z_{(1-\alpha/2)}$ (where $z_{(1-\alpha/2)} = 1.96$ for $\alpha=0.05$ or 2.57 for $\alpha=0.01$). Like the t-test, this is a two-tailed test and modifications can be made in the decision rule to test directional hypotheses with a one-tailed test.

The one-sample case can be used to test the previous question about fairness of a particular coin. If a coin is tossed 20 times and 13 heads are the result, is it a fair coin? As seen earlier the hypotheses are:

$$H_0: \ P_{heads} = 0.50$$
$$H_1: \ P_{heads} \neq 0.50$$

In this case the $\hat{p}$ is 13/20 or 0.65, P_0 equals 0.50 and n is 20. The calculation would be as follows:

$$z = \frac{0.65 - 0.50}{\sqrt{\dfrac{(0.50)(0.50)}{20}}} = \frac{+0.15}{0.11} = 1.36$$

Because the calculated z-value is less than the critical value of 1.96, we fail to reject the hypothesis, and we assume that the coin is fair and the difference between the observed 0.65 and expected 0.50 was due to random error. What if we had more data and the results were still the same? The z-test is an excellent example of the importance of sample size. Figure 14.1 shows the same proportional differences with an increasing number of observations. Note that if these results appeared with more than 47 or 48 tosses the results would be significant at 95% confidence and the null hypothesis would be rejected. If the same proportional difference exists with over 75 tosses H_0 can be rejected with 99% confidence.

Similar to one-sample t-tests, confidence intervals can also be created for the z-test of proportions:

$$P_0 = \hat{p} \pm Z_{(1-\alpha/2)} \sqrt{\frac{P_0(1-P_0)}{n}} \qquad \text{Eq. 14.3}$$

The interval indicates the possible range of results, with 95% confidence. With the above example, the hypotheses would continue to be:

$$H_0: \ \hat{p} = 0.50$$
$$H_1: \ \hat{p} \neq 0.50$$

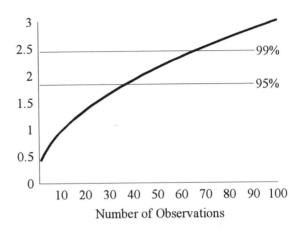

Figure 14.1 Effects of sample size on z-test results.

and the interval would be:

$$P_0 = 0.65 \pm 1.96 \sqrt{\frac{(0.50)(0.50)}{20}}$$

$$P_0 = 0.65 \pm 0.22$$

$$0.43 < P_0 < 0.87$$

Therefore, based on a sample of only 20 tosses, with 95% confidence, the probability of tossing a head is between 0.43 and 0.87. The outcome of 0.50 is a possible outcome, therefore H_0 cannot be rejected.

z-test of Proportions - Two-sample Case

In the two-sample case, proportions from two levels of a discrete independent variable are compared and the hypothesis under test is that the two proportions for the population are equal.

$$H_0: \quad P_1 = P_2$$
$$H_1: \quad P_1 \neq P_2$$

If the two populations (P_1 and P_2) are equal, then the best estimation of that population proportion would be the weighted average of the sample proportions:

$$\hat{p}_0 = \frac{n_1\,\hat{p}_1 + n_2\,\hat{p}_2}{n_1 + n_2} \qquad \text{Eq. 14.4}$$

This estimate of the population proportion is then used in the denominator of the z-ratio (Eq. 14.1) and the numerator is the difference between the two sample proportions:

$$z = \frac{\hat{p}_1 - \hat{p}_2}{\sqrt{\dfrac{\hat{p}_0(1 - \hat{p}_0)}{n_1} + \dfrac{\hat{p}_0(1 - \hat{p}_0)}{n_2}}} \qquad \text{Eq. 14.5}$$

In these two equations, $\hat{p}_1$, $\hat{p}_2$ are sample proportions and n_1, n_2 are the sample sizes. The decision rule for a two-tailed z-test would be, with $\alpha = 0.05$, reject H_0, if $z > z_{(1-\alpha/2)} = 1.96$ or $z < -1.96$.

To illustrate this test assume the following fictitious clinical trial. To possibly improve the survival rate for protozoal infections in AIDS patients, individuals with newly diagnosed infections were randomly assigned to treatment with either zidovudine alone or a combination of zidovudine and trimethoprim. Based on the following results did either therapy show a significantly better survival rate?

Zidovudine alone - 24 out of 94 patients survived, $\hat{p}_Z = 0.255$

Zidovudine with trimethoprim- 38 out of 98 patients survived, $\hat{p}_{ZT} = 0.388$

Is there a significant difference between 0.255 and 0.388 based on less than 200 patients? The best estimate of the population proportion, if there is no difference between the two samples, is calculated from the two weighted sample proportions:

$$\hat{p}_0 = \frac{94(0.255) + 98(0.388)}{94 + 98} = .323$$

The null hypothesis would be that there was not a significant difference between the two groups of patients in the proportion of patients surviving.

$$H_0: \quad P_Z = P_{Z\&T}$$
$$H_1: \quad P_Z \neq P_{Z\&T}$$

If the z-statistic is greater than +1.96 or less than -1.96, the researcher should reject the null hypothesis and conclude that there is a significant difference between the two groups. The computations would be:

$$z = \frac{0.255 - 0.388}{\sqrt{\dfrac{0.323(0.677)}{94} + \dfrac{0.323(0.677)}{98}}}$$

$$z = \frac{-0.133}{\sqrt{0.0023 + 0.0022}} = \frac{-0.133}{0.067} = -1.98$$

With $z = -1.98$ (which is smaller than the critical value of -1.96) the decision would be to reject H_0 and conclude that there was a significant difference in the results of the two treatments. In this case the patients receiving both zidovudine and trimethoprim have a significantly better survival rate.

z-tests for Proportions - Yates Correction for Continuity

In performing a z-test of proportions, the calculated z-value is based upon discrete, or discontinuous data, but as discussed in Chapter 6 the normal standardized distribution is based on a continuous distribution. Therefore, the calculated z-values are only an approximation of the theoretical z-distribution. Therefore, Yates (1934) argued that a more conservative approach was needed to estimate the z-statistic, which is more appropriate with the standardized normal distribution. In the two-sample case, the Yates correction for continuity is:

$$z = \frac{|\hat{p}_1 - \hat{p}_2| - \dfrac{1}{2}(\dfrac{1}{n_1} - \dfrac{1}{n_2})}{\sqrt{\dfrac{\hat{p}_0(1 - \hat{p}_0)}{n_1} + \dfrac{\hat{p}_0(1 - \hat{p}_0)}{n_2}}} \qquad \text{Eq. 14.6}$$

Because of the smaller numerator, this will result in a slightly smaller calculated z-value, and a more conservative estimate. Obviously, as the sample sizes become smaller and we know less about the true population, there will be a decrease in the calculated z-value and an even more conservative answer.

Using this correction for continuity, we can recalculate the previous AIDS treatment example, we were able to reject the null hypothesis and assumed that there was a better survival rate with the combination therapy. However, with Yates correction:

$$z = \frac{|0.255 - 0.388| - \frac{1}{2}(\frac{1}{94} + \frac{1}{98})}{\sqrt{\frac{0.323(0.677)}{94} + \frac{0.323(0.677)}{98}}}$$

$$z = \frac{0.133 - 0.01}{\sqrt{0.0023 + 0.0022}} = \frac{0.123}{0.067} = 1.84$$

we fail to reject H_0 and our decision is the opposite of the original test. With $z = 1.84$, the researcher cannot reject H_0 and must conclude there was no significant difference in the results of the two treatments.

Similarly, Yates correction can be applied to the one-sample case (i.e., the previous example of tossing a fair coin):

$$z = \frac{|p - P_0| - \frac{1}{n}}{\sqrt{\frac{(P_0)(1 - P_0)}{n}}}$$

Eq. 14.7

Obviously the larger the amount of information (n), the smaller the correction factor. Recalculation of our previous example gives:

$$z = \frac{|0.65 - 0.50| - \frac{1}{20}}{\sqrt{\frac{(0.50)(0.50)}{20}}} = \frac{0.10}{0.11} = 0.91$$

We still fail to reject H_0, but the calculated z-value is much smaller (0.91 compared to 1.36).

Proportion Testing for More Than Two Levels of a Discrete Independent Variable

What if there are more than two levels of the discrete independent variable? Could the z-test of proportions be expanded beyond only two levels of the discrete independent variable? In these cases, it is best to establish a

contingency table based on the frequency associated with each outcome. For example, assume in the previous zidovudine/trimethoprim study that there were actually four levels of treatment. The frequencies could be presented in the following table of outcomes:

	Zidovudine alone	Zidovudine/ trimethoprim	Zidovudine/ drug A	Zidovudine/ drug B
Lived	24	38	24	6
Died	70	60	86	51

In this case a more appropriate test would be a chi square test of independence, where the interrelationship is measured between the survival rate and type of drug therapy received to determine if the two variables are independent of each other. This test will be discussed in the next chapter.

Reference

Yates, F. (1934). "Contingency tables involving small numbers and the χ^2 test," Royal Statistical Society Supplement 1(series B):217-235.

Suggested Supplemental Readings

Bolton, S. (1997). Pharmaceutical Statistics: Practical and Clinical Applications, Marcel Dekker, Inc., New York, pp. 162-168.

Daniel, W.W. (1991). Biostatistics: A Foundation for Analysis in the Health Sciences, John Wiley and Sons, New York, pp. 120-125.

Glantz, S.A. (1987). Primer of Biostatistics, McGraw-Hill, New York, pp. 111-119.

Example Problems

1. During production runs, historically a specific dosage form is expected to have a defect rate of 1.5%. During one specific run, a sample of 100 tablets was found to have a defect rate of 4.8%. Does this differ significantly from what would normally be expected?

2. During initial Phase I and II studies, the incidence of nausea and vomiting

of a new cancer chemotherapeutic agent was 36% for 190 patients, while 75 control patients receiving conventional therapy experience nausea and vomiting at a rate of 55%.

    a. Is there a significant difference between the incidence of nausea and vomiting between these two drug therapies?

    b. Did the new agent produce a significantly lower incidence of nausea and vomiting?

3. During the development of a final dosage form, the frequency of defects were analyzed to determine the effect of the speed of the tablet press. Samples were collected at 80,000 (lower) and 120,000 (higher) units per hour. Initially 500 tablets were to be collected at each speed, unfortunately due to an accident only 460 tablets were retrieved at the higher speed. Based on the following results were there any significant differences between the two tablet press speeds?

Speed	n	# of defects
Low	500	11
High	460	17

4. During pre-approval clinical trials with a specific agent, it was found that the incidence of blood dyscrasia was 2.5%. In a later Phase IV study involving 28 patients, two developed blood dyscrasia. Is this outcome possible or is there something unique about the population from which the sample was taken for this last clinical trial?

5. A nursing home experiments with two different drug distribution systems. Units are randomly assigned to receive one of the two systems. After two months of implementation, surveyors observe the entire process from order entry to patient administration and recorded all medication errors. System A that is a traditional unit dose system has 148 errors out of 12,455 dosages; where System B, which relies heavily on robotics, has 89 errors for 10,002 doses observed. Is there a significant difference between these two systems?

Answers to Problems

1. Production was run with an expected defect rate of 1.5%, but found a rate of 4.8% for 100 tablets.

Hypotheses: H_0: $\hat{p} = 0.015$

H_1: $\hat{p} \neq 0.015$

Decision rule: With $\alpha = 0.05$, reject H_0, if $z > z_{(1-\alpha/2)} = 1.96$ or $z < -1.96$.

Data: $P_0 = 0.015$; $\hat{p} = 0.048$; $n = 100$

Calculations:

$$z = \frac{\hat{p} - P_0}{\sqrt{\dfrac{P_0(1 - P_0)}{n}}}$$

$$z = \frac{0.048 - 0.015}{\sqrt{\dfrac{(0.015)(0.985)}{100}}} = \frac{0.033}{0.012} = 2.75$$

Decision: With $z > 1.96$, reject H_0, conclude that there is a significant difference between the sample and the expected proportion of defects.

Alternative - confidence interval:

$$P_0 = \hat{p} \pm Z_{(1-\alpha/2)} \sqrt{\frac{P_0(1 - P_0)}{n}}$$

$$P_0 = 0.048 \pm 1.96 \sqrt{\frac{(0.015)(0.985)}{100}} = 0.048 \pm 0.024$$

$$+0.024 < P_0 < +0.072$$

Decision: The outcome 0.015 does not fall within the interval, therefore reject H_0.

2.   Incidence of nausea and vomiting between two therapies.

   a.   Two-tailed, not predicting direction:

Hypotheses: H_0: $P_N = P_T$

                           H_0: $P_N \neq P_T$

Decision rule: With $\alpha = 0.05$, reject H_0, if $z > z_{(1-\alpha/2)} = 1.96$ or $z < -1.96$.

Calculations:

$$\hat{p}_0 = \frac{n_F \hat{N}_N + n_T \hat{p}_T}{n_N + n_T} = \frac{(190)(0.36) + (75)(0.55)}{190 + 75} = 0.413$$

$$1 - \hat{p}_0 = 1.00 - 0.413 = 0.587$$

$$z = \frac{0.36 - 0.55}{\sqrt{\dfrac{(0.413)(0.587)}{190} + \dfrac{(0.413)(0.587)}{75}}} = \frac{-0.19}{0.067} = -2.83$$

Decision: With $z < -1.96$ reject H_0, and conclude there is a significant difference between the incidence of nausea and vomiting between the new drug and traditional therapy.

b. One-tailed, predicting lower incidence with new agent:

Hypotheses: H_0: $P_N \geq P_T$

                           H_0: $P_N < P_T$

Decision rule: With $\alpha = 0.05$, reject H_0, if $z < z_{(1-\alpha)} = -1.64$.

Decision: The computed z-value was -2.83. With $z < -1.64$ reject H_0, and conclude that the newer agent causes a significant decrease in the incidence of nausea and vomiting compared to traditional therapy.

3. Defects at two different speeds for a tablet press.

Speed	n	# of defects
Low	500	11
High	460	17

$$\hat{p}_L = 11/500 = 0.022 \qquad\qquad \hat{p}_H = 17/460 = 0.037$$

Hypotheses: H_0: $P_L = P_H$
             H_1: $P_L \neq P_H$

Decision rule: With $\alpha = 0.05$, reject H_0, if $z > z_{(1-\alpha/2)} = 1.96$ or $z < -1.96$.

Calculations:

$$\hat{p}_0 = \frac{n_L\,\hat{p}_L + n_H\,\hat{p}_H}{n_L + n_H} = \frac{(500)(0.022) + (460)(0.037)}{500 + 460} = 0.029$$

$$1 - \hat{p}_0 = 1.00 - 0.029 = 0.971$$

$$z = \frac{\hat{p}_L - \hat{p}_H}{\sqrt{\dfrac{\hat{p}_0(1-\hat{p}_0)}{n_L} + \dfrac{\hat{p}_0(1-\hat{p}_0)}{n_H}}}$$

$$z = \frac{0.022 - 0.037}{\sqrt{\dfrac{0.029(0.971)}{500} + \dfrac{0.029(0.971)}{460}}} = \frac{-0.015}{0.011} = -1.36$$

Decision: With the $z > -1.96$, fail to reject H_0, conclude that there is no significant difference in the defect rate based on the tablet press speed.

Yates Correction for Continuity:

$$z = \frac{|\hat{p}_1 - \hat{p}_2| - \dfrac{1}{2}\left(\dfrac{1}{n_1} + \dfrac{1}{n_2}\right)}{\sqrt{\dfrac{\hat{p}_0(1-\hat{p}_0)}{n_1} + \dfrac{\hat{p}_0(1-\hat{p}_0)}{n_2}}}$$

$$z = \frac{|0.022 - 0.037| - \dfrac{1}{2}\left(\dfrac{1}{500} + \dfrac{1}{460}\right)}{\sqrt{\dfrac{0.029(0.971)}{500} + \dfrac{0.029(0.971)}{460}}}$$

$$z = \frac{0.015 - 0.002}{0.011} = \frac{0.013}{0.011} = 1.18$$

Decision: With the $z < 1.96$, fail to reject H_0.

4. Incidence of a blood dyscrasia in a Phase IV clinical trail.

Hypotheses: H_0: $\hat{p} = 0.025$
$\qquad\qquad$ H_1: $\hat{p} \neq 0.025$

Decision rule: With $\alpha = 0.05$, reject H_0, if $z > z_{(1-\alpha/2)} = 1.96$ or $z < -1.96$.

Data: $P_0 = 0.025$; $\hat{p} = 2/28 = 0.071$; $n = 28$

Calculations:

$$z = \frac{\hat{p} - P_0}{\sqrt{\dfrac{P_0(1 - P_0)}{n}}}$$

$$z = \frac{0.071 - 0.025}{\sqrt{\dfrac{(0.025)(0.975)}{28}}} = \frac{0.046}{0.029} = 1.59$$

Decision: With $z < 1.96$, fail to reject H_0, and cannot conclude that the sample results are different from what was found with the original clinical trials.

Alternative - confidence interval:

$$P_0 = \hat{p} \pm Z_{(1-\alpha/2)} \sqrt{\frac{P_0(1 - P_0)}{n}}$$

$$P_0 = 0.071 \pm 1.96 \sqrt{\frac{(0.025)(0.975)}{28}} = 0.071 \pm 0.057$$

$$+0.014 < P_0 < +0.128$$

Decision: The outcome 0.025 falls within the interval, therefore H_0 cannot be rejected.

5. Error rates with two drug distribution systems.

$$\hat{p}_A = 148/12{,}455 = 0.0119 \qquad \hat{p}_B = 89/10{,}002 = 0.0089$$

Hypotheses: H_0: $P_A = P_B$
                H_1: $P_A \neq P_B$

Decision rule: With $\alpha = 0.05$, reject H_0, if $z > z_{(1-\alpha/2)} = 1.96$ or $z < -1.96$.

Calculations:

$$\hat{p}_0 = \frac{n_A\,\hat{p}_A + n_B\,\hat{p}_B}{n_A + n_B} = \frac{(12{,}455)(0.0119) + (10{,}002)(0.0089)}{12{,}455 + 10{,}002} = 0.0105$$

$$1 - \hat{p}_0 = 1.00 - .0105 = 0.9895$$

$$z = \frac{\hat{p}_1 - \hat{p}_2}{\sqrt{\dfrac{\hat{p}_0(1 - \hat{p}_0)}{n_1} + \dfrac{\hat{p}_0(1 - \hat{p}_0)}{n_2}}}$$

$$z = \frac{0.0119 - 0.0089}{\sqrt{\dfrac{(0.0105)(0.9895)}{12{,}455} + \dfrac{(0.0105)(0.9895)}{10{,}002}}} = \frac{0.003}{0.0014} = 2.14$$

Decision: With $z > +1.96$, reject H_0, and conclude that there is a significant difference in the error rate based on the drug distribution system used.

Note that Yates correction for continuity is not performed in this example because the large sample would result in only a 0.000089 reduction in the numerator and thus the same resultant z-value.

15

Chi Square Tests

The chi square tests are involved only with discrete variables. In the *goodness-of-fit test* there is one discrete variable. For the *test of independence,* two discrete variables are compared: one is usually independent (i.e., experimental vs. control group) and the other variable is dependent upon the first (i.e., cured vs. died). Chi square tests evaluate the importance of the difference between what is expected and what is observed.

Chi Square Statistic

Chi square (χ^2) can best be thought of as a discrepancy statistic. It analyzes the difference between observed values and those values that one would normally expect to occur. It is calculated by determining the difference between the frequencies actually observed in a sample data set and the expected frequencies based on probability. Some textbooks classify χ^2 as a nonparametric procedure because it is not concerned with distributions about a central point and does not require assumptions of homogeneity or normality.

In the previous chapter, the z-tests of proportion evaluated the results of a coin toss. This one-sample case was a measure of discrepancy, with the numerator representing the difference between the observed frequency (p) and the expected population results for a fair coin (P_O) (Eq. 14.2). With the z-tests in Chapter 14, we were concerned with proportions, or percents, and these were used with the appropriate formulas. With the chi square statistics, the frequencies are evaluated. The calculation involves squaring the differences between the observed and expected frequencies divided by the expected frequency. These results are summed for each cell or level of the discrete variable.

$$\chi^2 = \Sigma \frac{(f_O - f_E)^2}{f_E}$$

Eq. 15.1

This formula can be slightly rewritten as follows:

$$\chi^2 = \Sigma \left[\frac{(Observed - Expected)^2}{Expected} \right]$$

or

$$\chi^2 = \Sigma \frac{(O - E)^2}{E}$$

Eq. 15.2

Obviously, if all of the observed and expected values are equal for each level of the discrete variable the numerator is zero and the χ^2-statistic will be zero. Similar to the z-test, as the differences between the observed and expected frequencies increase, the numerator will increase and the resultant χ^2-value will increase. Because the numerator is squared, the resultant value must be equal to or greater than zero. Therefore at a certain point in the continuum from zero to positive infinity, the calculated χ^2-value will be large enough to indicate that the difference cannot be due to chance alone. Like the z-, t- and F-tests, critical values for the chi square distribution are presented in tabular form (Table B12, Appendix B). Like the t- and F-distributions, there is not one single χ^2 distribution, but a set of distributions. The characteristics of each distribution is dependant on the number of associated degrees of freedom. The first column on the left of Table B12 indicates the number of degrees of freedom (determination of which will be discussed later) and the remaining columns are the critical chi square values at different acceptable levels of Type I error (α).

The decision rule is written similar to previous tests. For example, assume we are dealing with four degrees of freedom and wish to have a 95% level of confidence. The decision rule would be: with $\alpha = 0.05$, reject H_0 if $\chi^2 > \chi^2_4(0.05) = 9.448$. If the calculated statistic derived from the formula (Eq. 15.2) is larger than the critical (9.448), the null hypothesis (the observed and expected values are the same) is rejected.

Chi Square for One Discrete Independent Variable

As seen in the previous chapter, the z-tests of proportions were limited to only one or two levels of a discrete independent variable. If the frequency counts are used (instead of proportions), a chi square test can be used and can be expanded to more than two levels. For example, assume that we wish to compare four lots of a particular drug for some minor undesirable trait (i.e., a blemish on the tablet coating). We randomly sample 1000 tablets from each batch and examine the tables for that trait. The results of the experiment are as follows:

<u>Number of Tablets with Blemishes</u>

Batch A	12
Batch B	15
Batch C	10
Batch D	9

A simple hypothesis for this data could be as follows:

H_0: The samples are selected from the same population
H_1: The samples are from different populations

The null hypothesis states that there is no significant difference between the four batches of drug based on the criteria tested. If there is no difference then they must be from the same sample population. In selecting the appropriate critical χ^2-value, the degrees of freedom is one less than number of levels of the discrete variable. Once again the K-1 levels are selected to correct for bias. In this example, since there are four batches being tested, the degrees of freedom is four minus one, or three. The decision rule, assuming 95% confidence is: with $\alpha = 0.05$, reject H_0 if $\chi^2 > \chi^2_3(0.05) = 7.815$. The value 7.815 is found in Table B12 at the intercept of the third row (degrees of freedom equal to three) and the second column of critical values ($\alpha = 0.05$). If there were no differences among the batches, we would expect to see the same results. Our best estimate of expected frequency is the average of the sample frequencies:

$$f_E = \frac{\Sigma \; frequencies \; per \; level}{number \; of \; levels} = \frac{\Sigma f_i}{k_i} \qquad \text{Eq. 15.3}$$

In this particular case:

$$f_E = \frac{12 + 15 + 10 + 9}{4} = 11.5$$

Therefore the χ^2 statistic would be calculated as follows:

	Observed	Expected	O-E	$(O-E)^2/E$
Batch A	12	11.5	+0.5	0.02
Batch B	15	11.5	+3.5	1.07
Batch C	10	11.5	-1.5	0.20
Batch D	9	11.5	-2.5	0.54
			$\chi^2 =$	1.83

Based on the results of the chi square test, with the calculated χ^2 less than 7.815, we fail to reject the null hypothesis. Therefore, our best guess is that they are from the same population, in other words, that there is no difference between the four batches.

Chi Square Goodness-of-fit Test

All chi square tests can be thought of as goodness-of-fit procedures because they compare what is observed to what is expected in a hypothesized distribution. However, the term goodness-of-fit is reserved for comparisons of a sample distribution to determine if the observed set of data is distributed as expected by a preconceived distribution. It is assumed that the sample distribution is representative of the population from which it is sampled. Sample observations are placed into mutually exclusive and exhaustive categories, and the frequencies of each category are noted and compared to expected frequencies in the hypothetical distribution. The following are examples of the use of this method for both normal and binomial distributions.

Goodness-of-fit for a Normal Distribution. The chi square goodness-of-fit test, can be used to determine if a sample is selected from a population which is normally distributed. The underlying assumption is that the sample distribution, because of random sampling, is reflective of the population from which it is sampled. Therefore, if the sample has characteristics similar to what is expected for a normal distribution, then one cannot reject the hypothesis that the population is normally distributed.

H_0:   Population is normally distributed
H_1: H_0 is false

Since many statistical procedures assume that sample data are drawn from normally distributed populations it is useful to have a method to evaluate this assumption. The chi squared test provides an excellent method, but should be restricted to sample sets with 50 or more observations. For example, using Sturges' Rule the distribution presented in Table 15.1 is created from the data presented in Chapter 4.

If the sample distribution is the best estimation of the population from which it was sampled, is the population in question normally distributed? Obviously, the greater the discrepancy between what is expected and what is actually observed, the less likely the difference is attributed to chance alone and the greater the likelihood that the sample is not from a normally distributed population. The test statistic would be Equation 15.2:

$$\chi^2 = \Sigma \left[\frac{(O - E)^2}{E} \right]$$

Degrees of freedom are based on the number of categories or class intervals and a number of estimated values. In order to calculate areas within a normal distribution one needs to know both the population mean and population standard deviation (Eq. 6.3):

$$z = \frac{x - \mu}{\sigma}$$

Calculation of z-values provides probabilities associated with the dividing points (boundaries) for our class intervals. The sample mean and standard deviation are the best available estimates of the population:

$$\overline{X} \approx \mu$$
$$S \approx \sigma$$

Therefore our best estimate of z-values would be an approximation based on our sample measurements:

$$z = \frac{x - \overline{X}}{S} \qquad \text{Eq. 15.4}$$

Because we are estimating two population parameters, each are subtracted from the number of levels of the independent discrete variable. One additional degree is subtracted to control for bias. Thus, degrees of freedom equals the number of cells minus three; one for the estimate of the population mean; one

Table 15.1 Distribution of C_{max} Data from Table 5.5

Interval Range	Frequency	
705.5-716.5	2	
716.5-727.5	6	
727.5-738.5	18	$\overline{X}$ = 752.9 mg
738.5-749.5	22	
759.5-760.5	35	S = 16.5 mg
760.5-771.5	28	
771.5-782.5	10	
782.5-793.5	4	
	125	

for the estimate of the population standard deviation and one for bias. In the above example, degrees of freedom equals eight levels minus three, or five degrees of freedom. The decision rule is: with α = 0.05, reject H_0 if $\chi^2 > \chi^2_{v=5}$ (.05) = 11.07.

Based on the discussion in Chapter 6, we can use the information presented about areas under the curve of a normal distribution to estimate the expected frequencies in each interval of this sample distribution if the population is normally distributed. For example, with a sample of 125 observations; if normally distributed, how many observations would be expected below 716.5 mg? The first step is to determine the z-value on a normal distribution representing 716.5 mg.

$$Z = \frac{x - \overline{X}}{S} = \frac{716.5 - 752.9}{16.5} = \frac{-36.4}{16.5} = -2.20$$

Looking at the standardized normal distribution (Table B2, Appendix B) the area under the curve between the mean and z = -2.20 is 0.4861. The proportion, or area under the curve, falling below the z-value is calculated by subtracting the area between the center and z-value from 0.5000 which represents all the area below the mean.

$$p(< 2.20) = 0.5000 - 0.4861 = 0.0139$$

The expected number of observations is the total number of observations multiplied by the proportion of the curve falling below z = -2.20:

$$E(<716.5) = 125(0.0139) = 1.74$$

Using this same method, it is possible to estimate the number of observations expected to be below 727.5 in a normal distribution (the greatest value in the second class interval).

$$Z = \frac{x - \overline{X}}{S} = \frac{727.5 - 752.9}{16.5} = \frac{-25.4}{16.5} = -1.54$$

$$p(<-1.54) = 0.5000 - 0.4394 = 0.0606$$

$$E(<727.5) = 125(0.0606) = 7.57$$

Continuing this procedure it is possible to calculate all areas below given points in the proposed normal distribution.

Interval Range	Expected Values Below the Largest Value in Each Class Interval
705.5-716.5	1.74
716.5-727.5	7.57
727.5-738.5	23.01
738.5-749.5	52.59
759.5-760.5	84.20
760.5-771.5	109.36
771.5-782.5	120.51
782.5-793.5	125.00

By default, if all the observations are represented under the area of the curve then the expected number of observations below the upper value of the highest interval must include all of the observations (in this case 125).

Unfortunately, we are interested in not only the areas below given points on the distribution, but also areas between the boundaries of the class intervals. Therefore, the number of observations expected between 716.5 and 727.5 is the difference between the areas below each point:

Expected (Range 716.5-727.5) = E(<727.5) - E(<716.5) = 7.57-1.74 = 5.83
Expected (Range 727.5-738.5) = E(<738.5) - E(<727.5) = 23.01-7.57 = 15.44

Using this same procedure it is possible to determine the expected results for the remaining categories and create a table. The expected amounts reflect a normal distribution.

Interval Range	Expected Values Below Level of Range	Expect Values Within Range
705.5-716.5	1.74	1.74
716.5-727.5	7.57	5.83
727.5-738.5	23.01	15.44
738.5-749.5	52.59	29.58
759.5-760.5	84.20	31.61
760.5-771.5	109.36	25.16
771.5-782.5	120.51	11.15
782.5-793.5	125.00	4.49
	$\Sigma =$	125

The chi square statistic is then computed comparing what is expected if the population distribution is normal to what was actually observed in the sample distribution. The greater the difference, the more likely one is to reject the hypothesis that the population represented by the sample is normally distributed. The chi square calculation is as follows:

Interval	Observed	Expected	(O-E)	$(O-E)^2/E$
705.5-716.5	2	1.74	0.26	0.039
716.5-727.5	6	5.83	0.17	0.005
727.5-738.5	18	15.44	2.56	0.424
738.5-749.5	22	29.58	-7.58	1.942
759.5-760.5	35	31.61	3.39	0.364
760.5-771.5	28	25.16	2.84	0.321
771.5-782.5	10	11.15	-1.15	0.119
782.5-793.5	4	4.49	-0.49	0.053
			$\chi^2 = \Sigma =$	3.267

Therefore, the decision is, with $\chi^2 < 11.07$, do not reject H_0 and conclude that we are unable to reject the hypothesis that the population is normally distributed. This process is laborious, but useful when evaluating data where it is important to determine if the population is normally distributed.

Goodness-of-fit for a Binomial Distribution. To illustrate the use of the chi square goodness-of-fit test for a binomial distribution, assume that four coins are tossed at the same time. This procedure is repeated 100 times. Based on the following results, are these "fair" coins?

0 heads	15 times
1 head	30 times
2 heads	32 times
3 heads	17 times
4 heads	6 times

From the discussion of probability in Chapter 2, using factorials, combinations and the binomial equation (Eq. 2.12), it is possible to produce the theoretical binomial distribution given a fair coin, p(head) = .50. For example the probability of tossing only one head is:

$$p(x) = \binom{n}{x} p^x q^{n-x}$$

$$p(1) = \binom{4}{1} (0.5)^1 (0.5)^3 = 0.25$$

A table can be produced for the probability of all possible outcomes. If the four coins are fair these would be the expected outcomes:

	p(x)	frequency for 100 times
0 heads	0.0625	6.25
1 head	0.2500	25.00
2 heads	0.3750	37.50
3 heads	0.2500	25.00
4 heads	0.0625	6.25

The comparison is made for the discrepancy between what was actually observed with 100 coin tosses and what was expected to occur. The hypotheses would be:

H_0: Population is a binomial distribution with p = 0.50
H_1: H_0 is false

and test statistic remains the same:

$$\chi^2 = \Sigma \left[\frac{(O - E)^2}{E} \right]$$

The decision rule is, with $\alpha = 0.05$, reject H_0 if $\chi^2 > \chi^2_{v=5-2}(0.05) = 7.82$. Here the degrees of freedom is based upon the number of discrete intervals minus two; one degree of freedom is subtracted because we are estimating the population proportions (p) and one is subtracted to prevent bias. The computation of the χ^2-value is as follows:

	Observed	Expected	(O-E)	(O-E)²/E
0 heads	15	6.25	8.75	12.25
1 head	30	25.00	5.00	1.00
2 heads	32	37.50	-5.50	0.81
3 heads	17	25.00	-8.00	2.56
4 heads	6	6.25	-0.25	0.01
			$\chi^2 =$	16.63

Based on the 100 coin tosses, the decision is with $\chi^2 > 7.82$, reject H_0, conclude that the sample does not come from a binomial distribution with p(head) = 0.50, the coins are not fair.

Chi Square Test of Independence

The most common use of the chi square test is to determine if two discrete variables are independent of each other. With this test we are concerned with conditional probability, what the probability is for some level of variable A given a certain level of variable B (Eq. 2.6)

$$p(A) \text{ given } (B) = p(A \mid B) = p(A \cap B)/p(B)$$

If the two discrete variables are independent of each other, then the probability of each level should be the same regardless of which B characteristic it contains.

$$P(A_1 \mid B_1) = P(A_1 \mid B_2) = P(A_1 \mid B_3) \ldots = P(A_1 \mid B_K) = P(A_1)$$

A contingency table is created where frequency of occurrences are listed for the various levels of each variable. The **contingency table** is used to determine whether two discrete variables are contingent or dependent on each other. This table has a finite number of mutually exclusive and exhaustive categories in the rows and columns. Such a design is a "K x J" contingency which has K rows, J columns and K x J cells. This bivariate table can be used to predict if two variables are independent of each other or if an association exists.

Levels of the First Variable

The hypothesis under test implies that there is no relationship (complete independence) between the two variables and that each are independent.

H_0: $P(B_1|A_1) = P(B_1|A_2) = P(B_1|A_3) \ldots = P(B_1|A_K) = P(B_1)$
           $P(B_2|A_1) = P(B_2|A_2) = P(B_2|A_3) \ldots = P(B_2|A_K) = P(B_2)$
           $\ldots$
           $P(B_K|A_1) = P(B_K|A_2) = P(B_K|A_3) \ldots = P(B_K|A_K) = P(B_K)$

H_1: H_0 is false

A simpler terminology for the two hypothesis would be:

H_0:   Factor B is independent of Factor A
H_1:   Factor B is related to Factor A

Thus, in the null hypothesis, the probability of B_1 (or B_2 ... or B_M) remains the same regardless of the level of variable A. If we fail to reject H_0, the independent variables have no systematic association and could also be referred to as **unrelated, uncorrelated** or **orthogonal variables.** Once again the test statistic is:

$$\chi^2 = \Sigma \left[\frac{(O-E)^2}{E} \right]$$

Much like the goodness-of-fit model, if there is complete independence the difference between the observed and expected outcomes will be zero. As the difference in the numerator increases the calculated χ^2-value will increase and eventually exceed a critical value, then the difference cannot be attributed to chance or random variability. To determine the critical value, the degrees of freedom are based on the number of rows minus one (K-1) times the number of columns minus one (J-1). This is based on the fact that if we had a contingency table such as the following:

	A_1	A_2	A_3	A_4	
B_1					100
B_2					200
B_3					100
	100	100	100	100	400

If we know the information for any six cells [(J-1)(K-1)] the remaining cells within the table would become automatically know; thus having no freedom to vary. With the following information for six cells (example bolded) the remaining cells could be easily determined and these last six cells have no freedom to change once the first six are identified.

	A_1	A_2	A_3	A_4	
B_1	**26**	**18**	10	46	100
B_2	43	**56**	**68**	33	200
B_3	**31**	26	22	**21**	100
	100	100	100	100	400

The decision rule is, with $\alpha = 0.05$, reject H_0 if χ^2 is greater than $\chi^2_{(J-1)(K-1)}(\alpha)$. In the case of four columns and three rows, the critical chi square value with $\alpha = 0.05$ from Table B12 is:

$$\chi^2_{(3)(2)}(\alpha) = \chi^2_6(\alpha) = 12.592$$

The expected value for any cell is calculated by multiplying its respective row sum times its respective column sum and dividing by the total number or the grand sum.

$$E = \frac{\Sigma C \cdot \Sigma R}{\Sigma Total}$$

Eq. 15.3

To illustrate this, the calculations for the expected values for a three by two contingency table would be:

(C1 x R1)/T	(C2 x R1)/T	(C3 x R1)/T	Σ = R1
(C1 x R2)/T	(C2 x R2)/T	(C3 x R2)/T	Σ = R2

$$\Sigma = C1 \qquad \Sigma = C2 \qquad \Sigma = C3 \qquad \Sigma\Sigma = T$$

For example, in a pharmacology study mice of various ages are administered a chemical proposed to induce sleep. After 30 minutes the animals are assessed to determine if they are asleep or awake (based on some predetermined criteria). The purpose of the study is to determine if the particular agent is more likely to induce sleep in different age groups. The study results are as follows:

	Asleep (C_1)	Awake (C_2)
3 months (R_1)	7	13
10 months (R_2)	9	11
26 months (R_3)	15	5

Simply stated, the hypothesis under test is that age does not influence sleep induction by the proposed agent being tested.

H_0: $P(C_1|R_1) = P(C_1|R_2) = P(C_1|R_3) = P(C_1)$
$\qquad P(C_2|R_1) = P(C_2|R_2) = P(C_2|R_3) = P(C_2)$
H_1: H_0 is false

Or simply stated:

H_0: Sleep is independent of the age of the mice
H_1: H_0 is false, a relationship exists

The decision rule is, with $\alpha = 0.05$, reject H_0 if $\chi^2 > \chi^2_{v=2}(.0.05) = 5.99$. A comparison of the observed and expected values are as follows:

Observed

	C_1	C_2	Σ
R_1	7	13	20
R_2	9	11	20
R_3	15	5	20
Σ	31	29	60

Expected

	C_1	C_2
	10.3	9.7
	10.3	9.7
	10.3	9.7

Calculation of the chi square statistic is:

$$\chi^2 = \frac{(7 - 10.3)^2}{10.3} + \frac{(13 - 9.7)^2}{9.7} + \frac{(9 - 10.3)^2}{10.3} + \ldots \frac{(5 - 9.7)^2}{9.7} = 6.94$$

The decision based on a sample of 60 mice is that with $\chi^2 > 5.99$, is to reject H_0 and conclude that age does influence the induction of sleep by this particular chemical. It appears that the agent has the greatest effect on the older animals.

For the chi square test of independence there are two general rules: 1) there must be at least one observation in every cell, no empty cells and 2) the expected value for each cell must equal or be larger than five. The chi square formula is theoretically valid only when the expected values are sufficiently large. If these criteria are not met, adjacent rows or columns should be combined so that cells with extremely small values or empty cells are combined to form cells large enough to meet the criteria. To illustrate this consider the following example of a multicenter study where patients were administered an experimental aminoglycoside for gram negative infections. The incidence of side effects are reported below.

Side Effects	Age in Years				
	<18	18-45	46-65	>65	
None	80	473	231	112	896
Mild	9	68	43	27	147
Moderate	2	24	8	8	42
Severe	1	5	3	6	15
Total	92	570	285	153	1100

Is there a significant difference in the incidence of side effects based upon the age of the patients involved in the study?

However, an examination of the expected values indicates that four cells fall below the required criteria of an expected value of at least five.

Side Effects	Age in Years				
	<18	18-45	46-65	>65	
None	74.94	464.29	232.15	124.62	896
Mild	12.30	76.17	38.08	20.45	147
Moderate	3.51	21.77	10.88	5.84	42
Severe	1.25	7.77	3.89	2.09	15
Total	92	570	285	153	1100

One method for correcting this problem would be to combine the last two rows (moderate and severe side effects):

	Age in Years				
Side Effects	<18	18-45	46-65	>65	
None	74.94	464.29	232.15	124.62	896
Mild	12.30	76.17	38.08	20.45	147
Moderate/Severe	4.76	29.54	14.77	7.93	57
Total	92	570	285	153	1100

This combination is more logical than combining the severe side effects with either the mild side effects or the absence of side effects. However, one cell still has an expected value less than five. The next logical combination would be the first two columns (ages <18 and 18-45 years old):

	Age in Years			
Side Effects	18-45	46-65	>65	
None	539.23	232.15	124.62	896
Mild	88.47	38.08	20.45	147
Moderate/Severe	34.30	14.77	7.93	57
Total	662	285	153	1100

This 3x3 design meets all of the criteria for performing a chi square analysis. The initial observed data would have the following appearance:

	Age in Years			
Side Effects	<46	46-65	>65	
None	553	231	112	896
Mild	77	43	27	147
Moderate/Severe	32	11	14	57
Total	662	285	153	1100

The hypotheses would be:

H_0: $P(S_1 \mid A_1) = P(S_1 \mid A_2) = P(S_1 \mid A_3) = P(S_1)$
$P(S_2 \mid A_1) = P(S_2 \mid A_2) = P(S_2 \mid A_3) = P(S_2)$
$P(S_3 \mid A_1) = P(S_3 \mid A_2) = P(S_3 \mid A_3) = P(S_3)$
H_1: H_0 is false

Or:

H₀: Severity of side effects is independent of age group
H₁: H₀ is false, a relationship exists

and the decision rule would be, with $\alpha = 0.05$, reject H₀ if $\chi^2 > \chi_4^2$ (0.05) = 9.49. Note the decrease from the original nine degrees of freedom (4-1 rows time 4-1 columns) to the new four degrees of freedom. The calculation for the chi square statistic would be:

$$\chi^2 = \frac{(553 - 539.23)^2}{539.23} + \frac{(231 - 232.15)^2}{232.15} + ... \frac{(14 - 7.93)^2}{7.93}$$

$$\chi^2 = 11.62$$

The decision is with $\chi^2 > 9.49$ reject H₀, conclude that there is a significant difference in side effects based on age.

If the chi square data for the test of independence is reduced to a 2x2 contingency table and the expected values are still too small to meet the requirements (no empty cells and an expected value of at least five per cell), then the **Fisher's exact test** can be employed. The Fisher's exact test will be discussed in Chapter 17 covering nonparametric tests.

Yates Correction for 2x2 Contingency Table

A 2 row by 2 column (2x2) contingency table could be set up as follows using the observed data:

a	b	a+b
c	d	c+d
a+c	b+d	n

Another way to calculate χ^2 in a 2x2 design (which would produce the identical results as Equation 15.2), is as follows:

$$\chi^2 = \frac{n(ad - bc)^2}{(a+b)(b+d)(a+b)(c+d)}$$ Eq. 15.5

As an example consider the following data. A new design in shipping containers for ampules is compared to the existing one to determine if the number of broken units can be reduced. One hundred shipping containers of each design are subjected to identical rigorous abuse and failures are defined as more than 1% broken ampules.

Results	New Container	Old Container	Total
Success	97	88	185
Failure	3	12	15
Totals	100	100	200

Do the data suggest the new design is an improvement over the one currently used?

In this case the expected values would be:

92.5	92.5
7.5	7.5

and the traditional calculation for the chi square statistic would be:

$$\chi^2 = \Sigma \frac{(O - E)^2}{E}$$

$$\chi^2 = \frac{(97 - 92.5)^2}{92.5} + \frac{(88 - 92.5)^2}{92.5} + \frac{(3 - 7.5)}{7.5} + \frac{(12 - 7.5)^2}{7.5} = 5.84$$

Using the alternate formula (Eq. 15.5), the same results are obtained:

$$\chi^2 = \frac{n(ad - bc)^2}{(a + b)(c + d)(a + c)(b + d)}$$

$$\chi^2 = \frac{200(97(12) - 3(88))^2}{(100)(100)(185)(15)}$$

$$\chi^2 = \frac{162000000}{27750000} = 5.84$$

In this particular example the hypotheses would be:

H_0:   Success or failure is independent of container style
H_1: H_0 is false

Or more accurately:

$$H_0: \quad P(S_1 \mid C_1) = P(S_1 \mid C_2) = P(S_1)$$
$$P(S_2 \mid C_1) = P(S_2 \mid C_2) = P(S_2)$$
$$H_1: \quad H_0 \text{ is false}$$

and the decision rule is with $\alpha = 0.05$, reject H_0 if $\chi^2 > \chi_1^2$ (0.05) = 3.84. Therefore, based on either formula the decision, since $\chi^2 > 3.84$ we would reject H_0, conclude that the rate of damage is not independent of the type of container used.

Similar to the discussion of the z-test for proportions, the calculated chi square value is based upon discrete, discontinuous data, but the chi square critical value is based on a continuous distribution. Therefore, the calculated chi square value is only an approximation of the theoretical chi square distribution and these approximations are good for larger numbers of degrees of freedom, but not as accurate for only one degree. Therefore, we must once again use a correction to produce a more conservative estimate. Yates correction for continuity also produces a smaller numerator and thus a more conservative estimate for the chi square statistic.

$$\chi^2_{corrected} = \frac{n(\mid ad - bc \mid - .5n\,)^2}{(a+b)(b+d)(a+b)(c+d)} \qquad \text{Eq. 15.6}$$

Recalculating the chi square statistic for the above example using Yates correction for continuity, the results are:

$$\chi^2_{corrected} = \frac{n(\mid ad - bc \mid - .5n\,)^2}{(a+b)(c+d)(a+c)(a+d)}$$

$$\chi^2_{corrected} = \frac{200[\mid (97)(12) - (3)(88)\mid - (.5)(200)\,]^2}{(100)(100)(185)(15)}$$

$$\chi^2_{corrected} = \frac{128000000}{27750000} = 4.61$$

Yates correction provides a more conservative chi square. If the above example were computed without Yates correction the resulting χ^2 would have equaled 6.88. In this particular case either finding would have resulted in the rejection of H_0.

Suggested Supplemental Readings

Bolton, S. (1997). Pharmaceutical Statistics: Practical and Clinical Applications, Marcel Dekker, Inc., New York, pp. 570-574.

Daniel, W.W. (1991). Biostatistics: A Foundation for Analysis in the Health Sciences, Second Edition, John Wiley and Sons, New York, pp. 531-551.

Dixon, W.J. and Massey, F.J. (1983). Introduction to Statistical Analysis. McGraw-Hill Book Company, New York, pp. 272-280.

Havilcek, L.L. and Crain, R.D. (1988). Practical Statistics for the Physical Sciences, American Chemical Society, Washington, DC, pp. 212-221.

Example Problems

1. There are certain requirements which discrete data must meet in order to be evaluated using the chi square test of independence. Seen below are several matrixes, do each meet the required criteria? If not, using the same data, modify the matrix to fulfill the required criteria (assume the levels of each variable are in an ordinal arrangement, D>C>B>A).

    a. Comparing Variable 1 and Variable 2

		Variable 1			
		A	B	C	D
	A	12	13	17	16
Variable 2	B	8	12	13	3
	C	4	2	0	0

    b. Comparing Variable 3 and Variable 4

		Variable 3		
		A	B	C
	A	6	8	1
Variable 4	B	13	2	5
	C	11	2	7
	D	5	5	2

    c. Comparing Variable 5 and Variable 6

Variable 5

		A	B	C
	A	12	6	17
Variable 6	B	17	15	14
	C	21	29	19

2. In an example presented earlier in this chapter, it was found that the average incidence of an undesirable trait (blemish on the tablet coat) was 11.5% for four batches of a particular drug. Samples of 30 tablets each are randomly selected during the next production run of the product, and the tablets are examined for blemishes. The results of the first 50 samples of 30 tablets each are as follows:

Number of Tablets with Blemished	Frequency
0	2
1	7
2	8
3	15
4	7
5	6
>5	5

Are these results what we might expect based on the information from the first four batches?

3. A pharmacist is evaluating the amount of time needed for nurse surveyors to observe drug delivery in 70 long-term care facilities. The median time required by the surveyors is 2.5 hours. The researcher wishes to know if the type of delivery system (unit dose vs. traditional) influences the amount of survey time required.

	Unit Dose	Traditional	Total
2.5 hr. or less	26	10	36
More than 2.5 hr.	14	20	34
Total	40	30	70

4. A survey was conducted of 100 randomly selected male and 100 randomly selected female pharmacists to measure their attitudes toward mandatory continuing education (MCE) requirements. Based on a series of questions an index was created which expressed the final results as either a positive or negative attitude toward MCE. It was found that 58 females and 37

males gave positive results. Was there a significant difference based on gender?

5. A medication, known to cause severe irritation to stomach mucosa, is tested with a series of special tablet coatings to prevent release until after the tablet has passed through the stomach. Three variations of the coating formula are tested on 150 fasted volunteers, randomly assigned to each group. The presence or absence of irritation, through endoscopic examination, is noted for each subject.

	GI Irritation	
	Present(P_1)	Absent(P_2)
Formula A	10	40
Formula B	8	42
Formula C	7	43

Was there a significant difference in the likelihood of irritation based on the coating formulas?

6. A series of measurements (n=275) are performed on the content of a particular dosage form. Using Sturge's rule the following intervals were created to represent this random sample which has a mean of 50.68 and a standard deviation of 4.24.

Interval	Frequency
38.55-41.25	3
41.25-43.95	12
43.95-46.65	33
46.65-49.35	60
49.35-52.05	59
52.05-54.75	56
54.75-57.75	42
57.45-60.15	8
60.15-62.85	2

Based on the sample results, could one assume that the population (batch) from which these samples were selected was normally distributed?

7. A manufacturer is experimenting with a new 50 mm diameter screw-type container using various amounts of torque for closure. The tightness of the containers are tested based on moisture permeability. From the data reported below, is there any significant difference in moisture level based

on the torque used to tighten the cap?

Moisture	Torque (inch-pounds) 21	24	27	30	
< 2000	26	31	36	45	138
≥ 2000	24	19	14	5	62
Total	50	50	50	50	200

8. An instrument manufacturer runs a series of disintegration tests to compare the pass/fail rate of a new piece of equipment. Tablets are sampled from a single batch of uncoated tablets. Two different temperatures are used and tested for compendia recommended times. Success is defined as all six tablets disintegrating in the disintegration equipment.

	Successes (R_1)	Failures (R_2)	
Higher Temperature (T_1)	96	4	100
Lower Temperature (T_2)	88	12	100
	88	16	200

Is there any relationship between the success/failure rate and the temperature used?

9. During a cholera outbreak in a war devastated country, records for one hospital were examined for the survival of children contracting the disease. These records also reported the children's nutritional status. Was there a significant relationship between their nutrition and survival rate?

	Nutritional Status Poor	Good
Survived	72	79
Died	87	32

Answers to Problems

1. The two criteria required in order to perform a chi square test of independence are: 1) there be no empty cells and 2) that the expected value for each cell must be ≥ 5.

a. Comparing Variable 1 and Variable 2 we find two empty cells (f=0) therefore this matrix fails the first criteria.

		Variable 1			
		A	B	C	D
	A	12	13	17	16
Variable 2	B	8	12	13	3
	C	4	2	0	0

If the variables are in some type of logical ordinal arrangement, the first step would be to combine levels B and C of Variable 2 and calculate the expected values of the new matrix and see if the expected values exceed 5.

		Variable 1				
		A	B	C	D	
Variable 2	A	12	13	17	16	58
	B	12	14	13	3	42
		24	27	30	19	100

The expected values are calculated by multiplying the respective margin valued and dividing by the total number of observations ($\Sigma R \Sigma C / N$).

Expected values:

		Variable 1				
		A	B	C	D	
Variable 2	A	13.92	15.66	17.40	11.02	58
	B	10.08	11.34	12.60	7.98	42
		24	27	30	19	100

In this case all the expected values are ≥ 5 therefore the matrix fulfills the required criteria.

b. With Variables 3 and 4 we note there are no empty cells, thus the only criterion we need to check is that all the expected values are sufficiently large.

Expected values: Variable 3

		A	B	C	
	A	7	5	3	15
Variable 4	B	9.33	6.67	4	20
	C	9.33	6.67	4	20
	D	9.33	6.67	4	20
		35	25	15	75

Unfortunately, all the expected values associated with level C in Variable 3 have expected values less than 5. The logical manipulation of the data would be to combine levels B and C of Variable 3 that will produce a 2x4 matrix which meets all the criteria for a chi square test of independence.

Observed Data

6	9
13	7
11	9
5	7

Expected Values

7	8
9.33	10.67
9.33	10.67
9.33	10.67

c. With Variable 5 and Variable 6 there are no empty cells and as can be seen below all the expected values are greater than 5. Therefore, the original data, without any modifications is sufficient to perform a chi square test of independence.

Variable 5

		A	B	C	
	A	11.67	11.67	11.67	35
Variable 6	B	15.33	15.33	15.33	46
	C	23	23	23	69
		50	50	50	150

2. Incidence of an undesirable trait in samples of 30 tablets each.

Hypotheses: H_0: Population is a binomial distribution with $p = 0.115$
H_1: H_0 is false

Decision rule: With $\alpha = 0.05$, reject H_0 if $\chi^2 > \chi^2_{v=7-2}(0.05) = 11.07$

Use the binomial distribution to calculate the probability of each occurrence:

$$p(x) = \binom{n}{x} p^x q^{n-x}$$

Example for 2 tablets with blemishes:

$$p(2) = \binom{30}{2}(.115)^2(.885)^{28} = 435(0.013)(0.033) = 0.187$$

the expected frequency for 2 tablets with blemishes in 50 samples is:

$$E(2) = (0.187)(50) = 5.64$$

Comparison of observed vs. expected:

Tablets with blemish	Observed	Expected	(O-E)	$(O-E)^2/E$
0	2	1.3	+0.7	0.38
1	7	5.0	+2.0	0.80
2	8	9.4	-1.4	0.21
3	15	11.3	+3.7	1.21
4	7	9.8	-2.8	0.80
5	6	6.7	-0.7	0.07
>5	5	6.5	-1.5	0.35
			$\chi^2 =$	3.82

Decision: With $\chi^2 < 11.07$, fail to reject H$_0$, conclude that the outcomes could result from chance alone.

3. Above and below the median time needed for nurse surveyors to observe drug deliveries.

Hypotheses: H$_0$: P(2.5 or less|UD) = P(2.5 or less|Trad) = P(2.5 or less)
P(>2.5|UD) = P(>2.5|Trad) = P(>2.5)
(time required is not influenced by delivery system)
H$_1$: H$_0$ is false

Decision Rule: With $\alpha = 0.05$, reject H$_0$ if $\chi^2 > \chi_1^2 (0.05) = 3.84$

Test statistic: (because of only one degree of freedom, use Yates correction)

$$\chi^2_{corrected} = \frac{n(|\,ad - bc\,| - .5n\,)^2}{(a+b)(b+d)(a+b)(c+d)}$$

Data:

	Unit Dose	Traditional	Total
2.5 hr. or less	26	10	36
More than 2.5 hr.	14	20	34
Total	40	30	70

Calculations:

$$\chi^2_{corrected} = \frac{70(\,|(26)(20) - (14)(10)| - .5(70)\,)^2}{(40)(30)(36)(34)}$$

$$\chi^2_{corrected} = \frac{70(\,|520 - 140| - 35\,)^2}{1468800} = \frac{70(345\,)^2}{1468800}$$

$$\chi^2_{corrected} = \frac{8331750}{1468800} = 5.67$$

Decision: With $\chi^2 > 3.84$, reject H_0 and conclude that the time required to do the nursing home surveys is dependent on the type of delivery system used in the facility.

4. Gender differences with respect to attitude toward mandatory continuing education.

Data: Out of 100 males and 100 females positive responses were:

Males	37
Females	58

Hypotheses: H_0: No difference between male and female pharmacists

                  H_1: Males and females responded differently

Decision rule: With $\alpha = 0.05$, reject H_0 if $\chi^2 > \chi^2_1(0.05) = 3.84$

Expected value:

$$f_E = \frac{\Sigma f_i}{n_i} = \frac{37 + 58}{2} = 47.5$$

Calculations:

	Observed	Expected	O-E	$(O-E)^2/E$
Males	37	47.5	-10.5	2.32
Females	58	47.5	+10.5	2.32
			$\chi^2 =$	4.64

Decision: With $\chi^2 > 3.84$, reject H_0 and conclude that there is a significant difference in the responses of pharmacists based on their gender, with female pharmacists more likely to have a positive attitude toward mandatory continuing education requirements.

5. Severe irritation to stomach mucosa compared with special tablet coatings.

	GI Irritation	
	Present(P_1)	Absent(P_2)
Formula A	10	40
Formula B	8	42
Formula C	7	43

Hypotheses: H_0: $P(P_1|F_A) = P(P_1|F_B) = P(P_1|F_C) = P(P_1)$
$\qquad\qquad\quad P(P_2|C_A) = P(P_2|C_B) = P(P_2|C_C) = P(P_2)$

$\qquad\qquad H_1$: H_0 is false

Decision rule: With $\alpha = 0.05$, reject H_0 if $\chi^2 > \chi_2^2 (0.05) = 5.99$

Observed				Expected		
10	40	50		8.33	41.67	50
8	42	50		8.33	41.67	50
7	43	50		8.33	41.67	50
25	125	150		25	125	150

Calculations:

$$\chi^2 = \sum \frac{(O - E)^2}{E}$$

$$\chi^2 = \frac{(10 - 8.33)^2}{8.33} + \frac{(40 - 41.67)^2}{41.67} + \ldots \frac{(43 - 41.67)^2}{41.67} = 0.66$$

Decision: With $\chi^2 < 5.99$, cannot reject H_0.

6. Content uniformity data.

   Sample mean = 50.68   Intervals = 9
   Sample S.D. = 4.24   df = 6
   n = 275

Hypotheses: H_0: Population is normally distributed
            H_1: H_0 is false

Decision rule: With $\alpha = 0.05$, reject H_0 if $\chi^2 > \chi_6^2 (0.05) = 12.59$

Example of the estimated value for interval 43.95-46.65:

$$Z = \frac{x - \mu}{\sigma} = \frac{43.95 - 50.68}{4.24} = \frac{-6.73}{4.24} = -1.59$$

$$p(<43.95) = 0.5000 - 0.4441 = 0.0559$$

$$E(<43.95) = 275(0.0559) = 15.37$$

$$Z = \frac{x - \mu}{\sigma} = \frac{46.65 - 50.68}{4.24} = \frac{-4.03}{4.24} = -0.95$$

$$p(<46.65) = 0.5000 - 0.3289 = 0.1711$$

$$E(<46.65) = 275(0.1711) = 47.05$$

Expected range (43.95-46.65) = E(<46.65) - E(<43.95)

Expected range (43.95-46.65) = 47.05 - 15.37 = 31.68

Interval	Observed	Expected	(O-E)	$(O-E)^2/E$
38.55-41.25	3	3.63	-0.63	0.109
41.25-43.95	12	11.74	+0.26	0.006
43.95-46.65	33	31.68	+1.32	0.055
46.65-49.35	60	56.98	+3.02	0.160
49.35-52.05	59	67.98	-8.98	1.186
52.05-54.75	56	56.65	-0.65	0.007
54.75-57.45	42	31.32	+10.68	3.642
57.45-60.15	8	11.47	-3.47	1.050
60.15-62.85	2	3.55	-1.55	0.677
			$\chi^2 = \Sigma =$	6.892

Decision: With $\chi^2 < \chi^2_{critical}$ cannot reject H_0 that the population is normally distributed.

7. A manufacturer is experimenting with a new 50 mm diameter screw-type container using various amounts of torque for closure. The tightness of the containers are tested based on moisture permeability. From the data reported below, is there any significant difference in moisture level based on the torque used to tighten the cap?

Moisture	Torque (inch-pounds)				
	21	24	27	30	
< 2000	26	31	36	45	138
≥ 2000	24	19	14	5	62
Total	50	50	50	50	200

Hypotheses:

H_0: $P(M_1|T_1) = P(M_1|T_2) = P(M_1|T_3) = P(M_1|T_4) = P(M_1)$
$P(M_2|T_1) = P(M_2|T_2) = P(M_2|T_3) = P(M_2|T_4) = P(M_2)$
H_1: H_0 is false

The null hypothesis stating that there the moisture observed is independent of the torque place upon the lid.

Decision rule: With $\alpha = 0.05$, reject H_0 if $\chi^2 > \chi_3^2 (0.05) = 7.81$

Expected values:

	Torque (inch-pounds)				
Moisture	21	24	27	30	
< 2000	34.5	34.5	34.5	34.5	138
≥ 2000	15.5	15.5	15.5	15.5	62
Total	50	50	50	50	200

Computation:

$$\chi^2 = \frac{(26 - 34.5)^2}{34.5} + \frac{(31 - 34.5)^2}{34.5} + ... \frac{(5 - 15.5)^2}{15.5}$$

$$\chi^2 = 18.43$$

Decision: With $\chi^2 > 7.81$ reject H_0, conclude that there is a significant difference in moisture level based on the amount of torque applied during closure.

8.   Disintegration results at two different temperatures.

	Successes (R_1)	Failures (R_2)	
Higher Temperature (T_1)	96	4	100
Lower Temperature (T_2)	88	12	100
	88	16	200

Hypotheses: H_0: $P(R_1 | T_1) = P(R_1 | T_2) = P(R_1)$
                           $P(R_2 | T_1) = P(R_2 | T_2) = P(R_2)$
            H_1: H_0 is false

Or, a null hypothesis that rate of successes in independent of temperature.

Decision rule: With $\alpha = 0.05$, reject H_0 if $\chi^2 > \chi_1^2 (0.05) = 3.84$

Computations (without Yates Correction):

$$\chi^2 = \frac{200[\ (96)(12) - (88)(4)\ ]^2}{(100)(100)(184)(16)}$$

$$\chi^2 = \frac{128,000,000}{29,440,000} = 4.35$$

Decision: With $\chi^2 > 3.84$, reject H_0 and conclude that there is a significant difference based on the temperature.

Yates' correction for 2x2 table:

$$\chi^2_{corrected} = \frac{n(\,|ad - bc| - .5n\,)^2}{(a+b)(c+d)(a+c)(a+d)}$$

$$\chi^2_{corrected} = \frac{200(\,|(96)(12) - (88)(4)| - .5(200)\,)^2}{(100)(100)(184)(16)}$$

$$\chi^2_{corrected} = \frac{200(\,800 - 100\,)^2}{29,440,000} = \frac{98,000,000}{29,440,000} = 3.329$$

Decision: With $\chi^2 < 3.84$, fail to reject H_0, conclude that there no significant difference in disintegration based on the temperature.

9. Survival during cholera outbreak vs. nutritional status

	Poor	Good	
Survived	72	79	151
Died	87	32	119
	159	111	270

Hypotheses: H_0: $P(S_1|N_1) = P(S_1|N_2) = P(S_1)$
$P(S_2|N_1) = P(S_2|N_2) = P(S_2)$
H_1: H_0 is false

The null hypothesis being that the survival rate is independent of the the nutritional status of the children.

Decision rule: With $\alpha = 0.05$, reject H_0 if $\chi^2 > \chi_1^2 (0.05) = 3.84$

Expected:

	Poor	Good	
Survived	88.9	62.1	151
Died	70.1	48.9	119
	159	111	270

Calculations:

$$\chi^2 = \Sigma \frac{(O - E)^2}{E}$$

$$\chi^2 = \frac{(72 - 88.9)^2}{88.9} + \frac{(79 - 62.1)^2}{62.1} + \frac{(87 - 70.1)^2}{70.1} + \frac{(32 - 48.9)^2}{48.9} = 17.77$$

Decision: With $\chi^2 > 3.84$, reject H$_0$, conclude that there is a significant difference in the survival rate based on the nutritional status

Yates' Correction for Continuity:

   a.   Without correction

$$\chi^2 = \frac{n(ad - bc)^2}{(a + b)(c + d)(a + c)(b + d)}$$

$$\chi^2 = \frac{270[(72)(32) - (87)(79)]^2}{(151)(119)(159)(111)} = 17.77$$

   b.   With correction

$$\chi^2_{corrected} = \frac{n(\,|ad - bc| - .5n\,)^2}{(a + b)(c + d)(a + c)(a + d)}$$

$$\chi^2_{corrected} = \frac{270(\,|(72)(32) - (87)(79)| - .5(270)\,)^2}{(151)(119)(159)(111)} = 16.74$$

In both cases, the null hypothesis is rejected and it is concluded that there is a significant relationship between nutrition and survival rate and that the two variables are not independent of each other.

16

Higher Order Tests
for Discrete Variables

The previous two chapters dealt with statistics associated with one and two discrete variables, the z-test of proportions and chi square test of independence. This chapter will focus on more applications associated with discrete outcomes. New terminology will be introduced (sensitivity and selectivity, relative risk and odds ratio) and related to conditional probability. In addition, the McNemar test, Cochran's Q test, Mantel-Haenszel test, the phi coefficient and the contingency coefficient will be presented as parallel tests to previous evaluations involving continuous variables as outcomes.

Conditional probability was important when we discussed the chi square test of independence in Chapter 15. Based on Equation 2.6 the probability of some level of variable A <u>given</u> a certain level of variable B was defined as

$$p(A) \text{ given } (B) = p(A \mid B) = p(A \cap B)/p(B)$$

and if the two discrete variables are independent of each other, then the probability of each level of A should be the same regardless of which B characteristic it contains.

$$P(A_1 \mid B_1) = P(A_1 \mid B_2) = P(A_1 \mid B_3) \ldots = P(A_1 \mid B_K) = P(A_1)$$

These points will be revisited in this chapter where more complex tests involving frequency data are discussed.

Sensitivity and Specificity

If we develop a specific test or procedure to identify a certain outcome or attribute, it is important that such a test produces the correct results. **Sensitivity** is defined as the probability that the method we use to identify a specific outcome will identify that outcome when it is truly present. If we are evaluating a diagnostic test for a medical condition, it will produce a positive result given the patient actually has the disease. In the case of chemical analysis, a method will detect a specific compound if that material is present. In contrast, **specificity** is the probability that the test or method will produce a negative result when the given outcome is not present. Once again, using the example of a diagnostic test, the test results are negative when the patient does not have the specific condition that the test is designed to detect. We can visually describe the results (similar to hypothesis testing in Chapter 7).

The Real World

		Positive	Negative
Test Results	Positive	Sensitivity	False Positive
	Negative	False Negative	Specificity

Like hypothesis testing, errors can occur in the lower left and upper right quadrants of our 2x2 table. Still using the diagnostic test as an example: 1) if the test is administered to a "healthy" person but produces a positive result for the specific condition, it would be called a **false positive result**; and 2) if administered to a person with the disease but it fails to detect the condition, it would be deemed a **false negative result**. Obviously, we want our test to have high sensitivity and specificity that would result in a low probability of either false positive or false negative results.

Before a diagnostic or analytical test is used in practice, it is important to evaluate the rates of error (false positive and negatives) which are experienced with the test. In the case of an analytical procedure, mixtures can be produced with and without the material that we wish to detect and then tested to determine whether or not the material is identified by the test.

Using a medical diagnostic test we can illustrate this process. Assume we have developed a simple procedure for identifying individuals with HIV-antibodies. Obviously we want our test to have a high probability of producing positive results if the person has the HIV infection (sensitivity). However, we want to avoid producing extreme anxiety, insurance complications, or even the potential for suicide, from a false positive result (1.0-p(specificity)). Therefore we pretest on a random sample of patients who have the presence or absence of HIV antibodies based on the current gold standard for this diagnostic procedure. Assume we start with 500 volunteers with 100 determined to be HIV-positive and the remaining 400 test as HIV-negative based on currently available procedures. We administer our diagnostic procedure and find the following results.

Study Volunteers

		HIV(+)(D)	HIV(-)($\overline{D}$)	
Results of Diagnostic Procedure	Positive (T)	90	8	98
	Negative ($\overline{T}$)	10	392	402
		100	400	500

Let us define the true diagnostic status of the patient with the letter D for the volunteers who are HIV(+) and $\overline{D}$ for volunteers who are HIV(-). We will also use the letter T to indicate the results from our new diagnostic procedure: T for a positive result and $\overline{T}$ for a negative result.

Suppose we randomly sample one of 100 HIV(+) volunteers. what is the probability that the person will have a positive diagnostic result from our test? Using conditional probability (Eq. 2.6) we calculate the results to be:

$$p(T \mid D) = \frac{p(T \cap D)}{p(D)} = \frac{.18}{.20} = .90$$

Thus, the sensitivity for a diagnostic test is 90%. In a similar manner, if we sample one patient from our 400 HIV(-) patients, what is the probability that our test result will be negative?

$$p(\overline{T} \mid \overline{D}) = \frac{p(\overline{T} \cap \overline{D})}{p(\overline{D})} = \frac{.784}{.800} = .98$$

In this example the specificity is 98%. Subtracting the results from the total for all possible outcomes (1.00), we can determine the probabilities of false positive or false negative results:

$$False\ positive = 1 - p(sensitivity) = 1 - .90 = .10$$

$$False\ negative = 1 - p(specificity) = 1 - .98 = .02$$

Identical results can be obtained by dividing the frequency within each cell by the sum of the respective column.

$$Sensitivity = \frac{90}{100} = .90$$

$$Specificity = \frac{392}{400} = .98$$

Using our previous layout for a 2x2 chi square design, it is possible to calculate the sensitivity and specificity of a test using the following formula:

<u>Real World</u>

		Present	Absent	
Test	Present	a	b	a+b
Results	Absent	c	d	c+d
		a+c	b+d	n

$$Sensitivity = \frac{a}{a+c} \qquad \text{Eq. 16.1}$$

$$Specificity = \frac{d}{b+d} \qquad \text{Eq. 16.2}$$

$$p(false\ positive\ results) = \frac{b}{b+d} \qquad \text{Eq. 16.3}$$

$$p(false\ negative\ results) = \frac{c}{a+c} \qquad \text{Eq. 16.4}$$

Bayes' Theorem

Let us take our previous example one step further. Based on our trial results with our diagnostic test, which has a sensitivity of 90% and selectivity of 98%, what is the probability that a person who has the HIV antibody in the general population will test positive with the new procedure? Assuming only our sample of 500 volunteers the answer would be:

$$p(D \mid T) = \frac{p(D \cap T)}{p(T)} = \frac{.18}{.196} = .918$$

Sensitivity and specificity are evaluators for the test procedure. However, we are more interested in the ability to detect a disease or condition based on the test results; specifically, the probability of disease given a positive test result (called the **predicted value positive** - PVP) and the probability of no disease given a negative test result (termed the **predicted value negative** - PVN). In other words, we are interested in the general population and want to know the probability that a person having the HIV antibody will test positive. We can calculate this using Bayes' theorem:

$$PVP = p(D \mid T) = \frac{p(T \mid D)p(D)}{p(T \mid D)p(D) + p(T \mid \overline{D})p(\overline{D})} \qquad \text{Eq. 16.5}$$

If this theorem is applied to our sample of 500 volunteers the result is the same:

$$PVP = \frac{(.90)(.20)}{(.90)(.20) + (.02)(.80)} = .918$$

Using this formula, if we know the sensitivity $\{p(T|D)\}$ and complement of the specificity $(1-p(\overline{T} \mid \overline{D}))$ diagnostic test, it can be applied to the general population if we have an estimate of the prevalence of a given disease. **Prevalence** is the probability of persons in a defined population having a specific disease or characteristic. For illustrative purposes, let us assume that the prevalence of HIV antibodies (D) is 5% in the general U.S. population. The calculation of the PVP is:

$$PVP = \frac{(.90)(.05)}{(.90)(.05) + (.02)(.95)} = .70$$

Thus, based on initial trials with our diagnostic test, there is a 70% chance that an individual with HIV antibodies will be identified using our test.

Extending Bayes' theorem, it is possible to determine the probability of having HIV antibodies given a negative diagnostic result or a PVN:

$$PVN = p(D \mid \overline{T}) = \frac{p(\overline{T} \mid D)p(D)}{p(\overline{T} \mid D)p(D) + p(\overline{T} \mid \overline{D})p(\overline{D})} \qquad \text{Eq. 16.6}$$

Using our example data with a population prevalence of .05, the PVN is:

$$PVN = p(D \mid \overline{T}) = \frac{(.10)(.05)}{(.10)(.05) + (.98)(.80)} = 0.006$$

There is a 0.6% chance of missing someone with HIV antibodies if we employ our new diagnostic procedure. Rewritten, Equations 16.5 and 16.6 could be stated as follows:

$$PVP = \frac{sensitivity \; x \; prevalence}{(sensitivity \; x \; prevalence) + [(1 - specificity) \; x \; (1 - prevalence)]} \qquad \text{Eq. 16.7}$$

$$PVN = \frac{[(1 - sensitivity) \; x \; prevalence]}{[(1 - sensitivity \; x \; prevalence)] + [(specificity) \; x \; (1 - prevalence)]} \qquad \text{Eq. 16.8}$$

Therefore, selectivity and sensitivity of a procedure can be applied to a known prevalence to predict the ability to detect specific outcomes. All four of these probabilities (sensitivity, selectivity, predicted value positive and predicted value negative) should be high to be useful for screening information.

Notice in the previous examples we were dealing with dichotomous results (pass or fail, present or absent). Such dichotomies will be used for the following tests that are expansions of the chi square test of independence.

McNemar's Test

The McNemar test can be used to evaluate the relationship or independence of paired discrete variables. The test involves dichotomous measurements (i.e., pass/fail, yes/no, present/absent) which are paired. The paired responses are constructed into a fourfold, or 2x2 contingency table and outcomes are tallied into the appropriate cell. Measurement can be paired on the same individuals or samples over two different time periods (similar to our previous use of the paired t-test in Chapter 8):

First Measurement

		Outcome 1	Outcome 2
Second Measurement	Outcome 1	a	b
	Outcome 2	c	d

Or subjects can be paired based on some predetermined and defined characteristic:

Characteristic B

		Outcome 1	Outcome 2
Characteristic A	Outcome 1	a	b
	Outcome 2	c	d

For example, if it were based on a yes/no response over two time periods, those individuals responding "yes" at both time periods would be counted in the upper left corner (cell a) and those answering "no" on both occasions would be counted in the lower right corner (cell d). Mixed answers, indicating changes in responses would be counted in the other two diagonal cells (b and c). If there was absolutely no change over the two time periods, we would expect that 100% of the results would appear in cells a and d. Those falling in cells c and b represent changes over the two measurements.

For the McNemar's test the statistic is as follows:

$$\chi^2_{McNemar} = \frac{(b-c)^2}{b+c} \qquad \text{Eq. 16.9}$$

As with Yate's correction of continuity more conservative approximation can be made for the McNemar test:

$$\chi^2_{McNemar} = \frac{(|b-c|-1)^2}{b+c} \qquad \text{Eq. 16.10}$$

The null hypothesis would be that there is no significant change between the two times or characteristics. Because we are dealing with a 2x2 contingency table, the degrees of freedom is one (rows-1 x columns-1). Thus we will compare our calculated statistic to a critical χ^2 with one degree of freedom or 3.84, (Appendix B, Table B10). If the $\chi^2_{McNemar}$ exceeds 3.84 we reject H_0 and assume a significant change between the two measurements (similar to our previous H_0: $\mu \neq 0$ in the paired t-test).

As an example, assume that 100 patients are randomly selected based on visits to a local clinic and assessed for specific behavior that is classified as a risk factor for colon cancer. The risk factor is classified as either present or absent. During the course of their visit and with a follow-up clinic newsletter, they are educated about the incidence and associated risks for a variety of cancers. Six months after the initial assessment patients are evaluated with respect to the presence or absence of the same risk factor. The following table represents the results of the study:

		Risk Factor Before Instruction		
		Present	Absent	
Risk Factor	Present	40	5	45
After Instruction	Absent	20	35	55
		60	40	100

The null hypothesis would be that the instructional efforts had no effect.

H_0:   Instruction did not influence presence of the risk factor
H_1: H_0 is false

The decision rule would be to reject H_0, of independence, if $\chi^2_{McNemar}$ greater than $\chi^2_1(1-\alpha) = 3.84$. The calculations would be:

$$\chi^2_{McNemar} = \frac{(b-c)^2}{b+c} = \frac{(5-20)^2}{5+20} = \frac{225}{25} = 9.0$$

Yate's correction of continuity would produce a more conservative estimation:

$$\chi^2_{McNemar} = \frac{(|b-c|-1)^2}{b+c} = \frac{(|5-20|-1)^2}{5+20} = \frac{196}{25} = 7.84$$

Either method would result in the rejection of H_0 and the decision that the instruction of patients resulted in a change in risk taking behavior.

Another way to think of McNemar's procedure is as a test of proportions, based on samples that are related or correlated in some way. The McNemar test does not require the computation of the standard error for the correlation coefficient. The computation, using the previous notations for a 2x2 contingency table is:

$$z = \frac{a-d}{\sqrt{a+d}} \qquad \text{Eq. 16.11}$$

where in large samples $\chi^2 = z^2$.

Cochran's Q Test

Cochran's Q test can be thought of as a complement to the complete randomized block design, discussed in Chapter 9, when dealing with discrete data. It is an extension of the McNemar test to three or more levels of the independent variable. Similar to the randomized complete block design discussed in Chapter 9, subjects or observations are assigned to blocks to reduce variability within each level of the independent variable. The design is used to create homogenous blocks. The data is set up so that each level of the independent variable represents a column and each row represents a homogeneous block. Similar to the randomized block design, subjects are assigned to blocks to reduce variability within each treatment level and subjects within each block are more homogeneous than subjects within the different blocks. As seen in Table 16.1, the blocking effect is represented by the row and each block contains results for each level of the independent variable. There is still only one observation per cell and this is reported as a pass (coded as 1) or fail (coded as 0) result. Each of the columns are summed (C) and the sum squared (C^2). Also, each block is summed (R) and the sum squared (R^2). Lastly, both the R and R^2 are summed producing $\sum R$ and $\sum R^2$. The formula for

TABLE 16.1 General Structure of a Randomized Block Design

	Levels of the Independent Variable				
	$\underline{C_1}$	$\underline{C_2}$	$\underline{C_k}$	$\underline{R}$	$\underline{R^2}$
Block b_1	x_{11}	x_{12} ...	x_{1k}	$\sum x_{1k}$	$\sum x_{1k}^2$
Block b_2	x_{21}	x_{22} ...	x_{2k}	$\sum x_{2k}$	$\sum x_{2k}^2$
Block b_3	x_{31}	x_{32} ...	x_{3k}	$\sum x_{3k}$	$\sum x_{3k}^2$
...	...	... ...	...	...	...
Block b_j	x_{j1}	x_{j2} ...	x_{jk}	$\sum x_{jk}$	$\sum x_{jk}^2$
C	$\sum x_{j1}$	$\sum x_{j2}$	$\sum x_{jk}$		
C^2	$\sum x_{j1}^2$	$\sum x_{j2}^2$ ...	$\sum x_{jk}^2$		
			$\sum R =$	$\sum\sum x_k$	
			$\sum R^2 =$	$\sum\sum x_k^2$	

Cochran's Q is:

$$Q = \frac{(k-1)\,[(k\sum C^2) - (\sum R)^2]}{k(\sum R) - \sum R^2} \qquad \text{Eq. 16.12}$$

where k is the number of levels of the discrete independent variable. The resultant Q-value is compared to the chi square critical value with K-1 degrees of freedom. If the Q-value exceeds the critical value there is a significant difference among the various levels of the independent variable.

As an example, a pharmaceutical company is trying to decide among four different types of gas chromatographs produced by four different manufacturers. To evaluate the performance of these types of equipment, ten laboratory technicians are asked to run samples and evaluate the use of each piece of equipment. They are instructed to respond as either acceptable (coded 1) or unacceptable (coded 0) for the analysis performed by the equipment. The results of their evaluations appear in Table 16.2. Is their a significant relationship between the manufacturer and technicians' evaluations?

Table 16.2 Evaluations for Various Types of Equipment

| Technician | Manufacturer | | | |
	A	B	C	D
1	0	1	0	1
2	0	0	0	1
3	1	0	0	1
4	0	1	0	1
5	0	0	1	0
6	0	0	1	1
7	0	0	0	1
8	0	1	1	1
9	0	0	0	1
10	1	0	0	1

The hypotheses being tested are:

H_0: Technician evaluations are independent of the equipment tested
H_1: H_0 is false

The decision rule is, with 95% confidence or α equal to 0.05, reject H_0 if Q is greater than $\chi^2_{(k-1)}(1-\alpha)$ which is 7.81 (k-1 = 3). The sum of columns and rows are presented in Table 16.3 and the calculation of Cochran's Q is as follows:

$$Q = \frac{(k-1)\,[(k \sum C^2) - (\sum R)^2]}{k(\sum R) - \sum R^2}$$

$$Q = \frac{(3)\,[(4)(103) - (17)^2]}{(4)(17) - 33} = \frac{369}{35} = 10.54$$

With Q greater than the critical value of 7.81, the decision is to reject the hypothesis of independence and assume that the type of equipment tested did influence the technicians' responses. Based on the Cs presented in Tables 16.2 and 16.3, manufacturer D's product appears to be preferred.

Table 16.3 Example of Cochran's Q Test

Technician	Manufacturer				R	R^2
	A	B	C	D		
1	0	1	0	1	2	4
2	0	0	0	1	1	1
3	1	0	0	1	2	4
4	0	1	0	1	2	4
5	0	0	1	0	1	1
6	0	0	1	1	2	4
7	0	0	0	1	1	1
8	0	1	1	1	3	9
9	0	0	0	1	1	1
10	1	0	0	1	2	4
C =	2	3	3	9		
$C^2 =$	4	9	9	81		

$$\Sigma R = \quad 17$$
$$\Sigma C^2 = 103 \qquad \Sigma R^2 = \qquad\qquad 33$$

Relative Risk

In the search for causes of specific diseases, epidemiologists are interested in the risks of certain behaviors or characteristics on the causes of these diseases. Outcomes (i.e., disease, disability, death) are compared against potential risk factors (i.e., predisposing characteristics, exposure to disease or pollutants, risk taking behavior). The design of such comparisons is presented below:

	Factor	No Factor
Outcome	a	b
No outcome	c	d

Using this design, a **cross sectional study** can be undertaken where an overall sample of the population is collected without regard for either the outcome or factors involved. For example, a cross section of the individuals in the Midwest are compared for the incidence of smoking and chronic lung disease. A second type of study, a **prospective study**, would involve sampling subjects with and without the risk factor and to evaluate the development of a certain condition or outcome over a period of time. For example, workers in a chemical production facility are divided into two groups: one group working unprotected in the existing conditions and the other group required to wear protective masks. After a period of time, workers in such a **follow-up** or **longitudinal study** would be evaluated on respiratory function tests. In these types of studies, individuals are evaluated for the risk of a particular outcome with exposure to the factor:

$$Risk\ of\ outcome\ with\ factor = \frac{a}{a+c} \qquad \text{Eq. 16.13}$$

and the risk of the outcome without exposure:

$$Risk\ of\ outcome\ without\ factor = \frac{b}{b+d} \qquad \text{Eq. 16.14}$$

The **relative risk** (RR) from exposure to the factor is the ratio between the two rates:

$$Relative\ Risk = \frac{\dfrac{a}{a+c}}{\dfrac{b}{b+d}} \qquad \text{Eq. 16.15}$$

Algebraically this can be simplified to:

$$Relative\ Risk = \frac{ab + ad}{ab + bc} \qquad \text{Eq. 16.16}$$

Relative risk can be any value greater than or equal to zero. If the RR = 1 there is no association between the factor and the outcome (independence). If the RR is greater than one this indicates a positive association or an increased risk that the outcome will occur with exposure to that factor. RR less than one is a negative association, or protection against the outcome. The relative risk is our best estimate of the strength of the factor-outcome association.

For example, suppose a cross sectional study was performed on a random sample of Midwesterners to determine the relative risk of developing a chronic lung disease for smokers versus non-smokers. First, it is important to have predefined criteria for labeling individuals as "smokers" and to classify

Table 16.4   Example of Relative Risk

		Risk Factor		
		Smokers	Non-smokers	
Chronic	Present	101	35	136
Lung Disease	Absent	51	313	364
		152	348	500

diagnostic criteria to define patients as having a chronic lung disease. With these criteria established, 500 individuals over 65 years of age are sampled and surveyed. The results are presented in Table 16.4. In this example the relative risk is:

$$RR = \frac{ab + ad}{ab + bc} = \frac{(101)(35) + (101)(313)}{(101)(35) + (35)(51)} = 6.60$$

A chi square analysis for our 2x2 table, with one degree of freedom, can be used to test the hypotheses associated with risk:

$$H_0: \quad RR = 1$$
$$H_1: \quad RR \neq 1$$

The null hypothesis is independence between the factor and the outcome. As they become closely related, the RR will increase and there is a greater likelihood that the difference is not due to chance alone and H_0 is rejected. In this example (Eq. 13.5):

$$\chi^2 = \frac{n(ad - bc)^2}{(a+b)(b+d)(a+b)(c+d)}$$

$$\chi^2 = \frac{500[(101)(313) - (35)(51)]^2}{(136)(364)(152)(348)} = 169.88$$

With a chi square greater than $\chi^2_1 = 3.84$, we can reject H_0 and assume that there is a significant association between smoking (as a risk factor) and chronic lung disease (the outcome).

Mantel-Haenszel Relative Risk

The Mantel-Haenszel relative risk ratio, some times referred to as the **Mantel-Haenszel common odds ratio,** is a method for calculating relative risk while controlling for a third potentially confounding variable. It involves stratification of our original data into levels for the third variable. The Mantel-Haenszel relative risk (RR_{MH}) is calculated as follows:

$$RR_{MH} = \frac{\sum \dfrac{a_i(c_i + d_i)}{N_i}}{\sum \dfrac{c_i(a_i + b_i)}{N_i}} \qquad \text{Eq. 16.17}$$

where a_i, b_i, ... N_i represent results at each individual strata or level. The test statistic produces an overall risk ratio controlling for the third variable. For example, consider gender as a possible confounding variable in our previous example of smoking and chronic lung disease. The results are presented below:

Gender	Chronic Lung Disease	Smoker	Non-smoker	Totals
Male	Yes	71	30	101
	No	27	97	124
		98	127	225
Female	Yes	30	5	35
	No	24	216	240
		54	221	275

For this example the relative risk of chronic lung disease in smokers, controlling for gender is:

$$RR_{MH} = \frac{\dfrac{71(27+97)}{225} + \dfrac{30(24+216)}{275}}{\dfrac{27(71+30)}{225} + \dfrac{24(30+5)}{275}} = \frac{65.31}{15.17} = 4.31$$

The results are interpreted similar to the RR discussed in the previous section. The next logical extension of this ratio is to determine if the original comparison is significant controlling for the possible confounding variable.

Mantel-Haenszel Chi Square

The Mantel-Haenszel test, sometimes referred to as the **Cochran-Mantel-Haenszel test**, can be thought of as a three-dimensional chi square test, where a 2x2 contingency table is associated with main factors in the row and column dimensions. However a third, possibly confounding variable, is added as a depth dimension in our design. This third extraneous factor may have k-levels and the resultant design would be 2x2xk levels of three discrete variables. In other words, we are comparing k different 2x2 contingency tables. Using the a,b,c,d labels as in the previous 2x2 designs, the Mantel-Haenszel compares each a_i (a_1 through a_k) with its corresponding expected value. The a_i is the observed value for any one level of the possible confounding variable. The statistic is:

$$\chi^2_{MH} = \frac{\left[\sum \frac{a_i d_i - b_i c_i}{n_i} \right]^2}{\sum \frac{(a+b)_i (c+d)_i (a+c)_i (b+d)_i}{(n_i - 1)(n_i^2)}}$$

Eq. 16.18

This can be modified to create a numerator that compares the observed and expected values for one cell of the 2x2 matrix and sums this comparison for each level of the confounding variable.

$$\chi^2_{MH} = \frac{\left[\sum \left(a_i - \frac{(a_i + b_i)(a_i + c_i)}{n_i} \right) \right]^2}{\sum \frac{(a+b)_i (c+d)_i (a+c)_i (b+d)_i}{n_i^2 (n_i - 1)}}$$

Eq. 16.19

The null hypothesis reflects independence between the row and column variable, correcting for the third extraneous factor. The calculated χ^2_{MH} is compared to the critical value $\chi^2_1(1-\alpha)$. If that value exceeds the critical value, the row and column factors are not independent and there is a significant relationship between the two factors.

For example, consider the previous example regarding relative risk of smoking and lung disease. Assume that we are concerned that the subjects environment might confound the finding. We decide to also evaluate the data based on home setting (i.e., urban, suburb, rural). Reevaluating the data, it is found that:

Site	Chronic Lung Disease	Smoker	Non-smoker	Totals
Urban	Yes	45	7	52
	No	16	80	96
		61	87	148
Suburban	Yes	29	10	39
	No	19	182	201
		48	192	240
Rural	Yes	27	18	45
	No	16	51	67
		43	69	112

Equation 16.14 can be simplified by modifying certain parts of the equation. For example the e_i (the expected value) for each confounding level of a_i is:

$$e_i = \frac{(a_i + b_i)(a_i + c_i)}{n_i}$$

Eq. 16.20

This is equivalent to stating that the sum of the margin for the row multiplied by the margin for the column divided by the total number of observations associated with the ith level is the expected value. This is the same way we calculated the expected value in the contingency table for a chi square test of independence. For example, for the suburban level the e_i is:

$$e_2 = \frac{(39)(48)}{240} = 7.8$$

This will be compared to the observed result ($a_2 = 29$) to create part of the numerator for Eq. 16.14. In a similar manner, a v_i can be calculated for the denominator at each level of the confounding variable:

$$v_i = \frac{(a_i + b_i)(c_i + d_i)(a_i + c_i)(b_i + d_i)}{n_i^2 (n_i - 1)}$$

Eq. 16.21

The v_i for the rural level is:

$$v_3 = \frac{(45)(67)(43)(69)}{(112)^2(112-1)} = 6.425$$

These intermediate results can be expressed in a table format:

	Urban	Suburban	Rural
a_i	45	29	27
e_i	21.43	7.80	17.28
v_i	8.23	5.25	6.42

and entered into the following equation:

$$\chi^2_{MH} = \frac{[\Sigma(a_i - e_i)]^2}{\Sigma v_i} \qquad \text{Eq. 16.22}$$

The results are

$$\chi^2_{MH} = \frac{[(45-21.43)+(29-7.80)+(27-17.28)]^2}{(8.23+5.25+6.42)} = \frac{(54.49)^2}{19.90} = 149.20$$

With the χ^2_{MH} greater than $\chi^2_i(1-\alpha)$ we reject the null hypothesis of no association between the two main factors controlling for the potentially confounding environmental factor. If the value would have been less than the critical χ^2 value we would have failed to reject the null hypothesis and assumed that the confounding variable affected the initial χ^2 results for the 2x2 contingency table.

A correction for continuity can also be made with the Mantel-Haenszel procedure:

$$\chi^2_{MH} = \frac{[\Sigma(a_i - e_i) - 0.5]^2}{\Sigma v_i} \qquad \text{Eq. 16.23}$$

In the previous example this correction would produce the expected, more conservative result:

$$\chi^2_{MH} = \frac{(54.49 - 0.5)^2}{19.90} = 146.47$$

In this case, either the Mantel-Haenszel test or the corrected version would produce a statistically significant result and rejection of the null hypothesis.

Phi Coefficient

In Chapter 12 the correlation coefficient was presented as a method for assessing the strength of a relationship between continuous variables. Modifications are available to measure relationships between discrete outcomes. The simplest would be a 2x2 chi square-type problem, where the levels of the two variables could be considered continuous in an assignment of 1 or 0 to these **dichotomous variables**. Called a **fourfold point correlation**, we can create a **phi coefficient** (ϕ) which measures the extent of the relationship between the two variables. The formula uses a layout similar to the ones presented earlier in this chapter and for the computational chi square statistic for a 2x2 design (Eq. 15.5):

a	b	a+b
c	d	c+d
a+c	b+d	n

The calculation of the phi coefficient is:

$$\phi = \frac{(b)(c) - (a)(d)}{\sqrt{(a+b)(c+d)(a+c)(b+d)}}$$

Eq. 16.24

For example, assume an equal number of males and females are treated with the same medication for a specific illness and the outcome is either success (the interpretation of ϕ is the same as Pearson's product-moment correlation) or failure.

	Success	Failure	
Males	30	20	50
Females	45	5	50
	75	25	100

The relationship between gender and response would be calculated as follows:

$$\phi = \frac{(20)(45) - (30)(5)}{\sqrt{(50)(50)(75)(25)}} = \frac{750}{2165.06} = 0.346$$

Thus, the ϕ-value is 0.346 and there is a weak correlation between gender and response, with women apparently responding proportionately better than men.

This process can be extended to dichotomous variables that have more than two categories. This **contingency coefficient** (C) utilizes the chi square contingency table and the statistic that is computed when comparing two discrete variables.

$$C = \sqrt{\frac{\chi^2}{\chi^2 + n}}$$

Eq. 16.25

Once again the significance of the C-value is interpreted the same as a correlation coefficient. For example in Chapter 15 it was found in a pharmacology experiment that the ages of mice and induction of sleep using a specific chemical were not independent of each other ($\chi^2 = 6.94$).

	Asleep (C_1)	Awake (C_2)
3 months (R_1)	7	13
10 months (R_2)	9	11
26 months (R_3)	15	5

The contingency coefficient would be:

$$C = \sqrt{\frac{6.94}{6.94 + 60}} = \sqrt{0.104} = .322$$

The results would be a weak correlation between the age of the mice and the induction of sleep.

Logistic Regression

Up to this point we have considered the effects of continuous independent variables and outcomes, which are measured as continuous dependent variables. What if the result is a binary, two-level discrete outcome (i.e., live or die)? Logistic regression analysis allows us to examine the relationship between a dependent discrete variable with two possible outcomes, and one or more independent variables. In logistic regression the independent variable(s) may be continuous or discrete. Also, unlike regression analysis, it may not be possible to order the levels of the independent variable. This method is especially useful in epidemiological studies involving a binary dependent variable, where we wish to determine the relationship between outcomes and exposure variables (i.e., age, smoking history, obesity, presence or absence of given pathologies). Such binary outcomes include the presence or absence of a disease state or the likelihood or odds of survival given a particular state. The use of odds, and odds ratios, for the evaluation of outcomes is one of the major advantages of logistic regression analysis.

The **odds ratio** (OR or θ) is a useful statistic for measuring the level of association in contingency tables. A 2x2 contingency table is constructed using the previously discussed notation:

	Outcome of Interest	Opposite Outcome
Independent Variable:		
Level 1	a	b
Level 2	c	d

The odds ratio can be calculated using the following equation:

$$OR = \theta = \frac{a}{b} \bigg/ \frac{c}{d} \qquad \text{Eq. 16.26}$$

which can be algebraically simplified to:

$$\theta = \frac{a \cdot d}{b \cdot c} \qquad \text{Eq. 16.27}$$

If θ is less than one, the outcome proportion for level one of the independent variable is greater than the proportion for level two. Conversely, if θ is greater than one, then the second level is greater than the proportion for the first level.

To illustrate odds ratio, and eventually logistic regression, consider the following example. Assume 156 patients undergoing endoscopy examinations, and based on predefined criteria, are classified into two groups based on the presence or absence of gastric ulcer(s). A majority of patients (105) are found to have gastric ulcers present and the remaining 51 are diagnosed as ulcer free. Researchers are concerned that smoking may be associated with the presence of gastric ulcers, through the swallowing of chemicals found in smoking products. These same individuals are further classified as either smokers or non-smokers. The results of the endoscopic examinations, based on the two variables

Table 16.5 Outcomes from Endoscopic Examinations

	Gastric Ulcer(s)		
	Present	Absent	
Smokers	60	23	83
Non-smokers	45	28	73
	105	51	156

are presented in Table 16.5. The odds ratio for having a gastric ulcer given that the person was a smoker is:

$$\theta_1 = \frac{a \cdot d}{b \cdot c} = \frac{60 \cdot 28}{45 \cdot 23} = 1.62$$

Thus, the odds or probability is much greater for a smoker requiring an endoscopic examination to exhibit a gastric ulcer. The outcomes seen in Table 16.5 represent a 2x2 contingency table similar to ones discussed and for which we already have several tests to analyze the data (i.e., chi square). Where the chi square tested the relationship between the two discrete variables, the odds ratio focuses on the likelihood that the act of smoking can be used as a predictor of an outcome of gastric ulcers. Unfortunately odds ratio are only concerned with 2x2 contingency tables. Logistic regression can be used when there are two or more levels of the independent variable.

If regression analysis were used on scores of 1 for success and 0 for failure using a fitted process, the resultant value would be interpreted as the predicted probability of a successful outcome. Unfortunately, with such an ordinal regression the outcomes or predicted probabilities could exceed 1 or fall below 0 (as discusses in Chapter 2, $0 \leq p(E) \leq 1$). In logistic regression, the equations involve the natural logarithm (ln) of the probabilities associated with the possible outcomes. These logarithms associated with the probabilites (or odds) are referred to as the **log odds** or **logit**.

$$\log it = ln \frac{\pi_{i1}}{\pi_{i2}} \qquad \text{Eq. 16.28}$$

Where π_{i1} is the probability of the first possible outcome of the dichotomous outcome (presence), π_{i2} is the probability of the second outcome (absence) at ith lead level of the predictor variable (smoking). These odds are based on the probabilities of being in any given cell of the matrix based on the total number of observations. The probability (π_{11}) of the presence of a gastric ulcer and being a heavy smoker is 60/156 = 0.385 and the second possible outcome for heavy smokers (π_{12} – absence of ulcer) is 23/156 = 0.147. The result would be the following probabilities, where the sum of all possible outcomes is one ($\sum p = 1.00$):

	Gastric Ulcer(s) Present	Absent
Smokers	0.385	0.147
Non-smokers	0.288	0.179

Therefore, for smokers the logit would be:

$$logit(S) = ln\frac{0.385}{0.147} = ln(2.62) = 0.96$$

and for non-smokers:

$$logit(S) = ln\frac{0.288}{0.179} = ln(1.61) = 0.48$$

By using the logit transformation the transformed proportion values can range from minus infinity and plus infinity (logit(1) = +∞, logit(.5) = 0, and logit(0) = -∞). In this particular example, the larger the logit value the greater the likelihood that the action (smoking) will serve as a predictor of the outcome (gastric ulcer).

	Gastric Ulcer(s) Present	Absent	Logit
Smokers	60	23	0.96
Non-smokers	45	28	0.48

We can also use the π values to calculate our odds ratio:

$$\theta = \frac{\pi_{11} \cdot \pi_{22}}{\pi_{12} \cdot \pi_{21}} \qquad \text{Eq. 16.29}$$

In this example the odds ratio is:

$$\theta = \frac{\pi_{11} \cdot \pi_{22}}{\pi_{12} \cdot \pi_{21}} = \frac{(0.385)(0.179)}{(0.288)(0.147)} = 1.62$$

The advantage of using the logistic regression analysis is we can expand the number of our levels of the independent variable to more than just two. Using the above example, assume that the researcher instead classified the smokers as light and heavy smokers and found the results in Table 16.6. Logits can be calculated for each of the levels seen in Table 16.6. For example the logit for heavy smokers would be:

$$log\, it(S) = ln\frac{19/156}{7/156} = ln\frac{0.122}{0.045} = ln(2.711) = 0.997$$

In this particular example, the larger the logit value the greater likelihood that the action (smoking) will serve as a predictor of the outcome (gastric ulcer). Listed below are the logit numbers for all three levels of smokers:

| | Gastric Ulcer(s) | | |
	Present	Absent	Logit
Heavy smokers	19	7	1.00
Light smokers	41	16	0.93
Non-smokers	45	28	0.48

What if the researchers are interested in a possible third confound variable, such as stress, alcohol intake or socioeconomic class? Multiple logistic regression offers procedures and interpretations similar to those found with multiple linear regression, except the transformed scale is based on the probability of success of a particular outcome. Also, many of the procedures used for multiple linear regression can be adapted for logistic regression analysis. Multiple logistic regression can be used to build models and assess the goodness-of-fit of the data to the proposed model. Application usually requires significant computer manipulation of the data and goes beyond the scope of this book. A more extensive introduction to the topic of multiple logistic regression can be found in Kleinbaum, et. al. (1982) and Forthofer and Lee (1995).

References

Forthofer, R.N. and Lee E.S. (1995). Introduction to Biostatistics: A Guide to Design, Analysis and Discovery, Academic Press, San Deigo, pp. 440-444.

Table 16.6 Outcomes from Endoscopic Examinations

	Gastric Ulcer(s)		
	Present	Absent	
Heavy smokers	19	7	26
Light smokers	41	16	57
Non-smokers	45	28	73
	105	51	156

Kachigan, S.K. (1991). Multivariate Statistical Analysis, second edition, Radius Press, New York, p. 181.

Suggested Supplemental Readings

Fisher, L.D. and van Belle, G. (1993). Biostatistics: A Methodology for the Health Sciences, John Wiley and Sons, Inc., New York, pp. 206-211.

Forthofer, R.N. and Lee E.S. (1995). Introduction to Biostatistics: A Guide to Design, Analysis and Discovery, Academic Press, San Deigo, pp. 104-107, 310-313, 440-444.

Havilcek, L.L. and Crain, R.D. (1988). Practical Statistics for the Physical Sciences, American Chemical Society, Washington, DC, pp. 83-93, 106-114, 209-212.

Ingelfinger, J.A., et al. (1994). Biostatistics in Clinical Medicine, McGraw-Hill, Inc. New York, pp. 16-17.

Kachigan, S.K. (1991). Multivariate Statistical Analysis, second edition, Radius Press, New York, p. 181.

Example Problems

1. Immediately after training on a new analytical method, technicians were asked their preference between the new method and a previously used, "old" method. Six months later, after the technicians had experience with the new method, they were resurveyed with respect to their preference. The results of the two surveys are presented below. Did experience with the new method significantly change their preferences?

		Preferred Method Before Experience		
		New	Old	
Preferred Method	New	12	8	20
After Experience	Old	3	7	10
		15	15	30

2. In Chapter 15, a piece of disintegration equipment showed different results based on the temperature under which the tests were run. Using the phi coefficient, how strong is the relationship between the temperature of the solution and the pass/fail rate of the test?

	Successes (R_1)	Failures (R_2)	
Higher Temperature (T_1)	96	4	100
Lower Temperature (T_2)	88	12	100
	184	16	200

3. Twenty volunteers were randomly assigned to a randomized three-way cross-over clinical trial involving the same topical medication presented in three different formulations (A,B and C). During each phase of the study volunteers were assessed for the presence or absence of erythema (redness) at the site of application. Was there any significant difference among the formulation for the incidence of erythema?

Volunteer	Formulation A	B	C	Volunteer	Formulation A	B	C
001	0	1	0	011	0	0	1
002	1	0	1	012	0	0	0
003	0	0	0	013	1	0	1
004	0	0	0	014	0	0	0
005	0	1	1	015	0	0	0
006	0	0	0	016	0	0	0
007	0	0	0	017	1	1	0
008	0	0	0	018	0	0	0
009	0	0	0	019	1	0	1
010	1	1	0	020	1	1	1

(code: 1 = erythema)

4. Returning to the first example in the problem set for Chapter 2, we employed 150 healthy females volunteers to take part in a multi-center

study of a new urine testing kit to determine pregnancy. One-half of the volunteers were pregnant, in their first trimester. Based on test results with our new agent we found the following:

		Study Volunteers		
		Pregnant	Not Pregnant	
Test Results for Pregnancy	Positive	73	5	78
	Negative	2	70	72
		75	75	150

What is the specificity and selectivity of our test and what is the likelihood of a pregnant volunteer experiencing a false negative result?

5. In one of the example problems in Chapter 15, an instrument manufacturer ran a series of disintegration tests to compare the pass/fail rate of a new piece of equipment at two extreme temperatures. The manufacturer decided to also evaluate the influence of paddle speed as a possible confounding factor. The test was designed to collect results at two speeds, defined as fast and slow. The results were as follows:

		Test Results		
Speed of Paddle	Temperature	Pass	Fail	Totals
Fast	39°C	48	2	50
	35°C	47	3	50
		95	5	100
Slow	39°C	48	2	50
	35°C	45	5	50
		93	7	100

Without Yate's correction for continuity there is a significant relationship between the temperature and proportion of test failures ($\chi^2 = 4.35$). Could the paddle speed be a confounding factor in the design?

6. During a cholera outbreak in a war devastated country, records for one hospital were examined for the survival of children contracting the disease. These records also reported the children's nutritional status. The charts of children were surveyed and first paired by sex, age, ethnic background and then information on survival was explored. Was there a significant

relationship between their nutrition and survival rate?

		Good Nutrition		
		Survived	Died	
Poor	Survived	52	10	62
Health	Died	45	28	73
		97	38	135

7. In an attempt to standardize a new analytical method across various nationalities and languages, the proposed method was tested at five laboratories in five different countries. Twelve identical samples were sent to each site and the laboratories were asked to pass or fail the samples based on the criteria specified with the new method. Based on the following results, was there a significant relationship between the outcome and the laboratory performing the test?

	Laboratory Result (1 = pass)				
Sample	A	B	C	D	E
101	0	1	1	1	0
102	1	0	1	1	1
103	0	0	0	0	0
104	1	1	1	1	1
105	1	1	1	1	1
106	1	0	1	1	0
107	1	0	0	1	1
108	1	1	1	1	1
109	1	1	1	1	1
110	1	1	1	1	1
111	1	0	1	1	1
112	1	1	1	1	1

8. A total of 750 women were followed for a period of ten years following radical mastectomy. A comparison of their survival rates versus whether or not there was axially node involvement at the time of the surgery is presented below:

		Nodal Involvement		
		Yes (+)	No (-)	
Outcome in	Dead	299	107	406
10 years	Alive	126	218	344
		425	325	750

a. Based on this one study, what is the relative risk of death within ten years following a mastectomy and positive nodes? Is the relationship between survival and node involvement statistically significant?

b. The researchers are concerned that the presence of estrogen receptors, because this factor (estrogen positive or estrogen negative patients) may have confounded the results of the study. Based on the following outcomes, what is the relative risk of death within 10 years and does estrogen receptor status appear to confound the results?

Estrogen Receptors	Outcome	Node(+)	Node(-)	Totals
Positive	Dead	179	26	205
	Alive	100	148	248
		279	174	453
Negative	Dead	120	81	201
	Alive	26	70	96
		146	151	297

9. In Chapter 15, it was found that the variables of torque of closure and moisture permeability were not independent of each other ($\chi^2 = 18.43$). Using a contingency coefficient, how strong is the relationship between these two variables?

Moisture	Torque (inch-pounds)				
	21	24	27	30	
< 2000	26	31	36	45	138
≥ 2000	24	19	14	5	62
Total	50	50	50	50	200

10. Modifying question 7 in Chapter 15, assume that containers which contained a moisture level <2000 are defined as "success." Using logistic regression, identify which amount of torque applied to the container closures would have the greatest likelihood of success?

Torque (inch-pounds):	Success (<2000)	Failure (≥2000)	
21	26	24	50
24	31	19	50
27	36	14	50
30	45	5	50
	138	62	200

Answers to Problems

1. Paired comparison between technicians' evaluations at two times - McNemar's test.

Hypotheses: H_0: Experience did not influence opinion of equipment
H_1: H_0 is false

Decision rule: With $\alpha = 0.05$, reject H_0, if $\chi^2_{McNemar} > \chi^2_1(1-\alpha) = 3.84$.

Calculations:

		Preferred Method Before Experience	
		New	Old
Preferred Method	New	12	8	20
After Experience	Old	3	7	10
		15	15	30

$$\chi^2_{McNemar} = \frac{(b-c)^2}{b+c}$$

$$\chi^2_{McNemar} = \frac{(8-3)^2}{8+3} = \frac{25}{11} = 2.27$$

Correction of continuity:

$$\chi^2_{McNemar} = \frac{(|b-c|-1)^2}{b+c}$$

$$\chi^2_{McNemar} = \frac{(|8-3|-1)^2}{8+3} = \frac{16}{11} = 1.45$$

Decision: Fail to reject H_0, conclude there was no significant change in method preference over the six month period.

2. Comparison of temperature and disintegration results.
    Variables: Discrete dichotomous variables (two measurement scales)

	Successes (R_1)	Failures (R_2)	
Higher Temperature (T_1)	96	4	100
Lower Temperature (T_2)	88	12	100
	184	16	200

Fourfold point correlations:

$$\phi = \frac{(b)(c) - (a)(d)}{\sqrt{(a+b)(c+d)(a+c)(b+d)}}$$

$$\phi = \frac{(4)(88) - (96)(12)}{\sqrt{(100)(100)(184)(16)}} = \frac{-800}{5425.86} = -0.147$$

Correlation results: $\phi = -0.147$, a "very weak" negative relationship between increasing temperature and successful disintegration results.

3. Comparison of three topical formulations - Cochran's Q.

Hypotheses: H_0:   Development of erythema is independent of the formulation used
            H_1: H_0 is false

Decision rule: With $\alpha = 0.05$, reject H_0 if $Q > \chi^2_2(1-\alpha) = 5.99$.

Computations:

	Formulation (1 = erythema)				
Volunteer	A	B	C	R	R^2
001	0	1	0	1	1
002	1	0	1	2	4
003	0	0	0	0	0
004	0	0	0	0	0
005	0	1	1	2	4
006	0	0	0	0	0
007	0	0	0	0	0
008	0	0	0	0	0
009	0	0	0	0	0
010	1	1	0	2	4
011	0	0	1	1	1
012	0	0	0	0	0
013	1	0	1	2	4
014	0	0	0	0	0
015	0	0	0	0	0
016	0	0	0	0	0
017	1	1	0	2	4
018	0	0	0	0	0
019	1	0	1	2	4
020	1	1	1	3	9
C =	6	5	6		
C^2 =	36	25	36		
				ΣR =	17
	ΣC^2 = 97			ΣR^2 =	35

$$Q = \frac{(k-1)\,[(k\,\Sigma C^2)-(\Sigma R)^2]}{k(\Sigma R)-\Sigma R^2}$$

$$Q = \frac{(2)\,[(3)(97)-(17)^2]}{(3)(17)-35} = \frac{4}{16} = 0.25$$

Decision: With $Q < 5.99$, fail to reject H_0 and conclude that erythema is independent of the formulation.

4.   Sensitivity, specificity and probability of a false negative result for a trial urine pregnancy test.

		Study Volunteers		
		Pregnant	Not Pregnant	
Test Results	Positive	73	5	78
for Pregnancy	Negative	2	70	72
		75	75	150

$$Sensitivity = \frac{a}{a+c} = \frac{73}{75} = .973$$

$$Specificity = \frac{d}{b+d} = \frac{70}{75} = .933$$

$$p(false\ negative\ results) = \frac{c}{a+c} = \frac{2}{75} = .027$$

5. Comparison of pass/fail rate with a piece of disintegration equipment at different temperatures, controlling for paddle speed - Mantel-Haenszel chi square.

Hypotheses: H_0: Temperature and failure rate are independent
(controlling for paddle speed)
H_1: H_0 is false

Decision rule: With $\alpha = 0.05$, reject H_0 if $\chi^2_{MH} > \chi^2_1(1-\alpha) = 3.84$.

		Test Results		
Speed of Paddle	Temperature	Pass	Fail	Totals
Fast	39°C	48	2	50
	35°C	47	3	50
		95	5	100
Slow	39°C	48	2	50
	35°C	45	5	50
		93	7	100

Intermediate steps for fast speed:

$$e_1 = \frac{(a_1+b_1)(a_1+c_1)}{n_1} = \frac{(50)(95)}{100} = 47.5$$

$$v_1 = \frac{(a_1+b_1)(c_1+d_1)(a_1+c_1)(b_1+d_1)}{n_1^2(n_1-1)}$$

$$v_i = \frac{(50)(50)(95)(5)}{100^2(99)} = \frac{1,187,500}{990,000} = 1.199$$

	Fast	Slow
a_i	48	48
e_i	47.5	46.5
v_i	1.2	1.6

Mantel-Haenszel chi square:

$$\chi_{MH}^2 = \frac{[\Sigma(a_i-e_i)]^2}{\Sigma v_i} = \frac{[(48-47.5)+(48-46.5)]^2}{1.2+1.6} = 1.43$$

Decision: Fail to reject H_0, conclude that the temperature and failure rates are independent.

6. Paired comparison between children based on nutritional status - McNemar's test.

Hypotheses: H_0:   Nutrition and survival are independent
                  H_1: H_0 is false

Decision rule: With $\alpha = 0.05$, reject H_0, if $\chi^2_{McNemar} > \chi^2_1(1-\alpha) = 3.84$.

		Good Nutrition		
		Survived	Died	
Poor	Survived	52	10	62
Health	Died	45	28	73
		97	38	135

Computations:

$$\chi_{McNemar}^2 = \frac{(b-c)^2}{b+c}$$

$$\chi^2_{McNemar} = \frac{(10 - 45)^2}{10 + 45} = \frac{1225}{55} = 22.27$$

Correction of continuity:

$$\chi^2_{McNemar} = \frac{(|b - c| - 1)^2}{b + c}$$

$$\chi^2_{McNemar} = \frac{(|10 - 45| - 1)^2}{10 + 45} = \frac{1156}{55} = 21.02$$

Decision: With $\chi^2_{McNemar} > 3.84$, reject H_0, conclude that there is a significant relationship between nutrition and survival rate.

7.   Comparison of laboratory results at five different sites - Cochran's Q.

Hypotheses: H_0: Development of passing the test is independent of laboratory
  H_1: H_0 is false

Decision rule: With $\alpha = 0.05$, reject H_0 if $Q > \chi^2_4(1-\alpha) = 9.49$.

Sample	A	B	C	D	E	R	R²
\multicolumn{8}{c}{Laboratory Result (1 = pass)}							
101	0	1	1	1	0	3	9
102	1	0	1	1	1	4	16
103	0	0	0	0	0	0	0
104	1	1	1	1	1	5	25
105	1	1	1	1	1	5	25
106	1	0	1	1	0	3	9
107	1	0	0	1	1	3	9
108	1	1	1	1	1	5	25
109	1	1	1	1	1	5	25
110	1	1	1	1	1	5	24
111	1	0	1	1	1	4	16
112	1	1	1	1	1	5	25
C =	10	7	10	11	9		
C² =	100	49	100	121	81		
					ΣR=	47	
					ΣR²=		209

Computations:

$$Q = \frac{(k-1)[(k\sum C^2) - (\sum R)^2]}{k(\sum R) - \sum R^2}$$

$$Q = \frac{(4)[(5)(451) - (47)^2]}{(5)(47) - 209} = \frac{184}{26} = 7.08$$

Decision: With $Q < 9.49$, fail to reject and conclude that the test outcome is independent of the laboratory in which the test is performed.

8. Survival ten years following radical mastectomy.

   a. Relative risk of death with positive node involvement:

		Nodal Involvement		
		Yes (+)	No (-)	
Outcome in	Dead	299	107	406
10 years	Alive	126	218	344
		425	325	750

$$RR = \frac{ab + ad}{ab + bc} = \frac{(299)(107) + (299)(218)}{(299)(107) + (107)(126)} = 2.14$$

Chi square test of significance:

Hypotheses: H_0: RR = 1
$\quad\quad\quad\quad\quad H_1$: RR $\neq$ 1

Decision rule: With $\alpha = 0.05$, reject H_0, if $\chi^2 > \chi^2_1(1-\alpha) = 3.84$.

Computations:

$$\chi^2 = \frac{n(ad - bc)^2}{(a+b)(b+d)(a+b)(c+d)}$$

$$\chi^2 = \frac{750[(299)(218) - (107)(126)]^2}{(406)(344)(425)(325)} = 103.92$$

Decision: With $\chi^2 > 3.84$, reject H_0, conclude there is a significant relationship between survival and presence or absence of positive nodes.

b. Relative risk of death with positive node involvement controlling for estrogen receptors:

$$RR_{MH} = \frac{\sum \dfrac{a_i(c_i + d_i)}{N_i}}{\sum \dfrac{c_i(a_i + b_i)}{N_i}}$$

$$RR_{MH} = \frac{\dfrac{179(100 + 148)}{453} + \dfrac{120(26 + 70)}{297}}{\dfrac{100(179 + 26)}{453} + \dfrac{26(120 + 81)}{297}} = \frac{136.78}{62.85} = 2.18$$

Significance of nodal involvement and death as an outcome controlling for the possible confounding factor of estrogen receptors.

Hypotheses: H_0: Nodal involvement and survival are independent (controlling for estrogen receptors)
                H_1: H_0 is false

Decision rule: With $\alpha = 0.05$, reject H_0 if $\chi^2_{MH} > \chi^2_1(1-\alpha) = 3.84$.

Calculations:

Intermediate steps for negative receptors:

$$e_2 = \frac{(a_2 + b_2)(a_2 + c_2)}{n_2} = \frac{(201)(146)}{297} = 98.8$$

$$v_2 = \frac{(a_2+b_2)(c_2+d_2)(a_2+c_2)(b_2+d_2)}{n_2^2(n_2-1)} = \frac{(201)(96)(146)(151)}{297^2(296)} = 16.3$$

	Positive	Negative
a_i	179	120
e_i	126.3	98.8
v_i	26.6	16.3

Mantel-Haenszel chi square:

$$\chi_{MH}^2 = \frac{[\Sigma(a_i - e_i)]^2}{\Sigma v_i} = \frac{[(179-126.3)+(120-98.8)]^2}{26.6+16.3} = 127.3$$

Decision: Reject H_0, conclude that survival and nodal involvement are related, controlling for estrogen receptors.

9. Comparison of torque of closure and moisture permeability where $\chi^2 = 18.43$.
    Variables: Discrete (2 x 4 contingency table)

Contingency coefficient:

$$C = \sqrt{\frac{\chi^2}{\chi^2+n}} = \sqrt{\frac{18.43}{18.43+200}} = \sqrt{0.084} = 0.290$$

Results: C = 0.290. a "weak" relationship between closure torque and moisture.

11. Logistic regression on four levels of torque:

Torque (inch-pounds):	Success (<2000)	Failure (≥2000)	
21	26	24	50
24	31	19	50
27	36	14	50
30	45	5	50
	138	62	200

Probabilities associated with each outcome:

Torque (inch-pounds):	Success (<2000)	Failure (≥2000)
21	.130	.120
24	.155	.095
27	.180	.070
30	.225	.025

Calculation of the logit for the 21 inch-pounds of pressure would be:

$$log\,it = ln\,\frac{\pi_{i1}}{\pi_{i2}}$$

$$logit(\,21\,) = ln\,\frac{.130}{.120} = ln(\,1.08\,) = 0.077$$

The logit for 30 inch-pounds would be:

$$logit(\,30\,) = ln\,\frac{.225}{.025} = ln(\,9.00\,) = 2.197$$

The results for all the logit calculations would be:

Torque (inch-pounds):	Success (<2000)	Failure (≥2000)	Logit
21	26	24	0.077
24	31	19	0.489
27	36	14	0.944
30	45	5	2.197

Based on the data available, it appears that there is an increasing likelihood of success as the torque increases during the sealing process.

17

Nonparametric Tests

Nonparametric statistical tests can be useful when dealing with extremely small sample sizes or when the requirements of normality and homoscedasticity cannot be met or assumed. These tests are simple to calculate, but are traditionally less powerful and the researcher needs to evaluate the risk of a Type II error. Often referred to as **distribution-free statistics**, nonparametric statistical tests do not make any assumptions about the population distribution. One does not need to meet the requirements of normality or homogeneity of variance associated with the parametric procedures (z-test, t-tests, F-tests, correlation and regression). Chi square tests are often cited as a distribution-free test, and have been covered in a previous chapter.

These tests usually involve ranking or categorizing the data and in doing such we decrease the accuracy of our information (changing from the raw data to a relative ranking). We may obscure true differences and make it difficult to identify differences which are significant. In other words, non-parametric tests require differences to be larger if they are to be found significant. We increase the risk that we will accept a false null hypothesis (Type II error). Therefore, nonparametric tests are generally considered to be less powerful than their parametric counterparts because of this greater chance of committing a Type II error. It may be to the researcher's advantage to tolerate minor doubts about normality and homogeneity associated with a given parametric test, rather than to risk the greater error possible with a nonparametric procedure.

Nonparametric tests have been slow to gain favor in the pharmaceutical community, but are currently being seen with greater frequency, often in parallel with the parametric counterparts. This is seen in the following example of a 1989 clinical trial protocol:

> If the variables to be analyzed are normally distributed and
> homogenous with respect to variance, a parametric analysis of
> variance which models the cross-over design will be applied.
> If these criteria are not fulfilled, suitable nonparametric tests
> will be used.

Nonparametric tests are relatively simple to calculate. Their speed and
convenience offers a distinct advantage over conventional tests discussed in the
previous chapters. Therefore, as investigators we can use these procedures as a
quick method for evaluating data.

This chapter will explore a few of the most commonly used nonparametric
tests which can be used in place of the previously discussed methods (i.e., t-
tests, F-tests, correlation) Nonparametric tests which analyze differences
between two discrete levels of the independent variable include the: 1)
Mann-Whitney U test and 2) median test. For comparing how paired groups of
data relate to each other, appropriate tests include: 1) Wilcoxon's signed-rank
test and 2) sign test. The analyses of variance models can be evaluated using:
1) the Kruskal-Wallis test or 2) Friedman two-way analysis of variance. When
criteria are not met for the chi square test of independence, the Fisher exact test
may be used. These nonparametric procedures are extremely valuable and in
many cases more appropriate when testing small sample sizes. Lastly, for
correlations, the Spearman rho test may be substituted.

Ranking of Information

Most nonparametric tests require that the data be ranked on an ordinal
scale. Ranking involves assigning the value 1 to the smallest observation, 2 to
the second smallest, and continuing this process until n is assigned to the
largest observation. For example:

Data	Rank	
12	1	
18	5	
16	3	$n = 5$
15	2	
17	4	

In the case of ties, the average of the rank values is assigned to each tied
observation.

Data	Rank	
12	1	
18	9	
16	6	
15	4	
17	7.5	n = 10
14	2	
15	4	
15	4	
17	7.5	
20	10	

In this example there were three 15s (ranks 3,4, and 5) with an average rank of 4 and two 17s (ranks 7 and 8) with an average rank of 7.5.

When comparing sets of data from different groups or different treatment levels (levels of the independent variable), ranking involves all of the observations regardless of the discrete level in which the observation occurs:

Group A (n=5)		Group B (n=7)		Group C (n=8)		Total (N=20)
Data	Rank	Data	Rank	Data	Rank	
12	3	11	2	15	8.5	
18	17.5	13	4.5	15	8.5	
16	12	19	19.5	17	15	
15	8.5	17	15	19	19.5	
17	15	16	12	18	17.5	
		15	8.5	16	12	
		14	6	13	4.5	
				10	1	
Σ =	56.0	Σ =	67.5	Σ =	86.5	ΣΣ = 210

Accuracy of the ranking process may be checked in two ways. First, the last rank assigned should be equal to the total N (in this example the largest rank was a tie between two observations (ranks 19 and 20), the average of which was 19.5. The second way to check the accuracy of the ranking procedure is the fact that the sum of all the summed ranks should equal N(N+1)/2, where N equals the total number of observations:

$$Sum\ of\ Summed\ Ranks = \sum\sum R_i = \frac{N(N+1)}{2} \qquad \text{Eq. 17.1}$$

In this case:

$$56.0 + 67.5 + 86.5 = 210 = \frac{20(21)}{2} = \frac{N(N+1)}{2}$$

Mann-Whitney U Test

The Mann-Whitney U test is a procedure for an independent variable that has two discrete levels and a continuous dependent variable (similar to the two-sample t-test). Data are ranked and a formula is applied. Note that the hypotheses are not concerned with the means of the populations. The parameters of normality and homogeneity of variance are not considered, where the t-test evaluated the null hypothesis the $\mu_1 = \mu_2$.

H_0: Samples are from the same population
H_1: Samples are drawn from different populations

The data are ranked and the sums of the ranks of the dependent variables is calculated for one level of the independent variable.

Data Level 1	Rank	Data Level 2	Rank
d_{11}	R_{11}	d_{21}	R_{21}
d_{12}	R_{12}	d_{22}	R_{22}
d_{13}	R_{13}	d_{23}	R_{23}
...	...	...	...
d_{1j}	R_{1j}	d_{2j}	R_{2j}
	ΣR_{1j}		

Either the first or second ranking could be used for the statistical sum of the ranks. The statistical values are calculated using the following two formulas where ΣR_{1j} is associated with n_1:

$$U = n_1 n_2 + \frac{n_1(n_1+1)}{2} - \sum_{i=1}^{1} R_{1j} \qquad \text{Eq. 17.2}$$

This U-value is applied to a second formula:

$$z = \frac{U - \frac{n_1 n_2}{2}}{\sqrt{\frac{n_1 n_2 \cdot [n_1 + (n_2+1)]}{12}}} \qquad \text{Eq. 17.3}$$

The calculated z-value is then compared to values in the normalized standard distribution (Table B2, Appendix B). If the calculated z-value is to the extreme of the critical z-value then H_0 is rejected. In the case of 95% confidence, the critical z-values would be either a -1.96 or +1.96. The numerator of the equation is similar to the z-test of proportions; we are comparing an observed U-value to an expected value that is the average of the ranks ($n_1 n_2/2$).

As an example of the Mann-Whitney U test, a pharmacology experiment was conducted to determine the effect of atropine on the release of acetylcholine (ACh) from rat neostriata brain slices. The measure of ACh release through stimulation was measured twice. Half of the sample received atropine before the second measurement. The ratio (stimulation 2 divided by stimulation 1) is as follows:

Control	Received Atropine
0.7974	1.7695
0.8762	1.6022
0.6067	1.0632
1.1268	2.7831
0.7184	1.0475
1.0422	1.4411
1.3590	1.0990

Is there a difference in the ratios between the control group and those administered the atropine? The hypotheses are:

H_0: Samples are from the same population
(i.e., no difference in response)
H_1: Samples are drawn from different populations
(i.e., difference in response)

The decision rule is, with $\alpha = .05$, reject H_0, if $|z| >$ critical $z_{(.975)} = 1.96$. The ranking of the data is presented in Table 17.1. A quick computational check for accuracy of the ranking shows that the ranking was done correctly:

$$\frac{N(N+1)}{2} = \frac{14(15)}{2} = 105 = 34 + 71$$

The computation of the test statistics would be:

$$U = n_1 n_2 + \frac{n_1(n_1+1)}{2} - \Sigma R_{1j}$$

Table 7.1 Sample Data for the Mann-Whitney U Test

Control	Rank	Received Atropine	Rank
0.7974	3	1.7695	13
0.8762	4	1.6022	12
0.6067	1	1.0632	7
1.1268	9	2.7831	14
0.7184	2	1.0475	6
1.0422	5	1.4411	11
1.3590	10	1.0990	8
$\Sigma =$	34	$\Sigma =$	71

$$U = (7)(7) + \frac{(7)(8)}{2} - 34 = 43$$

$$z = \frac{U - \frac{n_1 n_2}{2}}{\sqrt{\frac{n_1 n_2 \cdot [n_1 + (n_2 + 1)]}{12}}}$$

$$z = \frac{43 - \frac{(7)(7)}{2}}{\sqrt{\frac{(7)(7) \cdot [7 + 8)]}{12}}} = \frac{43 - 24.5}{7.83} = 2.36$$

Note that reversing Level 1 and Level 2 would produce identical results. In the above case the ΣR_{ij} is 71 and n_1 is 7:

$$U = (7)(7) + \frac{(7)(8)}{2} - 71 = 6$$

$$z = \frac{6 - \frac{(7)(7)}{2}}{\sqrt{\frac{(7)(7) \cdot [7 + 8)]}{12}}} = \frac{6 - 24.5}{7.83} = -2.36$$

The decision, either way, would be with $z > z_{critical} = 1.96$, reject H_0 and conclude that the samples are drawn from different populations and the response of the rat's neostriata release of ACh is affected by atropine.

Median Test

The median test may also be used for an independent variable with two discrete levels. This test utilizes the median for all of the data points tested. In many nonparametric statistics, the median is used instead of the mean as a measure of central tendency. The hypotheses are the same as the Mann-Whitney test.

H_0: Samples are from the same population
H_1: Samples are drawn from different populations

The first step is to create a 2 x 2 table using the *grand median* for all of the observations in both levels of the independent variable. As discussed previously, one valuable property of the median is that it is not affected by an outlier (extreme values).

	Group 1	Group 2	
Above the median	a	b	n = total observations
Below the median	c	d	

The calculated p-value is determined using a formula which incorporates a numerator of all the margin values (a+b, c+d, a+c and b+d) and a denominator involving each cell:

$$p = \frac{(a+b)!\,(c+d)!\,(a+c)!\,(b+d)!}{n!\,a!\,b!\,c!\,d!} \qquad \text{Eq. 17.4}$$

The decision rule is to reject H_0, if the calculated p is less than the critical p (α) in a normal standardized distribution, for example $\alpha = 0.05$.

As an example of the median test, the same data used for the Mann-Whitney U test will be considered. In this case the grand median is between data points 1.0632 and 1.0990 (ranks 7 and 8). The data for each level of the independent variable is classified as above or below the median and the results are presented in the following table:

	Control	Atropine	
Above the median	2	5	N = 14
Below the median	5	2	

In this example, all of the margin values (i.e., a+b) are seven and the computation of the probability of the occurrence is:

$$p = \frac{(2+5)!\,(2+5)!\,(5+2)!\,(2+5)!}{14!\,2!\,5!\,5!\,2!}$$

$$p = \frac{6.45 \times 10^{14}}{5.02 \times 10^{15}} = 0.128$$

With the calculated p = 0.128, there is a probability of this occurring 12.8% of the time by chance alone. We cannot reject H_0. The researcher cannot find a significant difference and must assume that the animals are drawn from the same population and there is no treatment effect.

Note that when using the Mann-Whitney test H_0 at the 0.05 level of significance, H_0 was rejected, but could not be rejected with the median test. If the same data is run using a t-test, the results are identical to the Mann-Whitney test:

Significance level:	0.1	0.05	0.01
Mann-Whitney U test	Reject H_0	Reject H_0	Accept H_0
Median test	Reject H_0	Accept H_0	Accept H_0
t-Test	Reject H_0	Reject H_0	Accept H_0

It appears that the median test is a slightly more conservative test than either the Mann-Whitney or t-tests, and more likely to result in a Type II error. This is due in part to the small amount of information available from the median test, results are dichotomized into above and below the median, and only two outcomes are possible.

Wilcoxon Matched-pairs Test

The Wilcoxon matched-pairs test offers a parallel to the matched-pair t-test discussed in Chapter 8. To accomplish this test, a traditional pre-posttest (before-after) table is constructed and the differences are calculated similar to the matched-pair t-test.

Subject	Before	After	d
1	67	71	+4
2	70	73	+3
3	85	81	-4
4	80	82	+2
5	72	75	+3
6	78	76	-2

The *absolute* differences (regardless of sign, positive or negative) are then ranked from smallest to largest.

Subject	Before	After	d	Rank |d|
1	67	71	+4	5.5
2	70	73	+3	3.5
3	85	81	-4	5.5
4	80	82	+2	1.5
5	72	75	+3	3.5
6	78	76	-2	1.5

Notice that the fourth and sixth subject have identical differences (even though the signs are different): therefore, they share the average rank of 1.5 (ranks 1 and 2). A T-value is calculated for the sum of the ranks associated with the *least frequent* sign (positive or negative).

Sub.	Before	After	d	Rank |d|	Rank associated with the Least Frequent Sign
1	67	71	+4	5.5	
2	70	73	+3	3.5	
3	85	81	-4	5.5	5.5
4	80	82	+2	1.5	
5	72	75	+3	3.5	
6	78	76	-2	1.5	1.5
				$T = \sum =$	7.0

Note in the above example that the third and sixth subjects were the only two with negative differences (the least frequent sign); therefore, their associated ranks were the only ones carried over to the last column and summed to produce the T-value. If all the signs are positive or negative then the T-value would be zero and no ranks would be associated with the least frequent sign.

A unique aspect of this test is that a certain amount of data may be ignored. If a difference is zero, the difference is neither positive or negative; therefore, a sign cannot be assigned. Thus, data associated with no differences are eliminated and the number of pairs (n) is reduced appropriately. To illustrate this point, note the example in Table 17.2. In this case n is reduced from 10 pairs to n = 8 pairs, because two of the results had zero differences. Also note that the least frequent sign was a negative, thus the T-value is calculated by summing only those rank scores with negative differences. The hypotheses for the Wilcoxon matched-pairs test are not concerned with mean differences, as seen with the t-test (where the null hypothesis was $\mu_d = 0$):

H_0: No difference between pre- and post-measurements
H_1: Difference between pre- and post-measurements

One simple calculation is to determine, under a zero change, the expected T-value or E(T) if there was no difference between the pre- and post-measuresments. The expected total for the ranks is E(Total) = n(n+1)/2. If H_0 is true then the total for each sign rank (+ or -) should be equal to half the total ranks (Eq. 17.1). Thus:

$$E(T) = \frac{n(n+1)}{2} \cdot \frac{1}{2} \quad or \quad E(T) = \frac{n(n+1)}{4} \qquad \text{Eq. 17.5}$$

Table 17.2 Example of Data for a Wilcoxon Matched-Pairs Test

Before	After	d	Rank $\lvert d \rvert$	Rank associated with least frequent sign
81	86	+5	6.5	
81	93	+12	8	
79	74	-4	4.5	4.5
80	80	0	-	
74	76	+2	3	
78	83	+5	6.5	
90	91	+1	1.5	
95	95	0	-	
68	72	+4	4.5	
75	74	-1	1.5	1.5
n = 8	$\sum =$	0		$T = \sum = 6$

The test statistic once again involves a numerator that compares the difference between an expected value and an observed result, in this case the T-value:

$$z = \frac{T - E(T)}{\sqrt{\dfrac{n(n+1)(2n+1)}{24}}}$$

Eq. 17.6

As with previous equations, if the observed and expected values are identical the numerator would be zero and the z-value would be zero. As the difference increases the z-value increases until it reaches a point of statistical significance with a given Type I error rate. In this procedure the decision rule is with a predetermined α, to reject H_0 if z is greater than $z(\alpha/2)$ from the normal standardized distribution (Table B2, Appendix B). For the above example the decision rule would be, with $\alpha = .05$, reject H_0 if $z > 1.96$ and the computations would be as follows:

$$E(T) = \frac{(8)(9)}{4} = 18$$

$$z = \frac{6 - 18}{\sqrt{\dfrac{8(9)(2(8)+1)}{24}}} = \frac{-12}{\sqrt{51}} = -1.68$$

The decision is with $z < 1.96$, we cannot reject H_0 and we are unable to find a significant difference between pre- and post-measurements.

Sign Test

The sign test is a second method for determining significant differences between paired observations and is based on the binomial distribution. It is among the simplest of all nonparametric procedures. Similar to the Wilcoxon test, differences are considered and any pairs with zero differences are dropped, and the n of the sample is reduced. A table for the pairs is constructed and only the sign (+ or -) is considered. Using the same example presented for the Wilcoxon test we find signs listed in Table 17.3. If there are no significant differences between the before and after measurements we would expect half the numbers to be positive (+) and half to be negative (-). Thus $p(+) = .50$ and $p(-) = .50$. If these was no significant difference between the before and after measurements, the null hypotheses would be that the proportion of positive and negative signs would be equal.

Table 17.3 Sample Data for a Sign Test

Before	After	d	Sign
81	86	+5	+
81	93	+12	+
79	74	-4	-
80	80	0	0
74	76	+2	+
78	83	+5	+
90	91	+1	+
95	95	0	0
68	72	+4	+
75	74	-1	-

H_0: No difference between measurement   or H_0: $p(+) = 0.50$
H_1: Difference between measurements exists H_1: $p(+) \neq 0.50$

The more the proportion of (+)s or (-)s differ from 0.50, the more likely that there is a significant difference and that the difference is not due to random error alone.

For samples less than 10 one can use the binomial distribution. Dropping the two zero differences the final number of paired observations is eight. What is the probability of six or more positive values out of eight differences, given that the probability of a positive value equals 0.50?

$$p(x) = \binom{n}{x} p^x q^{n-x}$$ Eq. 2.12

$$p(6 \ positives) = \binom{8}{6}(.50)^6(.50)^2 = 0.1092$$

$$p(7 \ positives) = \binom{8}{7}(.50)^7(.50)^1 = 0.0313$$

$$p(8 \ positives) = \binom{8}{8}(.50)^8(.50)^0 = 0.0039$$

$$p(> 5 \ positives) = \sum = 0.1444$$

Thus, there is almost a 15% chance that there will be six or more positive differences out of the 8 pairs by chance alone. Thus, we can not reject H_0.

For 10 or more pairs of observations, we can employ Yates' correction for continuity for the one sample z-test for proportions:

$$z = \frac{|p - P_0| - \dfrac{1}{n}}{\sqrt{\dfrac{(P_0)(1 - P_0)}{n}}} \qquad \text{Eq. 12.7}$$

where:

$$p = \frac{number \ of \ positives}{total \ number \ of \ pairs}$$

In this particular case:

$$p = \frac{6}{8} = .75$$

$$z = \frac{|.75 - .50| - \dfrac{1}{8}}{\sqrt{\dfrac{(.50)(.50)}{8}}} = \frac{.25 - .125}{\sqrt{.0313}} = 0.71$$

In a normal standardized distribution table (Table B2, Appendix B) the area below the point where $z = 0.71$ is .7611 (.5000 + .2611). Thus, the probability of being above $z = 0.71$ is .2389 and therefore not significant.

Kruskal-Wallis Test

Much as the F-test is an extension of the t-test, Kruskal-Wallis is an equivalent nonparametric extension of the Mann-Whitney U test for more than two levels of an independent discrete variable. The hypotheses are:

H_0: Samples are from the same population
H_1: Samples are drawn from different populations

Like the Mann-Whitney test, data are ranked and rank sums calculated, then a new statistical formula is applied to the summed ranks.

Level 1	Rank	Level 2	Rank	...	Level k	Rank
d_{11}	R_{11}	d_{21}	R_{21}	...	d_{k1}	R_{k1}
d_{12}	R_{12}	d_{22}	R_{22}	...	d_{k2}	R_{k2}
d_{13}	R_{13}	d_{23}	R_{22}	...	d_{k3}	R_{k3}
...	...	...	...	...	...	...
d_{1j}	$\underline{R_{1j}}$	d_{2j}	$\underline{R_{2j}}$	...	d_{kj}	$\underline{R_{kj}}$
	$\sum R_{1j}$		$\sum R_{2j}$			$\sum R_{kj}$

In this test the formula is:

$$H = \frac{12}{N(N+1)} \left[\sum \frac{(\sum R_{ij})^2}{n_j} \right] - 3(N+1) \qquad \text{Eq. 17.7}$$

The middle section of the equation involves the squaring of the individual sum of ranks for each level of the independent variable, dividing those by their respective number of observations and then summing these results. The decision rule in this test is to compare the calculated Kruskal-Wallis H-statistic with a χ^2-critical value from Table B12 in Appendix B. The degrees of freedom is based on the number of levels of the discrete independent variable minus one for bias (K-1).

For an example of the Kruskal-Wallis test, assume that three instruments located in different laboratories were compared to determine if all three instruments could be used for the same assay (Table 17.4). Was there a significant difference based on the following results (mg/tablet)? The hypotheses are:

H₀: Samples are from the same population
(no difference between instruments)
H₁: Samples are drawn from different populations

The data and associate ranks are presented in Table 17.4. The decision rule would be: with $\alpha = .05$, reject H₀, if $H > \chi^2_{k-1}(.95)$. With three discrete levels in our independent variable, the number of degrees of freedom is two and χ^2_2 equals 5.99. The calculations are as follows:

Table 17.4 Data for a Kruskal-Wallis Example

Instrument A		Instrument B		Instrument C	
Assay	Rank	Assay	Rank	Assay	Rank
12.12	8	12.47	14	12.20	10
13.03	18	13.95	21	11.23	1
11.97	7	12.75	16	11.28	2
11.53	3	12.21	11	12.89	17
11.82	6	13.32	19	12.46	13
11.75	5	13.60	20	12.56	15
12.25	12			11.69	4
12.16	9				
$\Sigma =$	68		101		62

$$H = \frac{12}{N(N+1)} \left[\Sigma \frac{(\Sigma R_{ij})^2}{n_j} \right] - 3(N+1)$$

$$H = \frac{12}{21(22)} \left[\frac{(68)^2}{8} + \frac{(101)^2}{6} + \frac{(62)^2}{7} \right] - 3(22)$$

$$H = 0.026(578.5 + 1700.2 + 549.1) - 66 = 7.52$$

The decision in this case is, with H > 5.99, reject H_0 and conclude that there is a significant difference among the three pieces of equipment and they are not equal in their assay results.

Some statisticians recommend a correction for ties (sharing of the same ranks) in the data, especially when there are a large number of such tied.

$$C = 1 - \left[\frac{\Sigma(t^3 - t)}{N^3 - N} \right]$$ Eq. 17.8

For example four sets of pair ties, and three sets of triplicate ties are:

$$4[(2)^3 - 2] + 3[(3)^3 - 3]$$

N equals the total number of observations. In this particular example, the correction would be as follows:

$$C = 1 - \left[\frac{4[(2)^3 - 2] + 3[(3)^3 - 3]}{(21)^3 - 21} \right]$$

$$C = 1 - \frac{96}{9240} = 1 - 0.0104 = 0.9896$$

The corrected H statistic (H') is:

$$H' = \frac{H}{C} \qquad\qquad \text{Eq. 17.9}$$

since the denominator will be less than 1, this correction will give a slightly higher value than the original H statistic. The decision rule is to reject H_0, if H' is greater than $\chi^2_{K-1}(1-\alpha)$, which is the chi square value from Table B12. In the example above, H' is:

$$H' = \frac{7.52}{0.9896} = 7.60$$

In most cases the adjustment is negligible. Unlike Yates corrections which produce a more conservative test statistic, the correction for ties produced a number more likely to find a significant difference and a more conservative approach would be to use the original H-statistic.

Friedman Two-way Analysis of Variance

The Friedman procedure can be employed for data meeting the design for the complete randomized block design (Chapter 9), but which fail to conform to the criteria for parametric procedures. The hypotheses test for differences in the various treatment levels controlling for the effects of blocking.

H_0:   No difference in the treatment levels
H_1:   A difference exists in the treatment levels

The summed ranks are used in the following formula:

$$\chi_r^2 = \frac{12}{nk(k+1)} \Sigma (R_j)^2 - 3n(k+1) \qquad \text{Eq. 17.10}$$

Where k represents the number of levels of the independent variable (treatments) and n the total number of rows (blocks). Critical values for small sample sizes (i.e., less than five blocks or rows) are available (Daniel, 1978). Larger sample sizes can be approximated from the standard chi square table for k-1 degrees of freedom. If the calculated χ_r^2 is greater than the critical χ^2 value (Table B12, Appendix B), then H_0 is rejected.

First, the treatment effect for the blocking variables is calculated by ranking each level of the column variable per row. For example if the column variable consisted of four levels, each row for the blocking variable would be ranked and assigned values 1,2,3 and 4 per row. Ties would be averages, similar to previous tests. The data is ranked separately for each row. Then the ranks associated with each column are summed (R_j) and applied to Eq. 17.10.

To illustrate this process, assume we are attempting to determine if there is any significant difference between the three formulas. To reduce inter-subject variability we administrer all three formulations to the same subjects (in a randomized order). The results are presented in Table 17.5. The hypothesis would be as follows:

H_0:   No difference exists between the two formulations
H_1:   A difference exists between the two formulations

Table 17.5   Results of Three Formulations Administered at Random to Twelve Volunteers

Subject	Formula A	Formula B	Formula C
1	125	149	126
2	128	132	126
3	131	142	117
4	119	136	119
5	130	151	140
6	121	141	121
7	129	130	126
8	133	138	136
9	135	130	135
10	123	129	127
11	120	122	122
12	125	140	141

Table 17.6 Example of the Freidman ANOVA for Data in Table 17.5

Subject	Formula A Data	Rank	Formula B Data	Rank	Formula C Data	Rank
1	125	1	149	3	126	2
2	128	2	132	3	126	1
3	131	2	142	3	117	1
4	119	1.5	136	3	119	1.5
5	130	1	151	3	140	2
6	121	1.5	141	3	121	1.5
7	129	2	130	3	126	1
8	133	1	138	3	136	2
9	135	2.5	130	1	135	2.5
10	123	1	129	3	127	2
11	120	1	122	2.5	122	2.5
12	125	1	140	2	141	3
$\Sigma =$		17.5		32.5		22

In this case the decision rule is to reject H_0 if the calculated χ_r^2 is greater than $\chi_2^2(.95)$ which equals 5.99 (note that n equals 12, which is large enough to use the critical value from the chi square table). Degrees of freedom for the chi square value is based on k-1 treatment levels. The ranking of the data is presented in Table 17.6 where the responses for each subject (block) is ranked independently of all other subjects. Finally the ranks are summed for each of the treatment levels (columns) and presented at the bottom of Table 17.6. The computation of the χ_r^2 is:

$$\chi_r^2 = \frac{12}{12(3)(4)} [(17.5)^2 + (32.5)^2 + (22)^2] - 3(12)(4)$$

$$\chi_r^2 = (0.0833)(1846.5) - 144 = 9.81$$

Therefore, with the calculated χ^2 greater than 5.99 we would reject H_0 and assume that there is a significant difference between formulations A, B and C.

Fisher's Exact Test

If data for a chi square test of independence is reduced to a 2x2 contingency table and the expected values are still too small to meet the requirements (at least five per cell), the Fisher's exact test can be employed (Fisher, 1936). This test is sometimes referred to as Fisher's four-fold test because of the four cells of frequency data. As described in Chapter 13, the 2x2 contingency table can be labeled as follows:

a	b	a+b
c	d	c+d

a+c   b+d   n

In this case the test statistic is identical to the median test:

$$p = \frac{(a+b)!\,(c+d)!\,(a+c)!\,(b+d)!}{n!\,a!\,b!\,c!\,d!}$$ Eq. 17.11

However, in this test, cells are based on the evaluation of two independent variables and not on estimating a midpoint based on the sample data.

Similar to the binomial equation, multiple tests are performed to determine the probability of the research data and additional probabilities are calculated for each possible combination to the extreme of the observed data.   These probabilities are summed to determine the exact likelihood of the outcomes. For example, assume the following data is collected:

3	7	10
7	3	10

10   10   20

The p-value is calculated for this one particular outcome; however, p-values are also calculated for the possible outcomes that are even more extreme with the **same fixed margins**:

2	8
8	2

1	9
9	1

0	10
10	0

Then the probabilities of all four possibilities are summed.

The decision rule compares this probability to a $p_{critical}$ (for example .05). If it is smaller than the $p_{critical}$, reject H_0 and conclude that the rows and columns are not independent.

To illustrate the use of this test, assume the following example. Twelve laboratory rats are randomly assigned to two equal-sized groups. One group serves as a control, while the experimental group is administered a proposed carcinogenic agent. The rats are observed for the development of tumors. The following results are observed:

	Tumor	No Tumor	
Experimental	4	2	6
Control	1	5	6
	5	7	12

Is the likelihood of developing a tumor the same for both groups? The hypotheses are:

H_0:   The group and appearance of a tumor are independent
H_1:   The two variables are not independent

The decision rule is, with $\alpha = 0.05$, reject H_0 if $p<0.05$. The computation for the probability of four tumors in the experimental group is:

$$p = \frac{(a+b)!\,(c+d)!\,(a+c)!\,(b+d)!}{n!\,a!\,b!\,c!\,d!}$$

$$p = \frac{6!\,6!\,5!\,7!}{12!\,4!\,1!\,2!\,5!} = 0.1136$$

For five tumors in the experimental group:

$$p = \frac{6!\,6!\,5!\,7!}{12!\,5!\,0!\,1!\,6!} = 0.0076$$

The probability of four or more experimental mice developing a tumor:

$$p(5) \;=\; .0076$$
$$p(4) \;=\; \underline{.1136}$$
$$.1212$$

Therefore the decision, with $p > 0.05$, is that H_0 cannot be rejected. It is assumed that the two variables are independent and that the incidence of tumor production is independent of the agent's administration.

Spearman Rank-Order Correlation

When continuous data are measured on an ordinal scale or if assumptions of population normality cannot apply to the data, the Spearman rank-order correlation, or Spearman rho, offers an alternate procedure to the correlation coefficient. Similar to other nonparametric tests, a procedure is used to rank the order of the observations for both variables and then the difference between the two ranks makes up part of the test statistic. As seen in the following example, a table (similar to Table 17.6) is created and the sum of the differences squared is inserted into the following formula:

$$\rho = 1 - \frac{6(\Sigma d^2)}{n^3 - n} \qquad \text{Eq. 17.12}$$

Unlike the correlation coefficient, which is concerned with the means for both the X and Y variables, here the investigator is interested in the correlation between the rankings.

To illustrate this process the previous data regarding volunteer heights and weights (Table 12.2) will once again be used. The results of the ranking process for each continuous variable is presented in Table 17.7. The computation for the Spearman rho is:

$$\rho = 1 - \frac{6(\Sigma d^2)}{n^3 - n} = 1 - \frac{6(4)}{6^3 - 6} = 1 - \frac{24}{210} = 0.886$$

A perfect positive or a perfect negative correlation will both produce a $\Sigma d^2 = 0$; therefore, the result will always be a positive number. Thus, this procedure

Table 17.7 Sample Data for Spearman Correlation

Subject	Observed Wgt.	Observed Hgt.	Ranked Wgt.	Ranked Hgt.	D	D^2
1	96.0	1.88	5	6	-1	1
2	77.7	1.80	2	3	-1	1
3	100.9	1.85	6	5	1	1
4	79.0	1.77	3	2	1	1
5	73.0	1.73	1	1	0	0
6	84.5	1.83	4	4	0	0
					$\Sigma d^2 =$	4

does not indicate the direction of the relationship. However, because the Spearman rho is used for small data sets, information can be quickly plotted on graph paper and the resulting scatter plot will indicate if the correlation is positive or negative. If the two continuous variables are normally distributed, the Pearson's correlation coefficient is more powerful than the test for Spearman correlation. Spearman's statistic is useful when one of the variables is not normally distributed or if the sample sizes are very small.

Kendall's tau or **Kendall's rank correlation** is another type of rank-order correlation that has many of the same characteristics as the Spearman rho. However, it is felt that the Spearman correlation is a better procedure (Zar, 1984) and for a larger n, Spearman is easier to calculate. More information about this test can be found in Bradley (Bradley, 1968).

Theil's Incomplete Method

As discussed in Chapter 16, linear regression models assume that the dependent variable is normally distributed. If the y-variable is not normally distributed, several non-parametric approaches can be used to fit a straight line through the set of data points. Possibly the simplest method is **Theil's "incomplete" method**.

As with most nonparametric procedures, the first step is to rank the points in ascending order for the values of x. If the number of points is odd and the middle point (the median) is deleted. An even number of data points is required. Data points are then paired based on their order - the smallest with the smallest above the median, the second smallest with second smallest above the median - until the last pairing represents the largest x-value below the median with the largest x-value.

For any pair of points, where $x_j > x_i$, the slope, b_{ij}, of a straight line joining the two points can be calculated as follows:

$$b_{ij} = \frac{(y_j - y_i)}{(x_j - x_i)} \qquad \text{Eq. 17.13}$$

These paired slope estimates are themselves ranked in ascending order and the median value becomes the estimated slope of the straight line which best fits all the data points. This estimated value of b is inserted into the straight line equation (y = a + bx) for each data point and each corresponding intercept is calculated (a = y - bx) for each line. These intercepts are then arranged in ascending order and the median is calculated as the best estimate of the intercept.

As an example, let us reconsider Problem 3 at the end of Chapter 16 that compared the various dosages and the *in vivo* response (AUC). The data is already rank ordered by the x-variable.

Length	Percent
100	1.07
300	5.82
600	15.85
900	25.18
1200	33.12

Because there is an odd number of measurements (n=5) the median is removed from the data base:

Point	Dosage	Percent
1	100	1.07
2	300	5.82
	~~600~~	~~15.85~~
3	900	25.18
4	1200	33.12

The slope of the lines are then calculated by the pairings of points 1 and 3, and 2 and 4. These slopes are:

$$b_{13} = \frac{25.18 - 1.07}{900 - 100} = \frac{24.11}{800} = 0.0301$$

$$b_{24} = \frac{33.12 - 5.82}{1200 - 300} = \frac{27.3}{900} = 0.0303$$

The median slope (b) is the average of the two slopes (0.0302). This measure is then placed in the formula for a straight line and the intercept is calculated for all three pairings.

$$a = y - bx$$

$$a_1 = 1.07 - (0.0302)(100) = -1.95$$

$$a_2 = 5.82 - (0.0302)(300) = -3.24$$

$$a_3 = 25.18 - (0.0302)(900) = -2.00$$

$$a_4 = 33.12 - (0.0302)(1200) = -3.12$$

The new intercept is the median for these four calculations, which is the average of the third and fourth ranked values:

$$Median\ intercept\,(a) = \frac{(-2.00) + (-3.12)}{2} = -2.56$$

These results are slightly different than the slope (0.0299) and intercept (-2.33) identified with the traditional linear regression model.

Theil's method offers three advantages over traditional regression analysis: 1) it does not assume that errors are solely in the y-direction; 2) it does not assume that the populations for either the x- or y-variables are normally distributed; and 3) it is not affected by extreme values (outliers). With respect to the last point, in the traditional least-squares calculation, an outlier might carry more weight than the other points and this is avoided with Theil's incomplete method.

References

Daniel, W.W. (1991). Biostatistics: A Foundation for Analysis in the Health Sciences, John Wiley and Sons, New York, pp. 723-724.

Fisher, R.A. (1936). Statistical Methods for Research Workers, Oliver and Boyd, London, pp. 100-102.

Zar, J.H. (1984). Biostatistical Analysis, second edition, Prentice Hall, Englewood Cliffs, NJ, p. 320.

Bradley, J.V. (1968). Distribution-free Statistical Tests, Prentice-Hall, Englewood Cliffs, NJ, pp. 284-287.

Suggested Supplemental Readings

Bradley, J.V. (1968). Distribution-Free Statistical Tests, Prentice-Hall, Inc., Englewood Cliffs, NJ.

Conover, W.J. (1980). Practical Nonparametric Statistics, John Wiley and Sons, New York.

Daniel, W.W. (1991). Biostatistics: A Foundation for Analysis in the Health Sciences, John Wiley and Sons, New York, pp. 576-624.

Gibbs, J.D. and Chakraborti, S. (1992). Nonparametric Statistical Inference, Marcel Dekker, Inc., New York.

Example Problems

Use the appropriate nonparametric test to answer all of the following questions.

1. Samples were taken from a specific batch of a drug and randomly divided into two groups of tablets. One group was assayed by the manufacturer's own quality control laboratories. The second group of tablets was sent to a contract laboratory for identical analysis.

Percentage of Labeled Amount of Drug

Manufacturer	Contract Lab
101.1	97.5
100.6	101.1
98.8	99.1
99.0	98.7
100.8	97.8
98.7	99.5

Is there a significant difference between the results generated by the two labs?

2. To evaluate the responsiveness of individuals receiving various commercially available benzodiazepines, volunteers were administered these drugs and subjected to a computerized simulated driving test. Twelve volunteers were randomly divided into four groups, each receiving one of three benzodiazepines or a placebo. At two week intervals they were crossed over to other agents and retested, until each volunteer had received each active drug and the placebo. Driving abilities were measured two hours after the drug administration (at approximately the C_{max} for the benzodiazepines), with the higher the score, the greater the number of driving errors. The following results were observed:

Benzo(A)	Benzo(B)	Benzo(C)	Placebo
58	62	53	50
54	55	45	51
52	58	48	53
62	56	46	57
51	60	58	61
55	48	61	49
45	73	52	50
63	57	51	60
56	64	55	40
57	51	48	47
50	68	62	46
60	69	49	43

3. Following training on content uniformity testing, comparisons were made between the analytical result of the newly trained chemist with those of a senior chemist. Samples of four different drugs (compressed tablets) were selected from different batches and assayed by both individuals. The results are listed below:

Sample Drug, Batch	New Chemist	Senior Chemist
A,42	99.8	99.9
A,43	99.6	99.8
A,44	101.5	100.7
B,96	99.5	100.1
B,97	99.2	98.9
C,112	100.8	101.0
C,113	98.7	97.9
D,21	100.1	99.9
D,22	99.0	99.3
D,23	99.1	99.2

4. Three physicians were selected for a study to evaluate the length of stay for patients undergoing a major surgical procedure. All these procedures occurred in the same hospital and were without complications. Eight records were randomly selected from patients treated over the past twelve months. Was there a significant difference, by physician, in the length of stay for these surgical patients?

| | Days in the Hospital | |
Physician A	Physician B	Physician C
9	10	8
12	6	9
10	7	12
7	10	10
11	11	14
13	9	10
8	9	8
13	11	15

5. Two groups of physical therapy patients were subjected to two different treatment regimens. At the end of the study period, patients were evaluated on specific criteria to measure percent of desired range of motion. Do the results listed below indicate a significant difference between the two therapies at the 95% confidence level?

Group 1	Group 2
78	75
87	88
75	93
88	86
91	84
82	71
87	91
65	79
80	81
	86
	89

6. A study was undertaken to determine the cost effectiveness of a new treatment procedure for peritoneal adhesiolysis. Twelve pairs of individuals who did not have complications were used in the study, and each pair was matched on degree of illness, laboratory values, sex, and age. One member of each pair was randomly assigned to receive the conventional treatment, while the other member of the pair received the new therapeutic intervention. Based on the following data, is there sufficient data to conclude at a 5% level of significance that the new therapy is more cost effective than the conventional treatment?

Cost in Dollars

Pair	New	Conventional
1	11,813	13,112
2	6,112	8,762
3	13,276	14,762
4	11,335	10,605
5	8,415	6,430
6	12,762	11,990
7	7,501	9,650
8	3,610	7,519
9	9,337	11,754
10	6,538	8,985
11	5,097	4,228
12	10,410	12,667

7. In preparing to market an approved tablet in a new package design, the manufacturer tests two different blister packs to determine the rates of failure (separation of the adhesive seal) when stored at various temperatures and humidities. One thousand tablets in each of two conditions were stored for three months and the number of failures were observed:

	40 degrees 50% relative humidity	60 degrees 50% relative humidity
Blister pack A	2	5
Blister pack B	6	6

Is there a significant relationship between the storage conditions and the frequency of failures based on the blister pack used?

8. After collecting the data for the preliminary study to determine if a new antihypertensive agent could lower the diastolic blood pressure in normal individuals (presented earlier as Table 8.3 and evaluated using a matched pair t-test), the researcher was concerned about his assumptions and sample size. Is there a significant change in blood pressure using a nonparametric procedure?

Subject	Before	After
1	68	66
2	83	80
3	72	67
4	75	74
5	79	70
6	71	77
7	65	64
8	76	70
9	78	76
10	68	66
11	85	81
12	74	68

9. Pharmacists were randomly assigned to two volunteer groups. Each group was administered a continuing education program by either live lecture in a group or as isolated learners through a one-way video and two-way audio system. Based on the following final examination results, did either group obtain significantly better test scores?

Live	Remote	
96	82	86
91	89	73
81	85	88
75	78	84
80	90	71
85	83	76
	88	97
	69	

10. Acme Chemical and Dye received from the same raw material supplier three batches of the oil at three different production sites. Samples were drawn from drums at each location and compared to determine if the viscosity was the same for each batch. Was there any difference?

Viscosity Batch A	Viscosity Batch B	Viscosity Batch C
10.23	10.24	10.25
10.33	10.28	10.20
10.28	10.20	10.21
10.27	10.21	10.18
10.30	10.26	10.22

11. Twelve healthy male volunteers received a single dose of various strengths of an experimental anticoagulant. Was there any significant relationship between the dosage and corresponding prothrombin time using the Spearman rho correlation?

Subject	Dose (mg)	Prothrombin Time (seconds)
1	200	20
2	180	18
3	225	20
4	205	19
5	190	19
6	195	18
7	220	19
8	175	17
9	215	20
10	185	19
11	210	19
12	230	20

Answers to Problems

1. Comparison of results from a contract laboratory and manufacturer's quality control laboratory.
   Independent variable: manufacturer vs. contract laboratory (discrete)
   Dependent variable: assay results (ranked to ordinal scale)
   Statistical test: Mann-Whitney U

Percentage of labeled amount of Drug

Manufacturer	Rank	Contract Lab	Rank
101.1	11.5	97.5	1
100.6	9	101.1	11.5
98.8	5	99.1	7
99.0	6	98.7	3.5
100.8	9	97.8	2
98.7	3.5	99.5	8
$\Sigma R =$	44		33

Hypotheses: H_0: Samples are from the same population
            H_1: Samples are drawn from different populations

Decision rule: With $\alpha = 0.05$, reject H_0, if $|z| >$ critical $z_{(.975)} = 1.96$

Calculations:

$$U = n_1 n_2 + \frac{n_1(n_1+1)}{2} - \Sigma R_{1j} = (6)(6) + \frac{(6)(7)}{2} - 44 = 13$$

$$Z = \frac{U - \dfrac{n_1 n_2}{2}}{\sqrt{\dfrac{n_1 n_2 \cdot [n_1 + (n_2+1)]}{12}}}$$

$$Z = \frac{13 - \dfrac{(6)(6)}{2}}{\sqrt{\dfrac{(6)(6) \cdot [6+7)]}{12}}} = \frac{13 - 18}{6.24} = -0.80$$

Decision: With $z < 1.96$, fail to reject H_0, fail to show a significant difference between the results from the two laboratories.

2. Benzodiazepines and responses to a computerized simulated driving test.
Independent variable: drugs or placebo (discrete, 4 levels)
Dependent variable: driving score (based on ordinal ranks)
Statistical test: Kruskal-Wallis

Benzo (A)	Rank	Benzo (B)	Rank	Benzo (C)	Rank	Placebo	Rank
45	3.5	48	9	45	3.5	40	1
50	14	51	17.5	46	5.5	43	2
51	17.5	55	26	48	9	46	5.5
52	20.5	56	28.5	48	9	47	7
54	24	57	31	49	11.5	49	11.5
55	26	58	34	51	17.5	50	14
56	28.5	60	37	52	20.5	50	14
57	31	62	42	53	22.5	51	17.5
58	34	64	45	55	26	53	22.5
60	37	68	46	58	34	57	31
62	42	69	47	61	39.5	60	37
63	44	73	48	62	42	61	39.5
$\Sigma=$	322		411		240.5		202.5

Check for ranking: $\Sigma\Sigma = 1,176 = (48)(49)/2 = N(N+1)/2$

Decision rule: With $\alpha = .05$, reject H_0 if $H > \chi^2_3(.95) = 7.81$.

Calculations:

$$H = \frac{12}{N(N+1)} \left[\Sigma \frac{(\Sigma R_{ij})^2}{n_j} \right] - 3(N+1)$$

$$H = \frac{12}{48(49)} \left[\frac{(322)^2}{12} + \frac{(411)^2}{12} + \frac{(240.5)^2}{12} + \frac{(202.5)^2}{12} \right] - 3(49)$$

$$H = (0.0051)(30954.27) - 147 = 10.87$$

Decision: With $H > 7.81$, reject H_0 and conclude that the samples were not drawn from the same population.

3.   Comparisons between the analytical results of the newly trained chemist and senior chemist.
Independent variable: two time periods (each sample serves as own control)
Dependent variable: Assay results (ranked to ordinal scale)
Test statistic: Wilcoxon matched-pairs test or Friedman two-way analysis of variance

Hypotheses: H_0: No difference between the two chemists
                  H_1: Difference exists between the two chemists

a.   Wilcoxon matched-pairs test

Decision rule: With $\alpha = 0.05$, reject H_0 if $|z| > 1.96$.

Data (Table 17.8)

Calculations:

$$E(T) = \frac{n(n+1)}{4} = \frac{(10)(11)}{4} = 27.5$$

Table 17.8 Data and Ranking Associated with Comparison of Two Chemists for the Wilcoxon Matched-Pairs Test

Sample Batch	New Chemist	Senior Chemist	D	Rank d	Rank associated with least frequent sign
A,42	99.8	99.9	0.1	1.5	
A,43	99.6	99.8	0.2	4	
A,44	101.5	100.7	-0.8	9.5	9.5
B,96	99.5	100.1	0.6	8	
B,97	99.2	98.9	-0.3	6.5	6.5
C,112	100.8	101.0	0.2	4	
C,113	98.7	97.9	-0.8	9.5	9.5
D,21	100.1	99.9	-0.2	4	4
D,22	99.0	99.3	0.3	6.5	
D,23	99.1	99.2	0.1	1.5	
					$T = \Sigma = 29.5$

$$Z = \frac{T - E(T)}{\sqrt{\dfrac{n(n+1)(2n+1)}{24}}}$$

$$Z = \frac{29.5 - 27.5}{\sqrt{\dfrac{10(11)(21)}{24}}} = \frac{2}{\sqrt{96.25}} = 0.20$$

Decision: Using the Wilcoxon matched-pairs test, the result is a z < 1.96. Thus we fail to reject H_0 and fail to show a significant difference in the assay results for the two scientists.

b. Friedman two-way analysis of variance - data (Table 17.9)

Decision rule: With $\alpha = 0.05$, reject $\chi_r^2 > \chi_1^2 = 3.84$.

Calculations:

$$\chi_r^2 = \frac{12}{nk(k+1)} \Sigma(R_j)^2 - 3n(k+1)$$

Table 17.9 Data and Ranking Associated with Comparison of Two Chemists for the Friedman Two-way Analysis of Variance

Sample, Batch	New Chemist Data	Rank	Senior Chemist Data	Rank
A,42	99.8	1	99.9	2
A,43	99.6	1	99.8	2
A,44	101.5	2	100.7	1
B,96	99.5	1	100.1	2
B,97	99.2	2	98.9	1
C,112	100.8	1	101.0	2
C,113	98.7	2	97.9	1
D,21	100.1	2	99.9	1
D,22	99.0	1	99.3	2
D,23	99.1	1	99.2	2
$\Sigma =$		14		16

$$\chi_r^2 = \frac{12}{10(2)(3)} [(14)^2 + (16)^2] - 3(10)(3)$$

$$\chi_r^2 = (0.02)(452) - 90 = 0.40$$

Decision: Using the Friedman two-way analysis of variance, the result is a $\chi_1^2 < 3.84$. Thus we fail to reject H_0 and fail to show a significant difference in the assay results for the two scientists.

4. Evaluation of length of stay for patients of three physicians.
   Independent variable: physicians (discrete, 3 levels)
   Dependent variable: length of patient stays (ranked to ordinal scale)
   Statistical test: Kruskal-Wallis test

Hypothesis:

H_0: Physicians are from the same population (no difference in stays)
H_1: Physicians are different in required lengths of stay

Decision rule: With $\alpha = 0.05$, reject H_0 if $H > \chi^2_2(.95) = 5.99$.

Days in the Hospital:

MD-A	Rank	MD-B	Rank	MD-C	Rank
9	8.5	10	13	8	5
12	19.5	6	1	9	8.5
10	13	7	2.5	12	19.5
7	2.5	10	13	10	13
11	17	11	17	14	23
13	21.5	9	8.5	10	13
8	5	9	8.5	8	5
13	21.5	11	17	15	24
$\Sigma R =$	108.5	$\Sigma R =$	80.5	$\Sigma R =$	111.0

Calculations:

$$H = \frac{12}{N(N+1)}\left[\Sigma \frac{(\Sigma R_{ij})^2}{n_j}\right] - 3(N+1)$$

$$H = \frac{12}{24(25)}\left[\frac{(108.5)^2}{8} + \frac{(80.5)^2}{8} + \frac{(111.0)^2}{8}\right] - 3(25)$$

$$H = 0.02(1471.53 + 810.03 + 1540.13) - 75 = 1.43$$

Decision: With $H < 5.99$, do not reject H_0 and conclude that no significant difference was identified for length of stay for patients of physicians A, B or C.

5. Comparison of two physical therapy regimens.
   Independent variable: two physical therapy regimens (discrete)
   Dependent variable: percent range of motion (ranked to ordinal scale)
   Statistical test: Mann-Whitney U test

   Hypotheses: H_0: Samples are from the same population
   $\qquad\qquad$ H_1: Samples are drawn from different populations

   Decision rule: With $\alpha = 0.05$, reject H_0, if $|z| > $ critical $z_{(.975)} = 1.96$

Group 1	Ranks	Group 2	Ranks
78	5	75	3.5
87	13.5	88	15.5
75	3.5	93	20
88	15.5	86	11.5
91	18.5	84	10
82	9	71	2
87	13.5	91	18.5
65	1	79	6
80	7	81	8
		86	11.5
		89	17
$\sum R =$	86.5	$\sum R =$	123.5

Calculations:

$$U = n_1 n_2 + \frac{n_1(n_1+1)}{2} - \sum R_{ij}$$

$$U = (9)(11) + \frac{(9)(10)}{2} - 86.5 = 57.5$$

$$Z = \frac{U - \dfrac{n_1 n_2}{2}}{\sqrt{\dfrac{n_1 n_2 \cdot [n_1 + (n_2+1)]}{12}}}$$

$$Z = \frac{57.5 - \dfrac{(9)(11)}{2}}{\sqrt{\dfrac{(9)(11) \cdot [9+12)]}{12}}} = \frac{57.5 - 49.5}{13.16} = 0.61$$

Decision: With $z < 1.96$, fail to reject H_0 and fail to show a significant difference between the two types of physical therapy.

6.   Study evaluating cost effectiveness of a new treatment for peritoneal adhesiolysis.

Independent variable: treatment received
(each pair serves as its own control)
Dependent variable: costs (based on ordinal ranks)
Test statistic: Wilcoxon matched-pairs test or Friedman two-way
. analysis of variance

Hypotheses: H_0: No difference between the two treatments
H_1: Difference between the two treatments

a. Wilcoxon matched-pairs test

Decision rule: With $\alpha = 0.05$, reject H_0 if $|z| > 1.96$.

Data:

Cost in Dollars				Sign Associated with least
New	Conventional	d	Rank d	frequent sign
11,813	13,112	+1,299	4	
6,112	8,762	+2,650	11	
13,276	14,762	+1,486	5	
11,335	10,605	-730	1	1
8,415	6,430	-1,985	6	6
12,762	11,990	-772	2	2
7,501	9,650	+2,149	7	
3,610	7,519	+3,909	12	
9,337	11,754	+2,417	9	
6,538	8,985	+2,447	10	
5,097	4,228	-869	3	3
10,410	12,667	+2,257	8	

$$\Sigma = T = 12$$

Calculations:

$$E(T) = \frac{n(n+1)}{2} \cdot \frac{1}{2} \quad or \quad E(T) = \frac{n(n+1)}{4}$$

$$E(T) = \frac{(12)(13)}{4} = 39$$

$$Z = \frac{T - E(T)}{\sqrt{\dfrac{n(n+1)(2n+1)}{24}}}$$

$$Z = \frac{12 - 39}{\sqrt{\dfrac{12(13)(25)}{24}}} = \frac{-27}{\sqrt{162.5}} = 2.11$$

Decision: Using the Wilcoxon matched-pairs test, the result is a z > 1.96; therefore reject H_0, conclude that the new treatment is more cost effective than the conventional one.

b. Friedman two-way analysis of variance – data (Table 17.10

Decision rule: With $\alpha = 0.05$, reject $\chi_r^2 > \chi_1^2 = 3.84$.

Calculations:

$$\chi_r^2 = \frac{12}{nk(k+1)} \Sigma(R_j)^2 - 3n(k+1)$$

Table 17.10 Data and Ranking Associated with Comparison of Two Chemists for the Friedman Two-way Analysis of Variance

Pairing	New Data	Rank	Conventional Data	Rank
1	11,813	1	13,112	2
2	6,112	1	8,762	2
3	13,276	1	14,762	2
4	11,335	2	10,605	1
5	8,415	2	6,430	1
6	12,762	2	11,990	1
7	7,501	1	9,650	2
8	3,610	1	7,519	2
9	9,337	1	11,754	2
10	6,538	1	8,985	2
11	5,097	2	4,228	1
12	10,410	1	12,667	2
$\Sigma =$		16		20

$$\chi_r^2 = \frac{12}{12(2)(3)} [(16)^2 + (20)^2] - 3(12)(3)$$

$$\chi_r^2 = (0.16)(656) - 108 = 1.33$$

Decision: Using the Friedman two-way analysis of variance, the result is a $\chi_1^2 < 3.84$. Thus we fail to reject H_0, fail to show a significant difference. Note this difference is the opposite of the Wilcoxon test on the same data. The Friedman test counted the positive and negative differences, whereas Wilcoxon measured the magnitude of the differences when the intermediate ranks were assigned.

7. Comparisons of two blister packs stored under different conditions.
   Independent variable: Storage conditions (discrete)
   Dependent variable: Type of blister pack (discrete)
   Test statistic: Fisher exact test (cell A has an expected value < 5)

	40 degrees 50% relative humidity	60 degrees 50% relative humidity	
Blister pack A	2	5	7
Blister pack B	6	6	12
	8	11	19

Hypothesis: H_0: Blister pack and storage conditions are independent
H_1: The two variables are not independent

Decision rule: With $\alpha = 0.05$, reject H_0 if $p(>2) > 0.05$.

Calculations:

a. $p(2)$ of two failures with blister pack A

$$p = \frac{(a+b)! (c+d)! (a+c)! (b+d)!}{n! \, a! \, b! \, c! \, d!}$$

$$p = \frac{7! \, 12! \, 8! \, 11!}{19! \, 2! \, 5! \, 6! \, 6!} = 0.256$$

b. p(1) of one failure with blister pack A

$$p = \frac{7! \, 12! \, 8! \, 11!}{19! \, 1! \, 6! \, 7! \, 5!} = 0.073$$

c. p(0) of no failures with blister pack A

$$p = \frac{7! \, 12! \, 8! \, 11!}{19! \, 0! \, 7! \, 8! \, 4!} = 0.006$$

Decision: The probability of two or less failures with blister pack A under independent conditions is 0.335 (0.256 + 0.073 + 0.006), therefore we cannot reject H_0 and assume that the frequency of failures by blister pack is independent of the storage conditions.

8. Comparisons between diastolic blood pressure before and after administration of a new drug.
    Independent variable: two time periods (each person serves as own control)
    Dependent variable: Assay results (ranked to ordinal scale)
    Test statistic: Wilcoxon matched-pairs test and sign test

    Hypotheses: H_0: No difference between pre- and post-blood pressures
                 H_1: Difference between pre- and post-blood pressures

    a. Wilcoxon matched-pairs test – data (Table 17.11)

    Decision rule: With $\alpha = 0.05$, reject H_0 if $|z| > 1.96$.

    Calculations:

$$E(T) = \frac{n(n+1)}{4} = \frac{12(13)}{4} = 39$$

Table 17.11 Data and Ranking Associated with Blood Pressure
Readings for the Wilcoxon Matched-Pairs Test

Subject	Before	After	d	Rank $\mid d \mid$	Rank associated with least frequent sign
1	68	66	-2	4	
2	83	80	-3	6	
3	72	67	-5	8	
4	75	74	-1	1.5	
5	79	70	-9	12	
6	71	77	+6	10	10
7	65	64	-1	1.5	
8	76	70	-6	10	
9	78	76	-2	4	
10	68	66	-2	4	
11	85	81	-4	7	
12	74	68	-6	10	

$$T = \Sigma = 10$$

$$Z = \frac{10 - 39}{\sqrt{\dfrac{12(13)(25)}{24}}} = \frac{-29}{\sqrt{162.5}} = -2.28$$

Decision: With $z < -1.96$, reject H_0, concluding that there is a significant decrease in the diastolic blood pressure with the new drug.

b. Sign test

Decision rule: With $\alpha = 0.05$, reject H_0 if $p < 0.05$

Data (Table 17.12)

Computations (binomial distribution):

$$p(0 \ negatives) = \binom{12}{0}(.50)^0(.50)^{12} = 0.00024$$

$$p(1 \ negative) = \binom{12}{1}(.50)^1(.50)^{11} = 0.00294$$

Table 17.12 Data and Ranking Associated with
Blood Pressure Readings for the Sign Test

Subject	Before	After	d	Sign
1	68	66	-2	-
2	83	80	-3	-
3	72	67	-5	-
4	75	74	-1	-
5	79	70	-9	-
6	71	77	+6	+
7	65	64	-1	-
8	76	70	-6	-
9	78	76	-2	-
10	68	66	-2	-
11	85	81	-4	-
12	74	68	-6	-

$$p(> 2\ negatives) = \Sigma = 0.00318$$

Decision: With $p < 0.05$, reject H_0, concluding that there is a significant decrease in the diastolic blood pressure with the new drug.

Computations (Yates correction formula):

Decision rule: With $\alpha = 0.05$, reject H_0 if $z > 1.96$.

$$p = \frac{1}{12} = 0.083$$

$$z = \frac{|.083 - .50| - \dfrac{1}{24}}{\sqrt{\dfrac{(.50)(.50)}{12}}} = \frac{.417 - .042}{\sqrt{.0208}} = 2.60$$

Decision: With $z < 1.96$, reject H_0 and conclude that there is a significant decrease in the diastolic blood pressure with the new drug.

9. Comparison of results for two delivery methods of continuing education.
   Independent variable: live vs. remote (discrete)
   Dependent variable: examination score (ranked to ordinal scale)
   Statistical test: Mann-Whitney U test

Hypotheses: H_0: Samples are from the same population
            H_1: Samples are drawn from different populations

Decision rule: With $\alpha = 0.05$, reject H_0, if $|z| >$ critical $z_{(.975)} = 1.96$

Live	Rank	Remote	Rank
96	20	82	9
91	19	89	17
81	8	85	12.5
75	4	78	6
80	7	90	18
85	12.5	83	10
		88	15.5
		69	1
		86	14
		73	3
		88	15.5
		84	11
		71	2
		76	5
		97	21
$\Sigma R =$	70.5	$\Sigma R =$	160.5

Calculations:

$$U = n_1 n_2 + \frac{n_1(n_1+1)}{2} - \Sigma R_{1j}$$

$$U = (6)(15) + \frac{(6)(7)}{2} - 70.5 = 40.5$$

$$Z = \frac{U - \frac{n_1 n_2}{2}}{\sqrt{\frac{n_1 n_2 \cdot [n_1 + (n_2 + 1)]}{12}}}$$

$$Z = \frac{40.5 - \frac{(6)(15)}{2}}{\sqrt{\frac{(6)(15) \cdot (6 + 16)}{12}}} = \frac{40.5 - 45}{12.84} = -0.35$$

Decision: With z < 1.96, fail to reject H_0, and fail to show a significant difference between the results from the two laboratories.

10. Comparison of a raw material at three different production sites.
    Independent variable: production site (discrete, 3 levels)
    Dependent variable: oil viscosity (ranked to ordinal scale)
    Statistical test: Kruskal-Wallis test

    Hypotheses: H_0: Samples are from the same population
                 H_1: Samples are drawn from different populations

    Decision rule: With $\alpha = 0.05$, reject H_0 if $H > \chi^2_2(.95) = 5.99$

Viscosity Batch A	Rank	Viscosity Batch B	Rank	Viscosity Batch C	Rank
10.23	7	10.24	8	10.25	9
10.33	15	10.28	12.5	10.20	2.5
10.28	12.5	10.20	2.5	10.21	4.5
10.27	11	10.21	4.5	10.18	1
10.30	14	10.26	10	10.22	6
$\Sigma =$	59.5		37.5		23

$$\Sigma\Sigma = 120 = (15)(16)/2 = N(N+1)/2$$

Calculations:

$$H = \frac{12}{N(N+1)} \left[\Sigma \frac{(\Sigma R_{ij})^2}{n_j} \right] - 3(N+1)$$

$$H = \frac{12}{15(16)} \left[\frac{(59.5)^2}{5} + \frac{(37.5)^2}{5} + \frac{(23)^2}{5} \right] - 3(16)$$

$$H = (0.05)(1095.10) - 48 = 6.76$$

Decision: With H > 5.99, reject H_0 and conclude that the samples were not drawn from the same population.

11. Comparison of strengths of an anticoagulant and prothrombin times.
    Independent variable: Continuous (amount of anticoagulant)
    Dependent variable: Continuous (prothrombin time)
    Statistical test: Spearman rho correlation

| | Observed | | Ranked | | | |
Subject	Dose	Ptime	Dose	Ptime	d	d^2
1	200	20	6	10.5	4.5	20.25
2	180	18	2	2.5	0.5	.25
3	225	20	11	10.5	-0.5	.25
4	205	19	7	6	-1	1
5	190	19	4	6	2	4
6	195	18	5	2.5	-2.5	6.25
7	220	19	10	6	-4	16
8	175	17	1	1	0	0
9	215	20	9	10.5	0.5	.25
10	185	19	3	6	3	9
11	210	19	8	6	-2	4
12	230	20	12	10.5	-1.5	2.25
					$\Sigma d^2 =$	63.5

Computation:

$$\rho = 1 - \frac{6(\Sigma d^2)}{n^3 - n}$$

$$\rho = 1 - \frac{6(63.5)}{12^3 - 12} = 1 - \frac{381}{1716} = .778$$

Decision: There is a strong positive correlation between the amount of anticoagulant and the prothrombin time.

18

Statistical Tests
for Bioequivalence

Up to this point, most of the statistical tests we have discussed are concerned with null hypotheses stating equality (i.e., Ho: $\mu_1=\mu_2$). These tests were designed to test for significant differences and by rejecting the null hypothesis, prove inequality. As discussed in Chapter 7, when finding a result that is not statistically significant we do not accept the null hypothesis, we simply fail to reject it. The analogy was presented of jurisprudence where the jury will render a verdict of "not guilty," but never "innocent." They failed to prove the client guilty beyond a reasonable doubt. Similarly, if our data fails to show a statistically significant difference exists, we do not prove equivalency. But what if we do want to show equality?

To address this topic several tests will be presented which are commonly used for bioequivalence testing in pharmacy. If we produce a new generic product, is it the same as the originator's product? Are we producing the same product from batch to batch, or are there significant variations between batches of our drug product? The tests presented in this chapter will help answer these questions.

Bioequivalence Testing

In order for an oral or injectable product to be effective it must reach the site of action in a concentration large enough to exert its effect. Bioavailability indicates the rate and/or amount of active drug ingredient that is absorbed from the product and available at the site of action. *Remington's Pharmaceutical Sciences*

(DiSanto, p.1451) defines bioequivalence as an indication "that a drug in two or more similar dosage forms reaches the general circulation at the same relative rate and the same relative extent." Thus, two drug products are bioequivalent if their bioavailabilities are the same and may be used interchangeably for the same therapeutic effect. In contrast to previous tests which attempted to prove differences, the objective of most of these bioequivalence statistics is to prove that two dosage forms are the same or at least close enough to be considered equal, beyond a reasonable doubt.

The measures of bioavailability are based upon measures of the concentration of the drug in the blood and we must assume that there is a direct relationship between the concentration of drug we detect in the blood and the concentration of the drug at the site of action. These usually involve the evaluation of the peak plasma concentration (C_{max}), the time to reach the peak concentration (T_{max}) and/or the area under plasma concentration-time curve (AUC). The AUC measures the extent of absorption and the amount of drug which is absorbed by the body, and the parameter most commonly evaluated in bioequivalence studies. Many excellent text books deal with the issues associated with measuring pharmacokinetic parameters - the extent of bioavailability and bioequivalence (Welling and Tse, 1995; Evans, Schentag and Jusko, 1992; Winter, M.E., 1994). The purpose of this discussion is to focus solely on the statistical manipulation of bioequivalence data.

There are three situations requiring bioequivalence testing: a) when a proposed marketed dosage form differs significantly from that used in the major clinical trials for the product; b) when there are major changes in the manufacturing process for a marketed product; and c) when a new generic product is compared to the innovator's marketed product (Benet and Goyan, 1995). Regulatory agencies allow the assumption of safety and effectiveness if the pharmaceutical manufacturers can demonstrate bioequivalence with their product formulations.

Experimental Designs for Bioequivalence Studies

Before volunteers are recruited and the actual clinical trial conducted, an insightful and organized study is developed by the principle investigator. As discussed in the Chapter 1, the first two steps in the statistical process is to identify the questions to be answered and the hypotheses to be tested (defined in the study objectives). Then the appropriate research design is selected (to be discussed below) and the appropriate statistical tests are selected. For in vivo bioavailability study, the FDA requires that the research design identify the scientific questions to be answered, the drugs(s) and dosage form(s) to be tested, the analytical methods used to assess the outcomes of treatment, and benefit-risk considerations involving human testing (21 *Code of Federal Regulations*, 320.25(b)).

Study protocols should not only include the objectives of the study, the patient inclusion and exclusion criteria, the study design, dosing schedules, and physiological measures; but also a statistics section describing the sample size, power determinations and the specific analyses which will be performed. These protocols are then review by an Institutional Review Board to evaluate the benefit-risk considerations regarding the volunteers. Two types of study designs are generally used for comparing the bioavailability parameters for drugs. Each of these designs employ statistics or modifications of statistics presented in previous chapters.

The first design is a **parallel group design** which is illustrated in Figure 18.1. In this design, volunteers are assigned to one of two "similar" groups and each groups receives only one treatment (either the test drug or the reference standard). In order to establish similar groups, volunteers are randomly assigned to one of the two groups using a random numbers table as discussed in Chapter Two. For example, assume that 30 healthy volunteers (15 per group) are required to compare two formulations of a particular product. Using a random numbers table, the volunteers (numbered 01 to 30) are assigned to one of the two groups (Table 18.1). Because of random assignment to the two treatment levels (groups), it is assumed that each set of volunteers is identical to the other (i.e., same average weight, average lean body mass, average physiological parameters). Therefore, any difference in the bioavailability measures are attributable to the drug formulation received. Results from this parallel design can be simply evaluated using a two sample t- test (Chapter 8). Also, if more that two formulations are involved, the volunteers can be randomly assigned to k treatment levels and the one-way analysis of variance can be employed (Chapter 9).

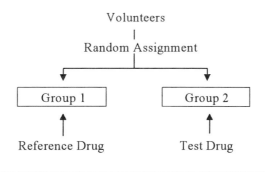

Figure 18.1 Parallel design involving two groups.

Table 18.1 Results of a Random Sample of 30 Volunteers for a Clinical Trial

Group 1			Group 2		
02	15	23	01	10	20
05	16	24	03	11	21
06	18	25	04	13	28
09	19	26	07	14	29
12	22	27	08	17	30

In the parallel group design each volunteer receives only one of the formulations of a drug. This design can be extremely useful for Phase II and Phase III clinical trials. It is easy to conduct and exposes volunteers to risk only once, but cannot control for inter-subject variability. The design is appropriate when there is an anticipated small inter-subject variability in response to the drug. To minimize patient risk, the parallel group design can be used for studies involving drugs with long elimination half-life and potential toxicity. Also the design can be employed with ill patients or those involving long periods to determine therapeutic response. However, the parallel group design is not appropriate for most bioavailability or bioequivalence studies. With inter-subject variability, unaccounted for in this design, it provides a less precise method for determining bioavailability differences.

To overcome some of the disadvantages of the parallel design, a second more rigorous approach is the **crossover study design**. In this design, volunteers are once again randomly assigned to two groups, but each group receives all the treatments in the study. In the case of the two formulations described above, each volunteer would receive both treatments. The order in which the volunteers received the formulations would depend on the group to which they were assigned (Figure 18.2). Using the same volunteer from our example in Table 18.1, if we employee a crossover study design, those subjects randomly assigned to Group 1 (volunteers 02, 05, 06, etc.) will first receive the reference drug (R). After an appropriate "washout" period, the same volunteers will receive the test drug (T). For those volunteers assigned to Group 2 the order of the drug will be reversed; with the test drug first, followed by the reference standard. In this simple two-period crossover study design (referred to as a standard 2 x 2 crossover design). The subjects in Group 1 receive an RT sequence and those in Group 2 a TR sequence. Note that every volunteer will receive both the test and reference drug.

The washout mentioned above is a predetermined period of time between the two treatment periods. It is intended to prevent any carry over of effects from the first treatment to the second treatment period. In this type of

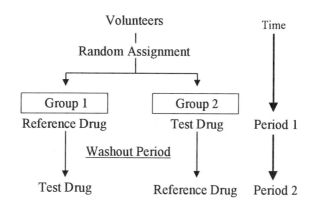

Figure 18.2 Two period crossover design for two groups.

Design, the washout period should be long enough for the first treatment to wear off. This washout period could be based on the half-live of the drug being evaluated. In five half-lives the drug can be considered removed from the body, with approximately 96.9% of the drug eliminated. Obviously, if the washout period is not sufficiently long there is a **carryover effect** and the second bioavailability measures will not be independent of the first measurements and would violate statistical criteria. Using well designed studies it is assumed that the washout period is sufficiently long enough to prevent any carryover effects.

In clinical trials, individual volunteers can contribute a large amount of variability to bioavailability measures. Thus the crossover design provides a method for removing inter-subject variability by having individuals serve as their own controls. The FDA recommend the a crossover design when evaluating pharmacokinetic parameters (21 *Code of Federal Regulations* 320.26(b) and 320.27(b)). In addition to having volunteers serving as their own controls and reduce inter-subject variability, these study designs also require fewer subjects to provide the same statistical power because the same volunteers are assessed for each treatment level.

Results from the crossover design presented on Figure 18.2 could be evaluated using either the a paired t-test (Chapter 8) or a complete randomized block design (Chapter 9). Once again, if more that two formulations are involved the volunteers can be randomly assigned to k treatment levels and the complete randomized block design can be used.

A third possible research design is a **balanced incomplete block design**. This last method overcomes several disadvantages associated with the complete randomized block design used in crossover studies. When there are more than two treatment levels, the "complete" crossover design may not be practical since such a design would involve an extended period of time, with several washout periods and an increased likelihood of volunteers withdrawing from the study. Also, such designs would involve a larger number of blood draws which increases the risk to the volunteers. An incomplete block design is similar to a complete block design, except not all formulations are administered to each block. The design is incomplete if the number of treatments for each block is less than the total number of treatments being evaluated in the study. Each block, or volunteer, is randomly assigned to a treatment sequence and the design is "balanced" if the resulting number of subjects receiving each treatment is equal. A complete discussion of this design is presented by Kirk (1968).

Selection of the most appropriate study design (parallel, crossover or balanced incomplete block design) depends on several factors. These include: 1) the objectives of the study; 2) the number of treatment levels being compared; 3) characteristics of the drug being evaluated; 4) availability of volunteers and anticipated withdrawals; 5) inter- and intra-subject variabilities; 6) duration of the sudy; and 7) financial resources (Chow and Liu, 1992).

Two-sample t-test Example

When pharmaceutical manufacturers and regulatory agencies began studying the bioequivalence of drug products, the general approach was to use a simple t-test or analysis of variance to evaluate plasma concentration-time curve (i.e., C_{max}, T_{max}, AUC). Since these traditional statistical tests (t-test and ANOVAs) were designed to demonstrate differences rather than similarities, they were incorrectly used to interpret the early bioequivalence studies. In the 1970s researchers began to note that traditional hypothesis tests were not appropriate for evaluating bioequivalence (Metzler, 1974).

Most of the statistical procedures involved with bioequivalence testing require that the data approximate a normality distribution. However, most of the bioavailability measures (AUC, t_{max}, and C_{max}) have a tendency to be positively skewed. Therefore, a transformation of the data may be required before analysis. The log transformation (geometric mean calculation presented in Chapter 5) on AUC is usually performed to remove the skewness. This log-transformed data is then analyzed using the procedures discussed below.

To illustrate the problems which exist when using some of our previous statistical tests, lets us take an example of a clinical trial comparing Acme Chemical's new generic antihypertensive agent to the innovators original product. This would portray the third situation cited previously by Benet. We

Table 18.2 Data from Two Randomly Assigned Groups (AUC in ng·hr/ml)

Acme Chemical (New Product)		Innovator (Reference Standard)	
61.3	91.2	80.9	70.8
71.4	80.1	91.4	87.1
48.3	54.4	59.8	99.7
76.8	68.7	70.5	62.6
60.4	84.9	75.7	85.0
Mean =	69.75	Mean =	78.35
S =	13.76	S =	12.79

design a very simple study to compare the two formulations of the same chemical entity, by administering them to two groups of randomly assigned volunteers. Only ten volunteers are assigned to each group. Our primary pharmacokinetic parameter of interest is the AUC (ng·hr/ml). The results of our *in vivo* tests are presented in Table 18.2.

If we use our traditional two-sample t-test as discussed in Chapter 8, the hypotheses would be:

$$H_0: \mu_1 = \mu_2$$
$$H_1: \mu_1 \neq \mu_2$$

The decision rule, base on α of 0.05 is to reject H_0 if $t > t_{18}(.025) = +2.104$ or $t < -t_{18}(.025) = -2.104$. The statistical analysis would be as follows:

$$S_p^2 = \frac{(n_1-1)S_1^2 + (n_2-1)S_2^2}{n_1+n_2-2} \qquad \text{Eq. 8.3}$$

$$S_p^2 = \frac{9(13.76)^2 + 9(12.79)^2}{18} \; 176.46$$

$$t = \frac{\overline{X_1} - \overline{X_2}}{\sqrt{\dfrac{S_P^2}{n_1} + \dfrac{S_P^2}{n_2}}} \qquad \text{Eq. 8.6}$$

$$t = \frac{69.75 - 78.35}{\sqrt{\dfrac{176.46}{10} + \dfrac{176.46}{10}}} = \frac{-8.60}{5.94} = -1.45$$

The result is that we fail to reject H_0 because the t-value is less than our critical value of -2.104. Therefore, with 95% confidence, we failed to prove a difference between the two formulations. However, at the same time we *did not* prove that the formulations were equal or identical.

Since in most cases the sample sizes are the same, we can make the following substitution for the demoninator in Eq. 8.6. However, if we do run into unequal sample sizes ($n_1 \neq n_2$) we can substitute the left side of equation for the standard error portion in any of the formulas discussed in this chapter.

$$\sqrt{\frac{S_P^2}{n_1} + \frac{S_P^2}{n_2}} = \sqrt{\frac{2S_p^2}{n}} \qquad \text{Eq. 18.1}$$

A potential problem exists with the Type II error in our statistical analysis. As discussed in Chapter 7, β is the error of failing to reject H_0 (equality) when there is a true difference between the formulations we are testing. As shown in Figure 7.5, with smaller sample sizes there is a greater likelihood of creating a Type II error. If an unethical entrepreneur wished to prove his product was equal to an innovator's drug, the easiest way to accomplish this would be to use very small sample sizes, apply traditional statistical methods, fail to reject H_0 and conclude that the two products were equivalent. To avoid such deceptions the FDA has developed guidelines to ensure adequate power in bioequivalence tests (i.e., 80/20 rule discussed below).

Power in Bioequivalence Tests

For most bioequivalence studies, the same size is usually 18-24 healthy normal volunteers. To detect a clinically important difference (20%), a power calculation is often performed prior to the study to determine the number of subjects needed to have the desired power (80%). For example, the following is a typical statement associated with a proposed protocol: "A sample size of 28 health males will be enrolled in this study to ensure study completion by at least 24 patients. Based on (a previous study sited) a sample size of 20 patients can provide at least 80% probability to show that the 90% confidence interval of the mean AUC value for the clinical lot of (test drug name) is within ±20% of the reference mean AUC value." Note that the investigators increased the sample size to ensure that there would be sufficient power once the data was collected.

Also, more than the required number of subjects are recruited to anticipate possible replacements for dropouts.

In the previous example we were unable to reject the null hypothesis that $\mu_1 = \mu_2$ based on 10 volunteers for each product. However, we might ask ourselves, if there was a difference between the two formulations, was our sample size large enough to detect a difference? In other words, was our statistical test powerful enough to detect a desired difference? Let us assume that we want to be able to detect a 10% difference from our reference standard ($78.35 \times 0.10 = 7.84 = \delta$). Using a formula extracted from Zar (1984), the power determination formula would be:

$$t_\beta \geq \frac{\delta}{\sqrt{\dfrac{2 S_p^2}{n}}} - t_{\alpha/2} \qquad \text{Eq. 18.2}$$

where $t_{\alpha/2}$ is the critical t-value for $\alpha = 0.05$, n is our sample size per level of our discrete independent variable and the resultant t_β is the t-value associated with our Type II error. To determine the power we will need to find the complement $(1-\beta)$ of Type II error. Using our data we find the following:

$$t_\beta \geq \frac{7.84}{\sqrt{\dfrac{2(176.46)}{10}}} - 1.96$$

$$t_\beta \geq \frac{7.84}{5.89} - 1.96 = 1.32 - 1.96 = -0.64$$

If we used a full t-table (for example *Geigy Scientific Tables* , 7th Ed. Ciba-Geigy Corp., Ardsley, NY, 1974, pp. 32-35), unlike the abbreviated version presented as Table B3 in Appendix B, we would find the probability associated with t-values with 18 degrees of freedom at p=.25 for t= -0.6884 and p=.30 for t= -0.5338. Through interpolation, a calculated t-value of -0.64 has a probability of 0.27. This represents the Type II error. The complement 0.73 (1-0.27), is the power associated with rejecting H_0 (bioequivalence) when in truth H_0 is false.

Let's further assume that we want to have at least 80% power to be able to detect a 10% difference between our two sets of tablets. We can modify the above formula to identify the appropriate sample size:

$$n \geq \frac{2S_p^2}{\delta^2}(t_\beta + t_{\alpha/2})^2 \qquad \text{Eq. 18.3}$$

If we look at the first column of Table B3 in Appendix B, the values listed for the various degrees of freedom represent our t-value for a one-tailed test with β=.20. In this case with would interpolate the t-value to be 0.862 for 18 degrees of freedom. The t($1-\alpha/2$) for 18 df is 2.10. Applied to our example:

$$n \geq \frac{2(173.46)}{(7.84)^2}(0.862 + 2.10)^2 \geq (5.64)(8.77) \geq 49.48$$

In this case, the sample size we should have used to ensure a power of at least 80%, to detect a difference as small as 10%, would have been a minimum of 50 volunteers per group.

Rules for Bioequivalence

To control the quality of bioequivalence studies the FDA has considered three possible standards: 1) the 75/75 rule; 2) the 80/20 rule; and 3) the $\pm$ 20 rule. The **75/75 rule** for bioequivalence requires that bioavailability measures for the test product be within 25% of those for the reference product (greater than 75% and less than 125%) in at least 75% of the subjects involved in the clinical trials (Federal Register, 1978). This rule was easy to apply and compared the relative bioavailability by individual subject, removing inter-subject variability. The rule was very sensitive when the size of the sample was relatively small, but was not valuable as a scientifically based decision rule. This 1977 rule was criticized for its poor statistical nature, was never finalized and was finally abandoned in 1980.

A more acceptable FDA criteria has focused on preventing too much Type II error and requires that manufacturer's perform a retrospective assessment of the power associated with their bioequivalence studies. In any study, there must be at least an 80% power to detect a 20% difference. In other words, this **80/20 rule** states that if the null hypothesis cannot be rejected at the 95% confidence level ($1-\alpha$), the sample size must be sufficiently large to have a power of at least 80% for a 20% difference to be detected between the test product and reference standard. (Federal Register, 1977). This 20% difference appears to have been an arbitrary selection to represent the minimum difference that can be regarded as clinically significant. Once again using the previous example, based on a pooled variance of 173.46, a desired difference of 20% (in this case 15.67 ng·hr/ml, 78.35 x 0.20 = δ), a Type I error rate of 0.05, and a Type II error rate of 0.20, the require sample size would be at least 12 volunteers per group.

$$n \geq \frac{2(173.46)}{(15.67)^2}(0.862 + 2.10)^2 \geq (1.41)(8.77) \geq 12.37$$

This seems like a dramatic drop in the amount of subjects required (at least 50 for a 10% difference and only 13 for a 20% difference), but it demonstrates how important it is to define the difference the researcher considers to be important (Table 18.3).

But even if we have enough power to detect a significant difference we still have failed to prove that the null hypothesis is true. Alternative tests are needed to work with the data presented. Similar to the approach used in Chapter 8 presenting the t-test, we will first use a confidence interval approach and then a hypothesis testing format to prove that even if there are differences between the new product and the reference standard, that difference falls within acceptable limits.

The last measure of bioequivalence, the ±20 **rule**, concerns the average bioavailability and states that the test product must be within 20% of the reference drug (between 80% and 120%). The ±20 rule appears to be most acceptable to the FDA. As will be seen in the following sections the ±20 rule can be tested by use of either a confidence interval or two one-tailed t-tests. These two methods are briefly introduced for comparisons for one test product to a reference standard. For a more in depth discussion of these tests and more complex bioequivalence tests, readers are referred to the excellent text by Chow and Liu (1992).

Creating Confidence Intervals

Considering our earlier discussion of the comparison of our new generic product to the innovator's product, we could write our hypotheses as follows, where the innovator's drug is referred to as the reference standard:

Table 18.3 Sample Size Required to Detect Various Differences with 80% Power Where the Reference Standard Mean is 78.35 (Table 18.2)

Difference	Minimum Sample Size
5	180
10	45
15	20
20	12
25	8
30	5

$$H_0: \; \mu_T = \mu_R$$
$$H_1: \; \mu_T \neq \mu_R$$

Where μ_T represents our new or "test" product and μ_R the "reference" or innovator's product. An alternative method for writing these hypotheses was seen in Chapter 8 when we discussed confidence intervals:

$$H_0: \; \mu_T - \mu_R = 0$$
$$H_1: \; \mu_T - \mu_R \neq 0$$

But, as discussed, we cannot prove true equality ($\delta = 0$). Rather we will establish an acceptable range and if a confidence interval falls with in those limits we can conclude that any difference is not therapeutically significant. Using this method for testing bioequivalence we create a confidence interval for the population difference:

$$\mu_T - \mu_R$$

Based on our sample results

$$\overline{X}_T - \overline{X}_R$$

Currently the FDA recommendations use a 90% confidence interval ($\alpha=0.10$). If the 90% confidence interval falls completely between 0.80 to 1.20, the two products are considered bioequivalence (an absolute difference less than 20%). With respect to a comparison of a test product to a reference standard, we want the test product to fall between 0.80 and 1.20:

$$0.80 < \mu_T - \mu_R < 1.20$$

As noted earlier in this chapter, pharmacokinetic parameters, such as Cmax and AUC often involve log transformations before the data is analyzed to ensure a normal distribution. The general formula for such a confidence interval would be:

$$\mu_T - \mu_R = (\overline{X}_T - \overline{X}_R) \pm t_{\upsilon(1-\alpha)} \sqrt{\frac{2S_p^2}{n}} \qquad \text{Eq. 18.4}$$

This is almost identical to Eq. 8.4 for the two-sample t-test. Because of formulas discussed later in this chapter, we will simplify the formula to replacing the sample difference with d and our standard error term with SE:

$$d = \overline{X}_T - \overline{X}_R \qquad \text{Eq. 18.5}$$

$$SE = t_\upsilon (1 - \alpha) \sqrt{\frac{2S_p^2}{n}} \qquad \text{Eq. 18.6}$$

If one thinks of this problem as an ANOVA with $\nu_1 = 1$ in Chapter 9, the MSW (mean square within) from the ANOVA table can be substituted for the S_p^2 term. Also, note that we are performing two one-tailed tests with 5% error loaded on each tail $(1-\alpha)$. Also, if the sample sizes are not equal the standard error portion of the equation can be rewritten as:

$$SE = t_\upsilon (1 - \alpha) \sqrt{\frac{S_p^2}{n_1} + \frac{S_p^2}{n_2}} \qquad \text{Eq. 18.7}$$

Using Eq. 18.4 through 18.7 we can create a confidence interval based on the same units of measure as the original data (i.e., AUC in ng.hr/ml). A better approach would be to calculate confidence intervals about the observed relative bioavailability between the test product and the reference standard; converting the information into percentages of the reference standard. With FDA's recommendation for at least 80% bioavailability in order to claim bioequivalence, the ratio of the two products are more often statistically evaluated than the differences between the AUCs.

$$80\% < \frac{\mu_T}{\mu_R} < 120\%$$

This ratio of bioavailabilities between 80 and 120% is an acceptable standard by the FDA and pharmaceutical regulatory agencies in most countries. The last step is to create a ratio between the change and the reference standard so outcomes can be expressed as percent of the reference standard:

$$Lower\ Limit = \frac{(d - SE) + \overline{X}_R}{\overline{X}_R} \times 100\% \qquad \text{Eq. 18.8}$$

$$Upper\ Limit = \frac{(d + SE) + \overline{X}_R}{\overline{X}_R} \times 100\% \qquad \text{Eq. 18.9}$$

Finally the resultant confidence interval is expressed as:

$$Lower\ Limit < \frac{\mu_T}{\mu_R} < Upper\ Limit \qquad \text{Eq. 18.10}$$

What we create is a confidence interval within which we can state with 95% confidence where the true population ratio falls based on our sample.

Applying these formulas to our previous example of Acme Chemical's generic and the Innovator's product, we find the following results:

$$SE = t_\nu(1-\alpha)\sqrt{\frac{2S_p^2}{n}} = (1.734)\sqrt{\frac{2(176.46)}{10}} = 10.30$$

$$d = \overline{X}_T - \overline{X}_R = 69.75 - 78.35 = -8.6$$

$$Upper\ Limit = \frac{(-8.6 + 10.3) + 78.35}{78.35} \times 100\% = 102.17\%$$

$$Lower\ Limit = \frac{(-8.6 - 10.3) + 78.35}{78.35} \times 100\% = 75.88\%$$

Thus, in this case, with 95% confidence, the true population ratio is between:

$$75.88\% < \frac{\mu_T}{\mu_R} < 102.17\%$$

This fails to meet the FDA requirement of falling within the 80% to 120% range. Therefore, we would conclude that the two products are not bioequivalent.

Comparison Using Two One-sided t-tests

The last method we will explore is to involve hypothesis testing to determine if we can satisfy the requirements for bioequivalence. As discussed previously, the absolute difference between the two products is less the 20% of the reference standard:

$$|\mu_T - \mu_R| < 20\% \ \mu_R$$

This method, proposed by Hauck and Anderson (1984), overcomes some of the negative aspects of the previous approaches by using a two one-sided t-tests to evaluate bioequivalence. In this case we deal with two null hypotheses which indicate outcomes outside of the acceptable differences for bioequivalency:

$$H_{01}: \mu_T - \mu_R \leq -20\%$$
$$H_{02}: \mu_T - \mu_R \geq +20\%$$

The two alternate hypotheses represent outcomes that fall short of the extremes:

$$H_{11}: \mu_T - \mu_R > -20\%$$
$$H_{12}: \mu_T - \mu_R < +20\%$$

Obviously, both of the null hypothesis must be rejected in order to prove:

$$80\% < \mu_T - \mu_R < 120\%$$

The equations for this two one-tailed test involves two θ's that define the "equivalence interval" where $\theta_1 < \theta_2$. In other words, θ_2 is always the upper equivalence limit and θ_1 the lower limit. In the case of equivalency being less than 20%, each theta (θ) represents a 20% difference in the units from which the data was collected: $\theta_2 = +20\%$ value and $\theta_1 = -20\%$ value. The Schuirmann's (1987) formulas for calculating the two one-sided t-tests are:

$$t_1 = \frac{(\overline{X}_T - \overline{X}_R) - \theta_1}{\sqrt{MS_E} \ \sqrt{2/n}} \qquad \text{Eq. 18.11}$$

$$t_2 = \frac{\theta_2 - (\overline{X}_T - \overline{X}_R)}{\sqrt{MS_E} \ \sqrt{2/n}} \qquad \text{Eq. 18.12}$$

These test H_{01} and H_{02} respectively. As with past tests of hypotheses, we establish a decision rule based on the sample size and a 95% confidence in our decision. Our decision rule is with $\alpha = 0.05$, reject H_{01} or H_{02} if $t > t_{df}(1-\alpha)$. Each hypothesis is tested with a Type I error of 0.05 (α). Traditionally we have tested out the hypothesis with a total α=.05; the procedure we actually use 1-2α rather than 1-α (Westlake, 1988). This would correspond to the 90% confidence intervals discussed in the previous section.

In this case theta represents our desired detectable difference (δ) and, as discussed previous, the MSE or MSW for only two levels of the discrete independent variable (v_1=1) is the same as S_p^2. Therefore, the equations can be rewritten as follows:

$$t_1 = \frac{(\overline{X}_T - \overline{X}_R) - \delta_1}{\sqrt{\frac{2S_p^2}{n}}} \qquad \text{Eq. 18.13}$$

$$t_2 = \frac{\delta_2 - (\overline{X}_T - \overline{X}_R)}{\sqrt{\frac{2S_p^2}{n}}} \qquad \text{Eq. 18.14}$$

Using our previous example and again assuming we wish to be able to detect a 20% difference for an innovator's product:

$$\delta = 78.35 \ x \ 0.20 = 15.67$$

Therefore, δ_1 = -15.67; δ_2 = +15.67, S_p^2 = 173.46 and our critical value through interpolation for $t_{18}(1-\alpha)$ is 1.73. The decision rule, with α=0.05, is to reject H_{01} or H_{02} if t > 1.73.

$$t_1 = \frac{(-8.6) - (-15.67)}{\sqrt{\frac{2(176.46)}{10}}} = \frac{7.07}{5.94} = 1.20$$

$$t_2 = \frac{15.67 - (-8.6)}{\sqrt{\frac{2(176.46)}{10}}} = \frac{24.27}{5.94} = 4.09$$

In this case we were able to reject H_{02} and prove that the difference was less than 120% (μ_{Test} - $\mu_{Reference}$ < +20%), but failed to reject H_{01}. We were not able to prove that μ_{Test} - $\mu_{Reference}$ was greater than 80%. Therefore, similar to our confidence interval in the previous section, we are unable to show bioequivalency between Acme's generic and the Innovator's reference standard.

Dissolution Testing

Dissolution tests provide an *in vitro* method to determine if products produced by various manufacturers or various batches from the same manufacturer are in compliance with compendia or regulatory requirements. For example, the *United States Pharmacopeia* (1985) states that aspirin tablets ($C_9H_8O_4$) must have "not less than 95% and not more than 105% of labeled amount of $C_9H_8O_4$." In addition, the tolerance level for dissolution testing is that "not less than 80% of the labeled amount of $C_9H_8O_4$ is dissolved in 30 minutes."

Dissolution profiles can be used to compare multiple batches, manufacturers, or production sites to determine if the products are similar with respect to percent of drug dissolved over given periods of time. The assumption made is that the rate of dissolution and availability will correlate to absorption in the gut and eventually similar effects at the site of action. This assumption can be significantly enhanced if manufacturers can establish an *in vivo-in vitro* correlation between their dissolution measures and bioavailability outcomes (FDA, 1997, p. 7).

Using aspirin tablets as an example, consider the two sets of profiles seen in Figure 18.3. All batches meet the dissolution criteria of 80% in 30 minutes, but the profiles vary. Are they the same or different enough to consider the batches not equivalent?

SUPAC-IR Guidance

To answer the question of equivalency in dissolution profiles the FDA has proposed a guidance for manufacturers issued as "Scale-up and Post-Approval Changes for Immediate Release Solid Oral Dosage Forms" (SUPAC-IR). This guidance is designed to provide recommendations for manufacturers submitting new drug applications, abbreviated new drug applications and abbreviated antibiotic applications for manufacturers who wish to change the process, equipment or production sites following approval of their previous drug submission (Federal Register, 1995). Previous evaluations involved single point dissolution tests (i.e., the previous aspirin monograph). The SUPAC-IR guidance can assist manufacturers with changes associated with: 1) scale-up procedures; 2) site changes in the manufacturing facilities; 3) equipment or process changes; and 4) changes in component or composition of the finished dosage form.

Under SUPAC-IR there are two factors which can be calculated: 1) a difference factor (f_1), and 2) a similarity factor (f_2). The published formulas are as follows:

$$f_1 = \left\{ \left[\sum |R_t - T_t| \right] \ / \ \left[\sum R_t \right] \right\} \cdot 100 \qquad \text{Eq. 18.15}$$

$$f_2 = 50 \, \text{Log} \left\{ \left[1 + \frac{1}{n} \sum (R_t - T_t)^2 \right]^{-0.5} \cdot 100 \right\} \qquad \text{Eq. 18.16}$$

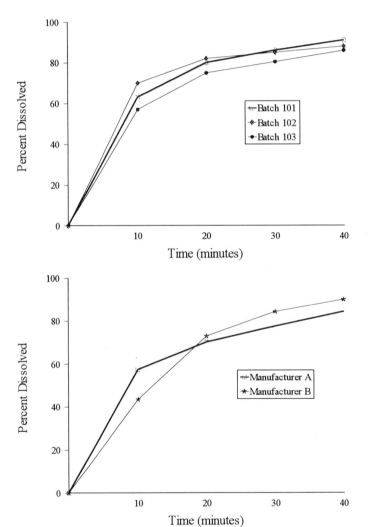

Figure 18.3 Examples of dissolution profiles.

where n is the number of time points in the dissolution profile, R_t is the percent dissolved for the reference standard at each time period, T_t is percent dissolved for the test product at the same time period, and log is the logarithm base 10. We will slightly rewrite these formulas to remove the negative, fractional root terminology:

$$f_1 = \frac{\sum |R_t - T_t|}{\sum R_t} \times 100$$

Eq. 18.17

$$f_2 = 50 \, \mathrm{Log} \left[\frac{1}{\sqrt{1 + \frac{1}{n}\sum (R_t - T_t)^2}} \times 100 \right]$$

Eq. 18.18

Table 18.4 Example of Data From Dissolution Tests on Two Drug Batches

Time (minutes):	15	30	45	60
	Batch Produced Using Original Equipment			
	63.9	85.9	85.4	93.6
	42.9	75.8	74.5	87.4
	58.1	77.3	83.2	86.4
	62.4	79.3	76.2	79.2
	52.5	74.5	90.3	94.5
	59.1	65.1	87.5	86.1
Mean:	56.48	76.32	82.85	87.87
SD:	7.74	6.79	6.29	5.61
RSD:	13.71	8.91	7.59	6.38
	Batch Produced Using Newer Equipment			
	78.5	85.6	88.4	92.9
	67.2	72.1	80.2	86.8
	56.5	80.4	83.1	85.4
	78.9	85.2	89.8	91.4
	72.3	84.1	85.4	94.1
	84.9	72.1	79.0	85.9
Mean:	73.05	79.92	84.32	89.42
SD:	10.13	6.33	4.35	3.83
RSD:	13.87	7.91	5.16	4.28

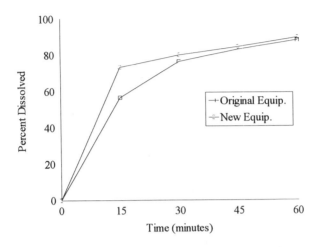

Figure 18.4 Dissolution profiles of data from Table 18.4.

The guidance for equivalency is that the f_1-value should be close to 0 (generally values less than 15) and the f_2-value should be close to 100, with values greater than 50 ensuring equivalency.

If the two dissolution profiles are exactly the same (one laying exactly over the second) the f_2 value will be 100. As the f_2-value gets smaller there is a greater difference between the two profiles. An f_2 of 50 represents a 10% difference, thus the SUPAC-IR guidance requires a calculated f_2-value between 50 and 100 for equivalency. As an example, consider the data presented in Table 18.4 and Figure 18.4 which show the results of dissolution tests performed on two batches of the same drug, one produced with the original equipment used for products NDA application, and the second with newer equipment. Are the following two profiles the same (less than a 10% difference) based on the f_1 and f_2 formulas proposed under SUPAC-IR?

Several criteria must be met in order to apply the f_1 and f_2 calculations (FDA, 1997). These include: 1) test and reference batches should be tested under exactly the same conditions, including the same time points; 2) only one time point should be considered after 85% dissolution for both batches; and 3) the "percent coefficient of variation" (what we've called the relative standard deviation in Chapter 5) at the earlier time points should be no more than 20% and at other time points should be no more than 10%. The rationale for these criteria is discussed by Shah and colleagues (1998).

Looking at the data presented in Table 18.4, our data fulfills all three criteria. Therefore, both the f_1 and f_2 statistics can be used to evaluate the equivalency of these two types of production equipment. To calculate certain values required by the statistics, we can create an intermediate table:

Time	R_t	T_t	$\lvert R_t\text{-}T_t \rvert$	$(R_t\text{-}T_t)^2$
15	56.48	73.05	16.57	274.56
30	76.32	79.92	3.60	12.96
45	82.85	84.32	1.47	2.16
60	87.87	89.42	1.55	2.40
$\Sigma=$	303.52	326.71	23.19	292.08

Using these numbers produces the following results:

$$f_1 = \frac{\sum \lvert R_t - T_t \rvert}{\sum R_t} \times 100 = \frac{23.19}{303.52} \times 100 = 7.64$$

$$f_2 = 50 \cdot \log \left[\frac{1}{\sqrt{1 + \dfrac{1}{n}\Sigma(R_t - T_t)^2}} \times 100 \right]$$

$$f_2 = 50 \cdot \log \left[\frac{1}{\sqrt{1 + \dfrac{1}{4}(292.08)}} \times 100 \right]$$

$$f_2 = 50 \cdot \log\,(11.62) = 50(1.06) = 53.3$$

In this example, f_1 is less than 15 and f_2 is greater than 50; therefore, we would conclude that the two dissolution profiles are not significantly different.

Although the tests presented in this chapter have focused strictly on bioequivalence, they provide us means for showing equivalence between levels of any discrete independent variables.

References

Federal Register (1977). 42: 1648.

Federal Register (1978). 43: 6965-6969.

Federal Register (1995). 60: 61638-61643.

FDA (1997). "Guidance for industry: dissolution testing of immediate release solid oral dosage forms" (BP1), Center for Drug Evaluation and Research, Food and Drug Administration, Rockville, MD, p. 9.

United States Pharmacopeia (1989). 22nd revision, United States Pharmacopeial Convention, Washington, DC, pp. 113-114.

Benet, L.Z. and Goyan, J.E. (1995). "Bioequivalence and narrow therapeutic index drugs" Pharmacotherapy 15:433-440.

DiSanto, A.R. (1990). "Bioavailability and Bioequivalency Testing" Chapter 76 in Remington's Pharmaceutical Sciences, 18th edition, Mack Publishing Company, pp. 1451-58.

Chow, S.C. and Liu, J.P. (1992). Design and Analysis of Bioavailability and Bioequivalence Studies, Marcel Dekker, Inc., New York.

Evans, W.E., Schentag, J.J. and Jusko, W.J. (eds), (1992). Applied Pharmacokinetics : Principles of Therapeutic Drug Monitoring, 3rd edition, Applied Therapeutics, Vancouver, WA.

Hauck, W.W. and Anderson, S. (1984). "A New Statistical Procedure for Testing Equivalence in Two-Group Comparative Bioavailability Trials" Journal of Pharmacokinetics and Biopharmaceutics 12:83-91.

Kirk, R.E. (1968). Experimental Design: Procedures for the Behavioral Sciences, Brooks/Cole Publishing, Belmont, CA, pp. 424-440.

Metzler, C.M. (1974). "Bioavailability: A problem in equivalence" Biometrics 30:309-317.

Schuirmann, D.J. (1987). "Comparison of the two one-sided tests procedure and the power approach for assessing the equivalence of average bioavailability" Journal of Pharmacokinetics and Biopharmaceutics 15:660.

Shah, V.P., et al. (1998) "In Vitro dissolution profile comparison – statistics and analysis of the similarity factor, f_2" Pharmaceutical Research 15:891-898.

Westlake, W.J. (1988). "Bioavailability and bioequivalence of pharmaceutical formulations" in Biopharmaceutical Statistics for Drug Development. Peace KE, ed. Marcel Dekker, New York, p.342.

Welling, P.G. and Tse, F.L.S. (1995). Pharmacokinetics, 2nd edition, Marcel Dekker, Inc., New York.

Winter, M.E. (1994). Basic clinical pharmacokinetics, 3rd edition, Mary Anne Koda-Kimble, M.A. and Lloyd Y. Young, L.Y. (eds), Applied Therapeutics, Vancouver, WA.

Zar, J.H. (1984). Biostatistical Analysis, 2nd ed., Prentice Hall, Englewood Cliffs, NJ, pp.134-136.

Supplemental suggested readings:

Hauck, W.W. and Anderson, S. (1984). "A New Statistical Procedure for Testing Equivalence in Two-Group Comparative Bioavailability Trials" Journal of Pharmacokinetics and Biopharmaceutics 12:83-91.

Rodda, B.E. (1990). "Bioavailability: design and analysis" in Statistical Methodology in the Pharmaceutical Sciences. Berry, D.A., ed., Marcel Dekker, New York, pp. 57-82.

Schuirmann, D.J. (1987). "Comparison of the two one-sided tests procedure and the power approach for assessing the equivalence of average bioavailability" Journal of Pharmacokinetics and Biopharmaceutics 15:657-680.

Schuirmann, D.J. (1990). "Design of bioavailability/bioequivalence studies" Drug Information Journal 15:315-323.

Shah, V.P., et al. (1998) "*In Vitro* dissolution profile comparison – statistics and analysis of the similarity factor, f_2" Pharmeutical Research 15:891-898.

Westlake, W.J. (1988). "Bioavailability and bioequivalence of pharmaceutical formulations" in Biopharmaceutical Statistics for Drug Development. Peace, K.E., ed. Marcel Dekker, New York, p.329-352.

Example Problems

1. In a clinical trial, data comparing Gigantic Drugs new generic product was
    compared with the Innovator's branded antipsychotic; both products
    contain the exact same chemical entity. One subject did not complete the
    study. The results were as follows:

	Innovator	Generic
Mean =	289.7	271.6
Standard Deviation =	18.1	20.4
n =	24	23

    Use the confidence interval approach and the two one-tailed t-tests to check for
    bioequivalence, assuming there should be less than a 10% difference between
    the two products.

2. Production of a certain product in two different countries (A and B) were
    compared to the manufacturer's original production site (standard).
    Dissolution data is presented in Table 18.5 and Figure 18.5. Visually it
    appears that site B has a profile closer to the reference standard, but do
    both of the foreign facilities meet the SUPAC-IR guidelines for similarity?

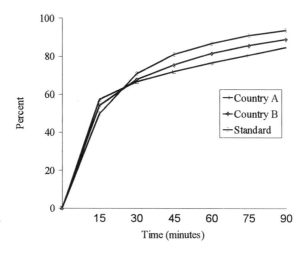

Figure 18.5 Dissolution profiles for two foreign countries.

Table 18.5 Dissolution Data (percent)

Time (minutes)	Country A	Country B	Standard
15	57.3	54.1	49.8
30	66.4	67.7	70.8
45	71.9	75.4	80.9
60	76.4	81.4	86.7
75	80.4	85.6	90.9
90	84.6	88.8	93.6

3. Tablets were randomly selected from a particular production batch, comminuted, mixed and the resultant powder divided into two equal quantities. Each of these two sample were sent to two laboratories for analysis. Each laboratory performed 30 assays on the mixtures.

Sample	Laboratory A	Laboratory B
Mean	98.84%	97.05%
S^2	15.71	12.44
S	3.96%	3.53%
n	30	30

Using the tests discussed for bioequivalence, do the following results show that there is a less than 5% difference in the outcomes for the assays at the two laboratories?

a. Based on a two sample t-test, was there a significant difference between the two laboratories? Was there a large enough sample to detect a 5% difference with 80% power?

b. Use the confidence interval approach and the two one-tailed t-tests method to check for bioequivalence, assuming there should be less than a 5% difference between the laboratories.

4. Presented in the lower half of Figure 18.3 are two dissolution profiles comparing the products produced by Manufacturer A and B. Using the data for those profiles presented below and the SUPAC-IR f_1 and f_2 formulas, is there a significant difference between these two products?

Time (minutes):	10	20	30	40
Manufacturer A	57.4	70.1	77.5	84.2
Manufacturer B	43.5	73.0	84.3	90.1

Answer to Problems

1. Clinical trial data comparing a new generic product to an Innovator's branded drug. Is there less than a 10% difference between the products?

	Innovator	Generic
Mean =	289.7	271.6
Standard Deviation =	18.1	20.4
n =	24	23

10% difference = 28.97 (δ=289.7 x 0.10)

Difference observed = 18.1 (289.7-271.6)

Pooled variance:

$$S_p^2 = \frac{(n_1 - 1) S_1^2 + (n_2 - 1) S_2^2}{n_1 + n_2 - 2} = \frac{23(18.1)^2 + 22(20.4)^2}{24 + 23 - 2} = 370.9$$

Standard error portion of the equations:

$$\sqrt{\frac{S_P^2}{n_1} + \frac{S_P^2}{n_2}} = \sqrt{\frac{370.9}{24} + \frac{370.9}{23}} = 5.62$$

a. Confidence interval

$$Lower\ Limit = \frac{(d - SE) + \overline{X}_R}{\overline{X}_R} \times 100\%$$

$$Lower\ Limit = \frac{(18.1 - 5.62) + 289.7}{289.7} \times 100\% = 104.3\%$$

$$Upper\ Limit = \frac{(d + SE) + \overline{X}_R}{\overline{X}_R} \times 100\%$$

$$Lower\ Limit = \frac{(18.1 + 5.62) + 289.7}{289.7} \times 100\% = 108.2\%$$

The limits of our estimated interval are:

$$Lower\ Limit < \frac{\mu_T}{\mu_R} < Upper\ Limit$$

$$104.3\% < \frac{\mu_T}{\mu_R} < 108.2\%$$

Therefore, we are 95% confident that we have equivalence because the difference is well within our criteria of $\pm 10\%$ and the true population ratio is somewhere between 104.3 and 108.2%.

b. Two one-tailed t-tests

Hypotheses: H_{01}: $\mu_T - \mu_R \leq 10\%$
H_{11}: $\mu_T - \mu_R > 10\%$

H_{02}: $\mu_T - \mu_R \geq 10\%$
H_{12}: $\mu_T - \mu_R < 10\%$

Decision rule: With $\alpha = 0.05$, reject H_{01} or H_{02} if $|t| > t_{45}(.95) \approx 1.679$

$$t_1 = \frac{(\overline{X}_T - \overline{X}_R) - \delta_1}{\sqrt{\frac{2S_p^2}{n}}} = \frac{18.1 - (-28.97)}{5.62} = 8.38$$

$$t_2 = \frac{\delta_2 - (\overline{X}_T - \overline{X}_R)}{\sqrt{\frac{2S_p^2}{n}}} = \frac{28.97 - 18.1}{5.62} = 1.93$$

Decision: Reject H_{01} and H_{02}, and conclude that there is a difference between the two populations are less than 10%.

2. To compare Country A and the "standard" original facility, the first step is to calculate the difference term in the denominator:

$$\Sigma(R_t - T_t)^2 = (49.8 - 57.3)^2 \dots + (93.6 - 84.6) = 453.95$$

The calculation of the remainder of the f_2 formula is as follows:

$$f_2 = 50 \cdot \log \left[\frac{1}{\sqrt{1 + \dfrac{1}{n} \Sigma(R_t - T_t)^2}} \; x \; 100 \right]$$

$$f_2 = 50 \cdot \log \left[\frac{1}{\sqrt{1 + \dfrac{1}{6}(453.95)}} \; x \; 100 \right]$$

$$f_2 = 50 \cdot \log (11.421) = 50 \cdot (1.058) = 52.9$$

Decision: With $f_2 > 50$ conclude that the two dissolution profiles are the same and that there is no significant difference between the product produced in Country A and the manufacturer's original production site.

To compare Country B and the "standard" original facility, the same process is used:

$$\Sigma(R_t - T_t)^2 = (49.8 - 54.1)^2 \dots + (93.6 - 88.8) = 137.56$$

$$f_2 = 50 \cdot \log \left[\frac{1}{\sqrt{1 + \dfrac{1}{6}(137.56)}} \; x \; 100 \right]$$

$$f_2 = 50 \cdot \log (20.444) = 50 \cdot (1.311) = 65.55$$

Decision: With $f_2 > 50$ conclude that the two dissolution profiles are the same and that there is no significant difference between the product produced in Country A and the manufacturer's original production site.

Note that Country B produced a higher f_2 and that confirms the visual assessment that the dissolution profile for Country B was closer to that of the original product.

3. Evaluation of tablet samples assayed by two separate laboratories to determine if there is a less than 5% difference in the outcomes for the assays.

Assay results based on percent label claim:

Sample	Laboratory A	Laboratory B
Mean	98.84%	97.05%
S^2	15.71	12.44
S	3.96%	3.53%
n	30	30
S_p^2		14.08

a. Two-sample t-test

Hypotheses: H_0: $\mu_A = \mu_B$
                H_1: $\mu_A \neq \mu_B$

Decision rule: With $\alpha = 0.05$. reject H_0 if $|t| > t_{58}(.975) \approx 2.002$.

$$t = \frac{\overline{X_1} - \overline{X_2}}{\sqrt{\dfrac{S_P^2}{n_1} + \dfrac{S_P^2}{n_2}}} = \frac{98.84 - 97.05}{\sqrt{\dfrac{14.08}{30} + \dfrac{14.08}{30}}} = \frac{1.79}{.969} = 1.85$$

Decision: Because t < 2.002, fail to reject H_0, and cannot prove a significant difference between Laboratory A and Laboratory B with 95% confidence.

Note that we have defined two terms to be used later, the standard error = 0.969 and the sample difference = -1.79, if Laboratory A is considered the reference standard.

Power determination: we will arbitrarily set our reference value as Laboratory A (98.84%) and the 5% difference is then 4.94 (δ = 98.84 x 0.05).

$$t_\beta \geq \frac{\delta}{\sqrt{\dfrac{2 S_p^2}{n}}} - t_{\alpha/2}$$

$$t_\beta \geq \frac{4.94}{\sqrt{\dfrac{2(14.08)}{30}}} - 1.96 = \frac{4.94}{0.969} - 2.002 = 3.10$$

With df=58, p(β) is less than 0.01; therefore, the power is greater than 0.99 (1-0.01). How many subjects would we have needed to have a power of greater than 80% to detect a 5% difference?

$$n \geq \frac{2S_p^2}{\delta^2}(t_\beta + t_{\alpha/2})^2$$

$$n \geq \frac{2(14.08)^2}{(4.94)^2}(0.085 + 2.002)^2 = 5.0$$

As few as 5 observations from Laboratory A and 5 from Laboratory B would have been sufficient to have 80% power to detect a 5% difference between the two laboratories.

b.   Confidence interval – where the standard error is 0.969 (the denominator in the power determination) and the observed difference (θ) is -1.79.

$$Lower\ Limit = \frac{(d - SE) + \overline{X}_R}{\overline{X}_R} \ x\ 100\%$$

$$Lower\ Limit = \frac{(-1.79 - 0.969) + 98.84}{98.84} \ x\ 100\% = 97.2\%$$

$$Upper\ Limit = \frac{(d + SE) + \overline{X}_R}{\overline{X}_R} \ x\ 100\%$$

$$Upper\ Limit = \frac{(-1.79 + 0.969) + 98.84}{98.84} \ x\ 100\% = 99.2\%$$

The limits of our estimated interval are:

$$Lower\ Limit\ <\ \frac{\mu_T}{\mu_R}\ <\ Upper\ Limit$$

$$97.2\%\ <\ \frac{\mu_T}{\mu_R}\ <\ 99.2\%$$

therefore, we are 95% confident that we have equivalency be the difference is well within our criteria of $\pm 5\%$.

Two one-tailed t-tests

Hypotheses: H_{01}: $\mu_A - \mu_B \leq 5\%$
              H_{11}: $\mu_A - \mu_B > 5\%$

              H_{02}: $\mu_A - \mu_B \geq 5\%$
              H_{12}: $\mu_A - \mu_B < 5\%$

Decision rule: With $\alpha = 0.05$, reject H_{01} or H_{02} if $|t| > t_{58}(.95) \approx 1.672$.

$$t_1 = \frac{(\overline{X}_A - \overline{X}_B) - \delta_1}{\sqrt{\frac{2S_p^2}{n}}} = \frac{1.79 - (-4.94)}{.969} = 6.94$$

$$t_2 = \frac{\delta_2 - (\overline{X}_A - \overline{X}_B)}{\sqrt{\frac{2S_p^2}{n}}} = \frac{4.94 - 1.79}{.969} = 3.25$$

Decision: Both H_{01} and H_{02} are rejected because $t > 1.672$. Therefore, conclude that $95\% < \mu_A - \mu_B < 105\%$.

4. Using the data presented for Figure 18.3 and the SUPAC-IR f_1 and f_2 formulas, is there a significant difference between these two products?

Time (minutes):	10	20	30	40	Σ
Manufacturer A (R)	57.4	70.1	77.5	84.2	289.2
Manufacturer B (T)	43.5	73.0	84.3	90.1	290.9
$|R\text{-}T| =$	13.9	2.9	6.8	5.9	29.5
$(R\text{-}T)^2 =$	193.21	8.41	46.24	34.81	282.67

$$f_1 = \frac{\Sigma|R_t - T_t|}{\Sigma R_t} \, x\, 100 = \frac{29.5}{290.9} \, x100 = 10.14$$

$$f_2 = 50 \cdot log\left[\frac{1}{\sqrt{1 + \frac{1}{n}\Sigma(R_t - T_t)^2}} \, x\, 100\right]$$

$$f_2 = 50 \cdot log\left[\frac{1}{\sqrt{1 + \frac{1}{4}(282.67)}} \, x\, 100\right] = 50 \cdot log\,(11.81) = 51.5$$

f_1 is less than 15 and the f_2 is above 50; we would conclude that the two profiles by the different manufacturers are not significantly different.

19

Outlier Tests

An outlier is an extreme data point which is significantly different from the remaining values in a set of observations. However, removal of an outlier is discouraged unless the data point can be clearly demonstrated to be erroneous. Rodda (1990) provided an excellent description of outliers when he described them as "... much like weeds; they are very difficult to define and are only called outliers because they are inconsistent with the environment in which they are observed." We need to use care in our decision making process to ensure that we remove the weed and not a budding piece of data.

Outliers on a Single Continuum

With both descriptive and inferential statistics it is common to report the center and spread of the sample data. An uncharacteristic observation could be either a valid data point that falls to one of the extreme tailing ends of our continuum or due to some error in data collection. In the latter case, this would be considered an outlier. Many detectable and undetectable effects could cause such an extreme measurement, including: 1) a temporary equipment malfunction; 2) a technician or observer misreading the result; 3) errors in data entry; 4) contamination; or 5) a very large or small measurement within the extremes of the distribution. With respect to the last point, an outlier does not necessarily imply that an error has occurred with the experiment, only that an extreme value has occurred. Vigilance is important with any data manipulation and an inspection of data for recording or transcribing errors is always warranted before the statistical analysis.

Another consideration is that an outlier could in fact be a legitimate observation in a strongly skewed distribution and represent a value at the extreme end of the longer tail. Various transformations on the data or ranking of the data can be used to minimize the effect of an outlier. This was pointed out in Chapter 17, when nonparametric statistics were described as less influenced by outliers than are traditional tests whose calculations are affected by measures of dispersion (variance and standard deviation).

Extreme values can greatly influence the most common measures of central tendency; they can greatly distort the mean and inflate the variance. This is especially true with small sample sizes. In contrast, the median and quartile measures are relatively insulated from the effects of outliers. For example consider the following assay results (in percents):

97, 98, 98, 95, 88, 99

Whether or not 88% is an outlier, it has an important effect on the mean and spread (range and variance) of the sample and can be termed an **influential observation** which will be discussed later in this chapter. Table 19.1 shows the impact this one observation can have on various measures of central tendency. As seen in Table 19.1, the extreme value pulls the mean in the direction of that value, increases the standard deviation by a factor of two, and the range is increased almost threefold. However, the median (97.5) is unaffected. This would also be true even if the lowest value were 78 or 68. As mentioned, the nonparametric tests rely on the ranking of observations and in many cases the median, and are less effected by outliers. In fact, using the various statistical tests listed below, 88% would not be rejected as an outlier. It would be considered only an influential observation.

A second example of assay results is presented below. In this case the more extreme value (86%) would be defined as an outlier, with 95% confidence using methods discussed later. In this particular sample there are only six tablets:

97, 98, 98, 95, 86, 99

For illustrative purposes, assume in this second case that these results were part of a larger sample of twelve tablets.

97, 98, 98, 95, 86, 99
98, 98, 97, 99, 98, 95

Table 19.1 Impact of a Potential Outlier on Measures of Central Tendency

	88% Included	88% Not Included
Mean	95.8	97.4
Standard Deviation	4.1	1.5
Range	11	4
Median	97.5	98

Without the outlier, both the first case and second case have approximately the same mean and standard deviation. Notice in Table 19.2, that the greater sample size "softens" the effect of the outlier. In the second case, 86% would not be identified as an outlier using the tests described in this chapter. If possible, additional measurements should be made when a suspect outlier occurs, particularly if the sample size is very small.

To test for outliers we need at least three observations. Naturally the more information we have (the larger the sample size), the more obvious an outlier will become, either visually or statistically. For a sample size as small as three observations there would need to be a wide discrepancy for one data point to be deemed an outlier. If an outlier is identified, it's important to try and identify the cause (i.e., miscalculation, data entry error, contamination). The identification of an outlier can lead to future corrective action in the process or research being conducted, but it can also serve as a potential source of new information about the population.

A simple technique to "soften" the influence of possible outliers is called **winsorizing** (Dixon and Masey, 1969). Using this process the two most extreme values, the largest value and the smallest value are changed to the value of their next closest neighbor $(x_1 \to x_2; x_n \to x_{n-1})$. For example, consider the following rank ordered set of observations, where 11 might be an outlier.

$$11,21,24,25,26,26,27,28,29,31$$

Table 19.2 Impact of a Potential Outlier on Measures of Central Tendency with Two Sample Sizes

	Case 1		
	86% Not Included	86% Included	Case 2
n	5	6	12
Mean	97.4	95.5	96.5
S.D.	1.5	4.8	3.5
Range	4	11	11
Median	98	97.5	98

Our suspected outlier would be replaced with the second lowest number. Also we would replace the largest value with the second largest:

$$\underline{21},21,24,25,26,26,27,28,29,\underline{29}$$

For the first set of data the mean and standard deviation are $\overline{24.8} \pm \overline{5.6}$ and for the winsorized data $\overline{25.6} \pm \overline{2.9}$. For this set of data the potential outlier has little impact (+3% change) on our sample mean. Although not a statistical test for outliers, winsorizing might provide a quick measure of the impact of extreme values on the measures of central tendency for our sample.

Plotting and Number of Standard Deviations from the Center

By using various plotting methods to display the data, outliers may become readily visible. For example, box-and-whisker plots are specifically designed to identify possible outliers (Figure 19.1). As discussed in Chapter 4, each of the "whiskers" or t-bars extending from the box equals three semi-interquartile ranges (SIQR) above and below the median. The SIQR being the distance between the upper or lower quartile and the median. Observations that fall above or below the whiskers can be identified as potential outliers. Potential outliers can also be observed using other graphic techniques including stem-and-leaf plots, histograms, line charts or point plots. In addition, scatter plots can be useful in identifying potential outliers involving two or more continuous variables.

An example of the box-whisker plots will be presented later when discussing residuals under the bivariate outliers section.

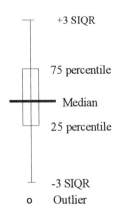

Figure 19.1 Box-and-whisker plot.

The "Huge" Rule

One method for detecting an outlier is to compare the means and standard deviations of the sample with and without the potential outlier. A general rule of thumb is to exclude a data point as an outlier if it is more than four standard deviations from the mean (Marascuilo, 1971). The rationale for this rule is that it is extremely unlikely ($p<0.00005$) to find values more than four standard deviations from the expected center of a distribution. The distance, in standard deviations, is measured between the mean and the potential outliers:

$$M = \frac{|x_i - \overline{X}|}{S} \qquad \text{Eq. 19.1}$$

where $\overline{X}$ and S are calculated from the sample data, ignoring the outlier value (x_i). If M > 4 then the data point is considered to be an outlier. To illustrate this rule of thumb test, consider the following observations:

99.3, 99.7, 98.6, 99.0, 99.1, 99.3, 99.5, 98.0,
98.9, 99.4, 99.0, 99.4, 99.2, 98.8, 99.2

Is the data point 98.0 an outlier considering this set of 15 observations? The mean and standard deviation are calculated. For the rule for huge error, the mean and standard deviation without 98.0 are used, and the number of standard deviations are calculated between the center and 98.0. These sample results are $\overline{X} = 99.17$ and $S = 0.29$. The calculation of the number of standard deviations from the mean for our potential outlier is:

$$M = \frac{|x_i - \overline{X}|}{S} = \frac{|99.17 - 98.0|}{0.29} = \frac{1.17}{0.29} = 4.03$$

Since 98.0 is more than 4.00 below the mean it is disregarded as an outlier. Several methods are used to statistically determine if observations are outliers or simply extremes of the population from which the sample is selected. The most commonly used statistics to detect univariate outliers (involving one discrete independent variable) are the Grubbs' test and the Dixon Q test and these will be discussed below. Others possible test's include: 1) Youden's test for outliers (Taylor, 1987); 2) Cochran's test for extreme values of variance (Taylor, 1987); and 3) studentized deleted residuals (Mason, 1989).

Grubbs' Test for Outlying Observations

Grubbs' procedure involves ranking the observations from smallest to largest ($x_1 < x_2 < x_3 \dots x_n$) and calculating the mean and standard deviation for all of the observations in the data set (Grubbs, 1969). One of the following formulas is used, depending upon whether x_1 (the smallest value) or x_n (the largest value), is suspected of being a possible outlier.

$$T = \frac{\overline{X} - x_1}{S} \quad or \quad T = \frac{x_n - \overline{X}}{S} \qquad \text{Eq. 19.2}$$

Due to these formulas, Grubbs' test is occasionally referred to as the **T procedure** or **T method**. This resultant T is compared to a critical value on Table B13 (Appendix B), based on the sample size (n) for a given α. The error level for interpreting the result of the Grubbs test is the same as our previous discussion of hypothesis testing. Once again α will represent the researcher controlled error rate. Assuming we use the 5% level (right column in Table B13), we may incorrectly reject an outlier one time in 20. If T is greater than the critical value, the data point may be rejected as an outlier. Using the previous example, the information is first ranked in ascending order (Table 19.3). The mean and standard deviations are then calculated. In this case we will calculate these measures with the proposed outlier included. The results are: $\overline{X} = 99.09$ and $S = 0.41$. Using Grubbs' test we first identify the critical value on Table B13 to be 2.409 for n=15 and α=.05. The calculation of the Grubbs' test is

$$T = \frac{\overline{X} - x_1}{S} = \frac{99.09 - 98.0}{0.41} = \frac{1.09}{0.41} = 2.66$$

Since our calculated value of 2.66 exceeds the critical value of 2.409, once again 98.0 is rejected as an outlier.

Dixon Q Test

A second method to determine if a suspected value is an outlier is to measure the difference between it and the next closest value and compare that difference to the total range of observations (Dixon, 1953). Various ratios of this nature (absolute ratios without regard to sign) make up the Dixon test for outlying observations or the Dixon Q test. Both Grubbs' and Dixon's Q assume that the population from which the sample is taken is normally distributed. The

Table 19.3	Sample Rank Ordered Data for Outlier Tests
	Value
x_1	98.0
x_2	98.6
x_3	98.8
...	98.9
	99.0
	99.0
	99.1
	99.2
	99.2
	99.3
	99.3
...	99.4
x_{n-2}	99.4
x_{n-1}	99.5
x_n	99.7

advantage of this test is that it is not necessary to estimate the standard deviation. First the observations are rank ordered (similar to Table 19.3):

$$x_1 < x_2 < x_3 < ... \ x_{n-2} < x_{n-1} < x_n$$

Formulas for the Dixon Q use ratios of ranges and subranges within the data. The ratios are used below, which depending on the sample size and whether x_1 (the smallest value) or x_n (the largest value) is suspected to be an outlier. If the smallest observation is suspected of being an outlier the following ratios are calculated:

Sample Size	Ratio	If x_1 is suspected	
$3 \leq n \leq 7$	τ_{10}	$\dfrac{x_2 - x_1}{x_n - x_1}$	Eq. 19.3
$8 \leq n \leq 10$	τ_{11}	$\dfrac{x_2 - x_1}{x_{n-1} - x_1}$	Eq. 19.4
$11 \leq n \leq 13$	τ_{21}	$\dfrac{x_3 - x_1}{x_{n-1} - x_1}$	Eq. 19.5

$$14 \leq n \leq 25 \qquad \tau_{22} \qquad \frac{x_3 - x_1}{x_{n-2} - x_1} \qquad \text{Eq. 19.6}$$

However, if the largest value is evaluated as the outlier a different, but parallel, set of ratios is used:

Sample Size	Ratio	If x_n is suspected	
$3 \leq n \leq 7$	τ_{10}	$\dfrac{x_n - x_{n-1}}{x_n - x_1}$	Eq. 19.7
$8 \leq n \leq 10$	τ_{11}	$\dfrac{x_n - x_{n-1}}{x_n - x_2}$	Eq. 19.8
$11 \leq n \leq 13$	τ_{21}	$\dfrac{x_n - x_{n-2}}{x_n - x_2}$	Eq. 19.9
$14 \leq n \leq 25$	τ_{22}	$\dfrac{x_n - x_{n-2}}{x_n - x_3}$	Eq. 19.10

The resultant ratio is compared to the critical values on Table B14 (Appendix B). If the calculated ratio is greater than the value in the table, the data point may be rejected as an outlier. Using the Dixon test for the data presented in Table 19.1, the critical value from Table B14 is $\tau = 0.525$, based on n=15 and $\alpha=.05$. The calculated Dixon ratio would be:

$$\frac{(x_3 - x_1)}{(x_{n-2} - x_1)} = \frac{98.8 - 98.0}{99.4 - 98.0} = \frac{0.8}{1.4} = 0.57$$

Because this calculated value of 0.57 exceeds the critical value of 0.525, we reject 98.0 as an outlier.

The Grubbs' and Dixon tests may not always agree regarding the rejection of the possible outlier, especially when the test statistic results are very close to the allowable error (i.e., 5% level). The simplicity of Dixon's test is of most benefit when small samples are involved and only one observation is suspected as an outlier. Grubbs' test requires more calculations (i.e., determining the sample mean and standard deviation), but is considered to be the more powerful of the two tests. Also, Grubbs' test can be used when there is more than one suspected outlier (Mason, p.512). As with any statistical test which measures the same type of outcomes, the researcher should select the outlier test he or she is most comfortable with before looking at the data.

As mentioned previously, both Grubbs' and Dixon's tests assume that the population from which the sample was taken is normal distributed. In the case of the Dixon's test with more than one outlier, the most extreme measurement will tend to be **masked** by the presence of other possible outliers. Masking occurs when two or more outliers have similar values. In a data set, if the two smallest (or largest) values are almost equal, an outlier test for the more extreme of the two values will not be statistically significant. This is especially true of sample sizes less than ten, where the numerator of the ratio is the difference between the two most extreme values. Only a test for both of these two smallest observations will be statistically significant. Plotting the data can sometimes avoid the masking problem.

Bivariate Outliers in Correlation and Regression Analysis

In the case of correlation and regression, where each data point represents values on different **axes**, an outlier is a point clearly outside the range of the other data points on the respective axis. Outliers may greatly effect the results of correlation and regression models. At the same time, many statistical tests for identifying multivariate outliers are prone to problems of masking, swamping or both; and no single method is adequate for all given situations. For our discussion we will focus only on the simplest situations where we are comparing only two continuous variables. Obviously problems will compound themselves as we add additional variables into our analyses.

In linear regression-type models, outliers generally do not occur in the independent variable, because the levels for this variable are selected by the researcher and can usually be controlled. Potential problems then exist only with the dependent or response variable. In contrast with a correlation model, where both variables can vary greatly, outliers may occur in either variable. The variables are sometime referred to as the **predictor variable** and the **response variable** depending on the focus of our investigation. For example, as the dose of a medication changes (predictor variable), what type of response do we see in the physiological response in laboratory animals (response variable)?

Let's first looking at the regression model where we can control the independent variable and are interested in possible outliers in the dependent (response) variable. Outlier detecting techniques are based on an evaluation of the residuals. The **residual** is the difference between the observed outcome (y_i) and the predicted outcome (y_c) based on the least square line that best fits the data ($r = y_i - y_c$). In Chapter 13, when evaluating if a linear relationship existed between our independent and dependent variable, we used residuals to explain the error with respect to the deviations about the regression line:

$$\Sigma(y_i - \overline{y})^2 = \Sigma(y_c - \overline{y})^2 + \Sigma(y_i - y_c)^2$$

$$SS_{total} = SS_{explained} + SS_{unexplained}$$

An outlier in linear regression is a data point that lies a great distance from the regression line. It can be defined as an observation with an extremely large residual.

To illustrate a potential outlier, consider the following example, where during one step in the synthesis of a biological product there is a brief fermentation period. The length (in hours) is evaluated to determine if changes in time period will influence the yield in units produced. The results of the experiment is presented in Table 19.4. If we perform a regression analysis (Table 19.5), as described in Chapter 13, we would reject the null hypothesis and conclude that there is a straight line relationship between our two variables. Therefore, we can draw a straight line through our data and graphically present it (Figure 19.2). Is the data point at the 4.5% concentration an outlier or simply an extreme measurement?

Table 19.4 Data and Residuals Presented in Figure 19.2

x	y_i	y_c	r
2.0	87.1	89.980	-2.840
2.5	95.2	93.165	+2.035
3.0	98.3	96.350	+1.950
3.5	96.7	99.535	-2.835
4.0	100.4	102.720	-2.320
4.5	112.9	105.905	+6.985
5.0	110.7	109.090	+1.610
5.5	108.5	112.275	-3.735
6.0	114.7	115.460	-0.760
			$\Sigma = 0.000$

Table 19.5 Regression Analysis for Figure 19.2

Source	SS	df	MS	F
Linear Regression	608.65	1	608.65	43.79
Residual	97.29	7	13.90	
Total	705.94	8		

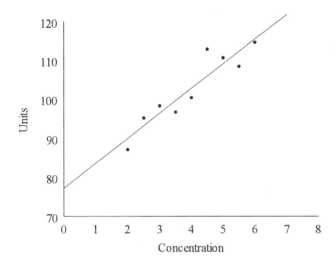

Figure 19.2 Data and best-fit line for yield vs. various concentrations.

Graphing techniques involving residuals can be useful in identifying potential outliers in one variable. For example if the box-and-whisker plot method were applied (Figure 19.3) to the residuals in Table 19.2 we would see that the residual of +6.985 seems to be an outlier. Note that the second largest residual −3.735 does not fall outside the lower whisker and would not be considered an outlier using the visual method.

A second method would be to create a scatter plot of the residuals against their corresponding outcomes (dependent variable), where the independent variable is on the x-axis and the residuals plotted on the y-axis. The residuals seen in Table 19.4 are used and plotted in Figure 19.3. Once again the residual +6.985 visually appears to be an outlier. Similar to univariate outliers, the plotting of residuals can help with subjective decisions about the possibility that a data point is an outlier.

Residual plots, like the one seen in Figure 19.4 should be a random scattering of points and there should be no systematic pattern. There should be approximately as many positive points as negative ones. Note in Table 19.4 that the sum of the residuals equals zero. Outliers are identified as points far above or below the center line. Instead of plotting the residuals (Figure 19.5), we can plot the **studentized residuals** which are calculated:

$$t = \frac{y_i - y_c}{\sqrt{MS_E}}$$

Eq. 19.11

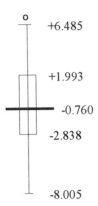

Figure 19.3 Box-and-whisker plot of residuals.

where MS_E is the $MS_{residual}$ taken off the ANOVA table used to test for linearity. These studentized values are scaled by the estimate of the standard error so their values follow a student t-distribution (Tables B3 and B4 in Appendix B). Use of the studentized residuals make systematic trends and potential outliers more obvious. Figure 19.5 shows the studentized residual plot of the same data seen in Figure 19.4. Note that the studentized value at 4.5% concentration does not exceed the critical t-value of $t_8(.975) = 2.306$; therefore, we cannot statistically reject this value as an outlier.

There are more objective statistical procedures available to evaluate such extreme points based on the residuals. A process know as **studentized deleted**

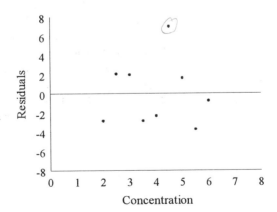

Figure 19.4 Scatter diagram showing residuals.

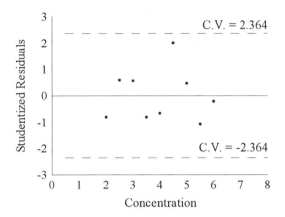

Figure 19.5 Scatter diagram studentized residuals.

residuals is a popular method for identifying outliers when there are multiple continuous variables. It involves deleting the outling observation and refitting the regression model with the remaining n-1 observations. By filling the model, it's possible to predict if the observation that was deleted from the data set was an outlier if the deleted residual was large. It requires calculations involving the standard error estimated for each deleted residual and are best handled through computer manipulation of the data. A detailed explanation of the studentized deleted residual method is found in Mason (1989, pp. 518-521).

For correlation problems, an outlier (represented by a pair of observations that are clearly out of the range of the other pairs) can have a marked effect on the correlation coefficient and often misleading results. Such a paired data point may be extremely large or small compared to the bulk of the other sample data. This does not mean that there should not be a data point that is greatly different from the other data points on one axis as long as there is a equal difference on the second axis, which is consistent with the remainder of the data. For example, look at the two dispersions in Figure 19.6. It appears that the single lone data point (A) on the left scatted diagram is consistent with the remainder of the distribution (as x increases, y also appears to increase). In contrast, point (B) is going in the opposite direction from the other sample points.

The problem occurs when one data point distorts the correlation coefficient or significantly changes the line of best-fit through the data points. The best check for a potential outlier is to remove the single observation and recalculate the correlation coefficient and determine its influence on the outcome of the sample. For

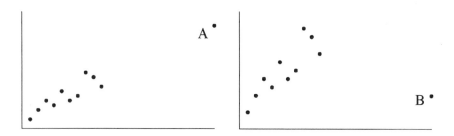

Figure 19.6 Examples of two correlation distributions.

example consider the data in Figure 19.7, where the data point at the extreme left side might be an outlier. Without the one point there is virtually no correlation (r=.07) and a best-fit line drawn between these points has slight positive slope (b=+0.426). However, if this point is added into our calculations, there is a "low" negative correlation (r=-.34) and our best-fit line changes to a negative slope (b= -0.686). One method for deciding to classify a data point as an outlier might be to collect more data to determine if the number is a true outlier or just an extreme value of a trend that was not noted in the original data.

Two additional problems may be seen with bivariate outliers. **Swamping** refers to several good data points that may be close to the suspected outlier and mask its effect. Using graphing techniques, it is possible to identify a cluster of data points and these might influence tests for outliers. **Influential observations** are data points

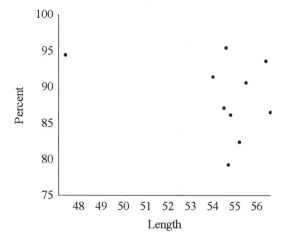

Figure 19.7 Possible outlier with a correlation example.

that have a pronounced influence on the position of the regression line. If removed, the remaining data can be refitted and the position of the regression line may shift by a significant amount. An outlier and an influential observation are not necessarily the same. Studentized deleted residuals may be helpful in identifying influential observations.

References

Dixon, W.J. (1953). "Processing data for outliers" Biometrics 1:74-89.

Dixon, W.J. and Massey, F.J. (1969). Introduction to Statistical Analysis, McGraw-Hill, New York, pp. 330-332.

Grubbs, F.E. (1969). "Procedures for detecting outlying observations in samples" Technometrics 11:1-21.

Marascuilo, L.A. (1971). Statistical Methods for Behavioral Science Research, McGraw Hill, New York, 1971, p. 199.

Mason RL, Gunst RF, Hess JL. (1989). Statistical Design and Analysis of Experiments, John Wiley and Sons, New York, pp. 518,526.

Rodda, B.E. (1990). "Bioavailability: design and analysis" in Statistical Methodology in the Pharmaceutical Sciences. Berry, D.A., ed., Marcel Dekker, New York, p. 78.

Taylor, J.K. (1987). Quality Assurance of Chemical Measures, Lewis Publishers, Chelsea, MI, p. 37-38.

Suggested Supplemental Readings

Bolton, S. (1997). Pharmaceutical Statistics: Practical and Clinical Applications, Marcel Dekker, Inc., New York, pp. 355-382, 675-684.

Mason RL, Gunst RF, Hess JL. (1989). Statistical Design and Analysis of Experiments, John Wiley and Sons, New York, pp. 510-527.

Example Problems

1. Is the data point 12.9 and outlier from the following set of observations?

$$12.3, 12.0, 12.9, 12.5, 12.4$$

2. The analytical laboratory at Acme Chemical assayed a solution that was assumed to be homogenous, but found the following assay results (in percent). Is 94.673 a possible outlier?

> 89.470, 94.673, 89.578, 89.096, 88.975, 89.204
> 85.765, 93.593, 89.954, 90.738, 90.122, 89.711

3. An experiment was designed to evaluate different theoretical concentrations of a particular agent. Based on HPLC analysis, the following recoveries were observed. Is the observation at 50% a possible outlier?

Theoretical %	% Recovered	Theoretical %	% Recovered
30	30.4	80	81.6
40	39.7	90	89.3
50	42.0	100	100.1
60	59.1	110	109.7
70	70.8	120	119.4

Answers to Problems

1. Outlier tests to evaluate 12.9:

   a. Rank order of data: 12.0, 12.3, 12.4, 12.5, 12.9

   b. Mean and standard deviation:

Without 12.9:	$\overline{X} = 12.3$	S = 0.22
With 12.9 included:	$\overline{X} = 12.42$	S = 0.33

   c. Rule for huge error

   $$M = \frac{|x_i - \overline{X}|}{S} = \frac{|12.3 - 12.9|}{0.22} = \frac{0.6}{0.22} = 2.73$$

   Decision with 2.73 < 4.00, do not reject 12.9 as an outlier.

   d. Grubbs' test - critical value with n=5 and α=.05 is 1.672.

   $$T = \frac{X_n - \overline{X}}{S} = \frac{12.9 - 12.42}{0.33} = \frac{0.48}{0.33} = 1.45$$

Decision with 1.45 < 1.672, do not reject 12.9 as an outlier.

e. Dixon test - with n=5 and α=.05, critical τ = 0.642.

$$\frac{(x_n - x_{n-1})}{(x_n - x_1)} = \frac{12.9 - 12.5}{12.9 - 12.0} = \frac{0.4}{0.9} = 0.44$$

Decision with 0.44 < 0.642, do not reject 12.9 as an outlier.

2. Outlier tests to determine if 94.673% is an outlier.

a. Rank order of data:

85.765, 88.975, 89.096, 89.204, 89.470, 89.578
89.711, 89.954, 90.122, 91.738, 93.593, 94.673

b. Mean/standard deviation:

Without 94.673:	$\overline{X}$ = 89.74	S = 1.90
With 94.673 included:	$\overline{X}$ = 90.16	S = 2.31

c. Rule for huge error

$$M = \frac{|x_i - \overline{X}|}{S} = \frac{|89.74 - 94.673|}{1.90} = \frac{4.93}{1.90} = 2.60$$

Decision with 2.60 < 4.00, fail to reject 94.673 as an outlier.

d. Grubbs' test - critical value with n=12 and α=.05 is 2.27.

$$T = \frac{x_n - \overline{X}}{S} = \frac{94.673 - 90.16}{2.31} = \frac{4.513}{2.31} = 1.95$$

Decision with 1.95 < 2.27, fail to reject 94.673 as an outlier.

e. Dixon test - with n=12 and α=.05, critical τ = 0.546.

$$\frac{(x_n - x_{n-2})}{(x_n - x_2)} = \frac{94.673 - 91.738}{94.673 - 88.975} = \frac{2.935}{5.698} = 0.515$$

Decision with 5.15 < 0.546, fail to reject 94.673 as an outlier.

3. Evaluation of HPLC analysis to determine if 50% is a possible outlier. Listed below are the results of the typical regression analysis table and the calculated slope and y-intercept for all the data, and the data excluding the potential outlier.

Outcomes:	With the potential outlier included	With the potential outlier excluded
n =	10	9
Σx =	750	700
Σy =	742.1	700.1
Σx^2 =	64,500	62,000
Σy^2 =	63,713.21	61,949.21
Σxy =	64,072	61,972
b =	+1.02	+0.99
a =	-2.29	+0.79

As can be seen, the proposed outlier does affect the slope and intercept point, but is this effect significant and should the 50% response be considered an outlier? Figure 19.7 shows a scatter plot for the HPLC data and the line of best fit. The results of the linear regression analysis would be as follows:

Source	SS	df	MS	F
Linear Regression	8583.30	1	8583.30	1170.98
Residual	58.67	8	7.33	
Total	8641.97	9		

The values on the line of best fit can be calculated using the formula $y_c = a + bx$. These values and the residuals associated with the difference between the data (y) and y_c is presented in Table 19.4. If the residuals are ranked from the lowest to the highest we find the following:

x	y_i	r	x	y_i	r
50	42.0	-6.71	100	100.1	+0.39
120	119.4	-0.71	40	39.7	+1.19
110	109.7	-0.21	70	70.8	+1.69
90	89.3	-0.21	30	30.4	+2.09
60	59.1	+0.19	80	81.6	+2.29

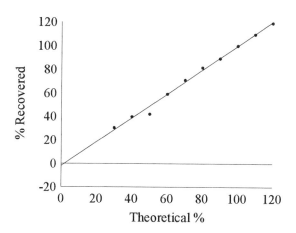

Figure 19.7 Scatter plot of HPLC outcomes.

Table 19.4 Residuals Presented in Figure 19.7

$\underline{x}$	$\underline{y_i}$	$\underline{y_c}$	$\underline{r}$
30	30.4	28.31	+2.09
40	39.7	38.51	+1.19
50	42.0	48.71	-6.71
60	59.1	58.91	+0.19
70	70.8	69.11	+1.69
80	81.6	79.31	+2.29
90	89.3	89.51	-0.21
100	100.1	99.71	+0.39
110	109.7	109.91	-0.21
120	119.4	120.11	<u>-0.71</u>
			$\Sigma = 0.000$

A box-and-whisker plot can be created with the median of +0.29 (average of fifth and sixth ranks), 25%ile of -0.21 (third rank) and 75%ile of +1.69 (eighth rank). In this case the whiskers would extend to -2.56 and +3.14. Clearly the value of -6.71 would be an outlier because it is located beyond the lower whisker. A studentized residuals plot can be created for each HPLC outcome. For example the value at 100% would be:

$$t = \frac{y_i - y_c}{\sqrt{MS_E}} = \frac{100.1 - 99.71}{\sqrt{7.33}} = 0.144$$

Each of the studentized residuals are plotted and the critical t-value is $t_{n-1}(1-\alpha/2)$ which is $t_9(.975)$ or 2.26.

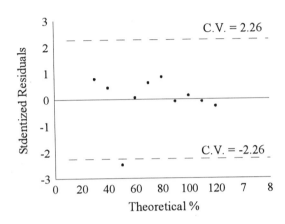

20

Statistical Errors
in the Literature

In the preface to this book, we discussed the need for a better understanding of statistics in order to avoid making research mistakes and to be better able to identify possible errors in published documents. It only seems fitting to conclude this book by reviewing the prevalence of these mathematical misadventures and identifying some of the most common types of statistical errors.

The purpose of this chapter is to point out errors in that can occur, not to criticize individual authors. It is doubtful that any of the errors described below were the result of intentional manipulation of findings or overt attempts to mislead the reader. More than likely, they are errors committed due to a misunderstanding or misinterpretation of the statistics used to evaluate the findings. Therefore, examples will be presented without reference to the specific author(s), journal article or publication referenced. However, the reader should appreciate that these are all actual errors which have occurred in refereed journals of medicine or pharmacy.

Errors and the Peer Review Process

In recent years the use of statistical analysis in published works has increased greatly, due in no small part to the ease, accessibility and power of modern desktop computers. This has also lead to an increase in the complexity of the procedures performed and reported in the literature. As noted by Altman (1991) there is an increasing trend to use statistics in the medical literature,

Table 20.1 Changes in the Use of Statistics in the Literature

	1978	1990
No statistics or descriptive only	27%	11%
t-tests	44%	39%
Chi square	27%	30%
Linear regression	8%	18%
Analysis of variance	8%	14%
Multiple regression	5%	6%
Non-parametric tests	11%	25%

From: Altman, D.G. (1991). "Statistics in medical journals: developments in the 1980s" Statistics in Medicine 10:1899.

which are usually not taught to medical students during their education and may not even be taught in postgraduate programs. He found a dramatic decrease between 1978 and 1990 in the percentage of papers which contained no statistics or only descriptive statistics (Table 20.1). The number of simple inferential statistics (i.e., t-test, chi square) remained the same and more complex statistics increased greatly during that time period. Earlier work by Felson and colleagues (1984), showed an even more dramatic increase in the use of statistics in Arthritis and Rheumatism, between the years 1967-68 and 1982 (Table 20.2)

As pointed out by Glantz (1980), few researchers have had formal training in biostatistics and "assume that when an article appears in a journal, the reviewers and editors have scrutinized every aspect of the manuscript, including the statistical methods." As he noted this assumption was usually not correct. Have things changed that much in the past 20 years? Are today's researchers any more knowledgeable of statistics, even though they now have

Table 20.2 Changes in the Use of Common Statistics

	1967-68	1982
t-tests	17%	50%
Chi square	19%	22%
Linear regression	1%	18%

From: Felson, D.T., et al. (1994). "Misuse of statistical methods in Arthritis and Rheumatism" Arthritis and Rheumatism 27:1020.

Table 20.3 Prevalence of Statistical Errors in the Literature (percent of articles with at least one statistical error)

Percent	Journal(s)	Reference
57	Canadian Medical Association Journal and Canadian Journal of Public Health - 1960	Badgley, 1961
60	Arthritis and Rheumatism -1967-68	Felson, 1984
42	British Medical Journal – 1976	Gore, 1976
44	Circulation -1977	Glantz,1980
45	British Journal of Psychiatry – 1977-78	White, 1979
66	Arthritis and Rheumatism -1982	Felson, 1984
65	British Journal of Anaesthesia -1990	Goodman and Hughes, 1992
74	American Journal of Tropical Medicine and Hygiene –1988	Cruess, 1989
54	Clinical Orthopaedics and Related Research, Spine, Journal of Pediatric Orthopaedics, Journal of Orthopaedic Research, Journal of Bone and Joint Surgery and Orthopedics – 1970-1990	Vrbos, 1993
75	Transfusion – 1992-1993	Kanter and Taylor, 1994
40	British Journal of Psychiatry – 1993	McGuigan, 1995

the power of very sophisticated software packages in their desktop computers? Most journals do not employ a statistician or involve a statistician in their review process. McGuigan (1995) noted than only a small portion of articles he reviewed (24% to 30%) employed a statistician as coauthors or acknowledge their help in papers. In fact, in the peer review process, colleagues reviewing articles submitted to journals probably have about the same statistical expertise as the authors submitting them.

Over the last several decades there have been several articles presented in the medical literature which report the incidence and types of error seen in publications (Table 20.3). In these papers statisticians review either all the articles published during a given time period (usually one year) in a specific periodical or randomly sample articles from a publication over a longer period. These errors are related to mistakes in the medical literature, because this is area where most of the research has been conducted. However, it is doubtful that the incidence of these errors is any less frequent in the pharmacy literature.

A problem to consider with the results presented in Table 20.3 was that most of these evaluations used different methods of assessing mistakes and there were no standardized criteria for defining statistical errors. Therefore, the same error may be defined differently or the researchers may have been focusing their attentions on different parameters for establishing such errors. As errors are discussed, citations will be made to the articles presented in Table 20.3 and the proportion of such errors identified by the various authors in their research of the medical literature.

Problems with Experimental Design

Many of the problems reported in the literature related to the design of the studies. Ultimately such experimental design problems will flaw statistical results. For example, many studies have inadequate or no control group as part if the design. These types of incidences were reported to be as high as 41% (McGuigan, 1995) and 58% (Glantz, 1980). Outcomes from various medical interventions are extremely difficult to evaluate without a control set of subjects to determine if the outcome would occur without the intervention.

As discussed in Chapter 3, there are two requirements for any statistical procedure, that 1) samples are selected or volunteers assigned by some random process and 2) each measurement is independent of all others (except in certain repeat measurement designs). Unfortunately McGuigan (1995) and Cruess (1989) found errors related to randomization in 43% and 12%, respectively, of the articles they evaluated. Also there was a disregard for statistical independence in 10% of the articles review by Gore and colleagues (1977) and 5% of those by Kanter and Taylor (1994).

In one research project it was found that 5% of studies fail to state a null hypotheses (McGuigan, 1995) and in a second study, questionable conclusions were drawn from the results in 47.5% of the articles evaluated (Vrbos, 1993). Excellent books exist on research design studies, especially Friedman and colleagues (1985), which are more effective in evaluating the desired outcomes.

Another problem, commonly seen in the methodology section of papers, is a failure to state and/or reference statistics used in the article. Failure to cite the specific statistics used were found in 41.5% of the articles reviewed by McGuigan (1995) and 13% of those by Kanter and Taylor (1994). In addition, studies of the medical literature found that many times conclusions were stated without any indication which statistical tests were performed (49% for Kanter and Taylor, 1994; and 35.7% for Vrbos, 1993).

Another common problem is a failure of authors to cite references for lesser known statistical procedures employed in their data analysis. Commonly used procedures (t-tests, ANOVA, correlation, linear regression and even some of the popular nonparametric tests) need not be referenced. But lesser used procedures should be referenced so readers can understand the inferential statistics involved. Nothing is more frustrating than to have a colleague or student ask about A-B-C statistical procedure; to search Medline for references to that test and find 10 to 15 articles mentioning the A-B-C test in the online abstract; to retrieve all the articles from the library; and to find that not one of the authors cite a source for the A-B-C test in the methodology sections. More than likely the A-B-C test was part of a printout involved with a sophisticated software package and referenced somewhere in that software's reference manual. Even referencing the software would help readers seeking more information about a specific test.

Standard Deviations versus Standard Error of the Mean

When reporting continuous data, it is important to describe the centers of the distribution and provide information about the dispersion of points around the center(s). Unfortunately, studies by Gore and colleagues (1977) and White (1979) reported inadequate description of basic data, including centers and dispersions in 16.1% and 12.9% of the articles they reviewed, respectively.

As discussed in Chapter 5, the standard deviation (S) measures dispersion of the sample and provides an estimate of the dispersion of the population from which the sample was taken. In contrast the standard error of the mean (SEM), or standard error (SE), is a measure of how all possible sample means might vary around the population mean. As seen in the following equation, the SEM will always be smaller that S.

$$SEM = \frac{S}{\sqrt{n}}$$

Because SEM is smaller, investigators will often report that value because it gives the perception of greater precision.

Often authors fail to state the measurement to the right of the ± symbol (7.1% from White's research, 1979; 13% for Felson, et al., 1984; and 25% for Kanter and Taylor, 1994). Is it the S or the SE, or even relative standard deviation (RSD)? If not stated the reader cannot adequately interpret the results. Even if the authors state in the methodology what is represented by the value to the right of the ± symbol, tables should still be self-explanatory, so readers can evaluate the results. For example, in an article evaluating serum lipid levels after long-term therapy with a calcium channel blocking agent, the author made the following statement: "After a mean treatment period of 5.3 years, total cholesterol and triglyceride levels were not significantly different from baseline, whereas the mean high-density lipoprotein cholesterol value increased significantly from 1.17 ± 0.41 nmol/L at the initiation of treatment to

1.39 ± 0.36 nmol/l at 5.3 years (P<0.05)." The findings were presented in a table and an abbreviated version of this table is presented in Table 20.4. Unfortunately, no where in the article did the author state whether the values to the right of the ± symbol in the table or the text represent the standard deviation or the standard error of the mean. Only after recalculating the statistics is it possible to determine that the values reflect the standard deviation. Looking solely at the HDL cholesterol data in Table 20.4, if the measure of dispersion was the standard deviation, a two-sample t-test produces a t-value of 2.705, p<0.003. In conteast, if the figure to the right of the ± symbol was the SEM, the two-sample t-test result would be t = 0.40, p>0.35. Thus, data in the original table represents the mean ± standard deviation. However, the only way to determine this is to actually recalculate the statistical outcome.

Another potential problem is using the standard deviation for non-normal data. As discussed in Chapter 6, the standard deviation reflects certain mathematical characteristics associated with normally distributed data. The median and quartiles are more appropriate measures for skewed distributions. However, McGuigan (1995) reported that 39 of the 164 papers he reviewed (24%) used the mean and standard deviation for describing skewed or ordinal data. This occurred with less frequency (19%) in the work by Kanter and Taylor (1994). An example of skewed data can be seen in a recent article comparing two drugs and their effects on the amount of eosinophile derived neurotoxin (EDN). Part of the results are presented in the upper half of Table 20.5 and the authors report that they "compared between treatment groups using t-tests." Also, "values of P < 0.05 were considered statistically significant." Note that the outcomes are reported as mean ± standard error. Converting the dispersion to standard deviations (S=SEM·√n) we find the results presented in the lower portion of Table 20.5. Note in all cases that the standard deviation is larger than the mean, indicating data which is positively

Table 20.4. Example of Failure to Identify S or SEM (n=45)

Parameter	Mean BaseLine Value	Mean Value at 4-8 years (mean, 5.3 yrs)
Total cholesterol (nmol/L)	7.17 ± 0.83	7.01 ± 0.92
HDL cholesterol (nmol/L)	1.17 ± 0.41	1.39 ± 0.36*
Triglycerides (nmol/L)	1.38 ± 0.63	1.35 ± 0.61

*Statistically significant increase (p<0.05).
HDL = high-density lipoprotein.

Table 20.5 Examples of Skewed Data Evaluated Using ANOVA

Original information cited in article (mean ± SE):

Nasal EDN (ng/ml)	Drug A (n=16)	Drug B (n=14)	Placebo (n=15)
Treatment day 1	245 ± 66	147 ± 49	275 ± 133
Treatment day 15	78 ± 34*	557 ± 200	400 ± 159

Data modified to reflect dispersion of the sample (mean ± SD)

Treatment day 1	245 ± 264	147 ± 183	275 ± 515
Treatment day 1	78 ± 136*	557 ± 748	400 ± 615

* P < 0.05 versus Drug B or placebo based on change from day 1 to day 15.

skewed. A nonparametric procedure or log transformation of the original data would have been the preferred method for analyzing the data.

Another problem with dispersions is to evaluate ordinal data by calculating a mean and standard deviation. This was identified in 25% of articles reviewed by Avram and colleagues (1985). An example of the use of parametric procedures to evaluate ordinal data is presented in a publication from the 1980s, where women who received lumpectomy or mastectomy for breast cancer were asked to rate their feelings of femininity. The authors used a simple three level ordinal scale (0 = no change, 1 = a little less feminine and 2 = moderately less feminine). Unfortunately, the authors took the responses, calculated means and standard deviations for women with lumpectomies versus those with mastectomies, and evaluated the data using a two sample t-test ("t=4.35, p<0.01" after 14 months). The more appropriate assessment would have been a chi square test of independence with frequencies of responses in each of the following cells:

	No change	A Little Less Feminine	Moderately Less Feminine
Lumpectomy			
Mastectomy			

Problems with Hypothesis Testing

We know from our previous discussions in Chapter 7, that the Type I error rate can be expressed as either α or p and provides the researcher with a certain degree of confidence $(1-\alpha)$ in their statistics. Unfortunately in Vrbos' (1993) review of the literature there was confusion over the level of significance or meaning of "p" in 46% of the articles.

A second problem, which appears less frequently, is assuming the null hypothesis is true simply because the researcher fails to reject the null hypothesis. Remember, as discussed in Chapter 7 that the null hypothesis is never proven, we only fail to reject it.

A third problem related to hypothesis testing is the failure to perform a prestudy power calculation or the failure to have an adequate sample size. This was observed in 50% of the articles reviewed by McGuigan (1995). For example, in a recent study comparing two routes of administration of a hematopoetic growth factor the authors reported the data in Table 20.6. Note the small sample size, n=4. If there was a significant difference (i.e., 20%) at the <100 U/Kg/wk dosage, how many subjects would be required to detect such a difference? The authors used an ANOVA to evaluate the results. Since there are only two levels of the independent variable, we can use the formula presented in Chapter 7 (Eq. 7.2) as a quick estimate of the number of subjects required to detect a 20% difference with 80% power. Performing the calculations found that the required number of subjects would be 188 per delivery system. This large number is due primarily to the large variance in the sample data.

The following is an example of a 1998 clinical trial protocol where the researchers have clearly attempted to control the Type II error rate. "A sample size of 28 healthy males will be enrolled in this study to ensure study completion by at least 24 patients. Based on (*a previous study)* a sample size of 24 patients can provide at least 80% probability to show that the 90% confidence interval of the mean AUC value for the clinical lot of *Drug B* is within ±20% of the reference (commercial lot) mean AUC value."

Readers should be cautious of papers that report unnecessarily small and overly exact probabilities. For example, in a 1988 publication the authors were reporting the difference in parasitic infection rates in children in a developing country and the change in the frequencies of infections before and after their particular intervention. The change reported "for prevalence in 1984 vs. 1985, $\chi^2 = 624$, df=1, $p<10^{-11}$)." In other words, the Type I error rate was less than 0.00000000001! This paper clearly overstates the obvious. A second example, illustrating probabilities which are too exact, comes from a 1993 article presenting volunteer demographics (Table 20.7). Good luck finding a statistical

Table 20.6 Comparison of Mean Posologies at the End (Day 120) of Study

Dosage	Time	IV Group (n=4)	SC Group (n=4)	Statistical Difference
>150 U/Kg/wk	Day 120	255 ± 131	138 ± 105	P <0.01
<100 U/Kg/wk	Day 120	69 ± 45	58 ± 43	ns

Table 20.7 Volunteer Demographics

	Group A	Group B
Age (yr)	67.4 ± 5.8	61.4 ± 8.6 *

* P=0.0539

table which provides a column for p = 0.0539! Also, note that the authors failed to indicate what the values were to the right of the ± symbol. In both cases, it appears that the authors were simply reporting results directly from the computer printout, without any attempt to apply a reasonable explanation to their results. This type of presentation of statistical results should warn the reader to read the article with extreme caution to ensure that the appropriate analysis was performed.

Problems with Parametric Statistics

As discussed in Chapter 8, the two additional underlying requirements for performing a parametric statistic (t-tests, F-tests, correlation and regression) are that the data: 1) come from populations which are normally distributed and 2) that sample variances (which are reflective of the population variances) be approximately equal (homogeneity of variance).

One common error is to perform a parametric test on data that is obviously skewed. The incidence of such mistakes range from 8% (Kanter and Taylor, 1994) and 17.7% (Gore, 1977) to as large as 54% (McGuigan, 1995). Note in the data cited in Table 20.5 that the standard deviations are greater than the means which would indicate that the data is positively skewed.

One method for correcting this problem is to transform the data so the resultant distribution is approximately normal; for example, the log transformation of data from a positively skewed distribution. This is illustrated in the statistical analysis section of a paper by Cohn and colleagues (1993), where they evaluate cardiac function: "Because values were extremely skewed to the right, the Holter monitor results were transformed using the logarithmic transformation..." Another approach would be to perform one of the nonparametric procedures.

A second type of error related to parametric and nonparametric procedures, confusing paired vs. unpaired data and performing an inappropriate statistical test (i.e., an ANOVA instead of a randomized block design or a paired t-test for unpaired data). Paired data obviously has advantages in that a person serves as their own control and it provides a more rigorous test, because we are evaluating changes within individual subjects. Kanter and Taylor (1994) noted that in 15% of the articles they studied that the wrong t-test (paired/unpaired) was used and McGuigan (1995) found that in 26% of the papers he studied that the type of t-test (paired/unpaired) was not mentioned. For example, in a recent article comparing the pharmacokinetic results between two time periods are presented in Table 20.8. As indicated in the table and the methodology section of the original paper, "the statistical analysis employed analysis of variance." As seen in Table 20.8 this clearly represents paired data (each subject serves as his own control, being measured at two separate time periods). The authors obviously established a decision rule and rejected the results for any $p < 0.05$. Recalculating the statistics we find the results to be even more significant than reported in the article: $F=12.09$, $df=1,14$, $p<0.005$. Obviously a two-sample t-test would produce the identical results: $t=3.48$, $df=14$, $p < 0.005$.

Table 20.8 Comparison of Eight Subjects Following a Single Oral Dose of a Drug at 10 and 22 Hours

| Subject | C_{max} ng/ml^{-1} | |
	10.00 h	22.00h
1	59.5	18.6
2	75.2	7.5
3	33.6	18.9
4	37.6	33.9
5	27.8	20.8
6	28.4	14.9
7	76.8	29.7
8	37.5	15.0
Mean (SD)	47.1 (20.4)	19.9 (8.4)*

* $P<0.05$ compared to 10.00 h (analysis of variance)

However, a more rigorous paired t-test shows that there is even less type I error when such a design is employed: paired-t = 3.41, df = 7, p < 0.0025. Unfortunately, in this particular example the author failed to observe the requirement of homogeneity of variance in order to perform an ANOVA. Note that $S^2_{10h} = 416.16$ and $S^2_{22h} = 70.60$ are not equal or even similar. Therefore the most appropriate statistic would have been a paired t-test looking at the difference for each subject or a nonparametric Wilcoxon Matched-pairs test, the results of such a procedure would be Z = 2.52, p < 0.02.

Another common error, discussed in Chapter 10, is the use of multiple t-tests to address a significant ANOVA where H_0: $\mu_1 = \mu_2 = \mu_3 ... = \mu_k$ is false. The compounding of the error using multiple t-tests was defined as experiment-wise error rate:

$$a_{ew} = 1 - (1 - \alpha)^C$$

To correct this problem post-hoc procedures were presented in Chapter 10. The incidence of this type of error has been fairly consistent at around one out of every four articles reviewed (27% for Glantz, 1980; 24% for Altman, 1991; and 22% for Kanter and Taylor, 1994). An example of the misinterpretation of data due to experiment-wise error is illustrated in a recent article evaluating different athletic mouth guards and their effect on air flow in young adults (ages 20-36). The author's findings are presented in Table 20.9. They concluded, based on this table, "that each of the three athletic mouth guards used in this study significantly reduced air flow (P<0.05) ... Similarly, peak expiratory flow rates were significantly reduced by the different mouth guards (P<0.05)." The authors clearly state in their table that the measure of dispersion is the standard deviation. Therefore, it's a relatively easy process to re-evaluate their data using the ANOVA formula presented in Chapter 9 and the post hoc procedures in Chapter 10. This re-evaluation finds that there was in fact a significant difference with respect to the mouth guards tested and the outcome measures for only the PEF. The calculated F-value was 4.85 where the critical F-value for 95% confidence is 2.53. In fact the outcome was significant with a p < 0.005. Assume the original hypothesis of equality was tested the ($\alpha = 0.05$), Scheffe *post hoc* pair-wise comparisons with the same error rate find that there were only two significant differences: no mouth guard > mouth guard 2 and no mouth guard > mouth guard 3. Unlike the authors' findings, there was no significant difference between the PEF for mouth guard 1 and no mouth guard. How could the author's have found a significant difference for all three mouth guards? If one calculates three separate two-sample t-tests comparing each mouth guard to no mouth guard, there is still no significant difference (t=1.05).

Table 20.9 Effects Three Different Mouth Guards on Air Flow (n=17)

	FEV$_1$ (liters)	PEF (l/min)
No mouth guard	3.46 (0.70)	508.65 (70.25)
Mouth guard 1	3.17 (0.16)†	472.88 (68.44) †
Mouth guard 2	2.97 (0.19) †	432.31 (78.99) †
Mouth guard 3	3.04 (0.86) †	428.38 (65.02) †

* Values represent means (s.d.); † values are significantly different (P<0.05; ANOVA) from the values recorded with no mouth guard.

It appears that, finding a significant ANOVA, the authors simply assumed that all the mouth guards provided significantly less air flow. Without a statement in the methodology section on how significant ANOVAs were evaluated, the question must remain unanswered.

Errors with the Chi Square Test of Independence

As discussed in Chapter 15 the chi square test of independence is used to evaluate the independence or relationship (lack of independence) between two discrete variables. Overall problems with chi square analysis were identified in 15% of the articles reviewed by McGuigan (1995).

Two criteria are required in order to perform this test: 1) there cannot be any empty cells (a cell within the matrix where the frequency equals zero); and 2) the expected value for each cell must be equal to or greater than five. A common mistake in the literature is to proceed with the statistical analysis even though one or both of these criteria are violated. An excellent example of this type of error appears in an article evaluating the practice of breast self-examination (BSE) in relationship to "susceptibility" scores (risk factors) for developing breast cancer. The authors concluded the following: "Forty-one (36%) participants with high susceptibility scores practiced BSE monthly or more frequently (Table 20.10). However, chi-square analysis showed no statistically significant difference in the level of perceived susceptibility of students and the frequency of BSE, $\chi^2(10)=13.1925$, p=.2131, $\alpha=.05$." Note that 24% (5/21) of the cells are empty. If we calculated the expected values for each cell under complete independence we would determine that 67% of the cells fail to meet the criteria of expected values greater or equal to five. Clearly the use of the chi square test of independence was inappropriate for this contingency table. If we modify the data by collapsing the cells in a logical order, we can create a matrix which fulfills the criteria required (Table 20.11).

Table 20.10 Original Table Reporting Susceptibility Scores and Annual Frequency of BSE

| | Perceived Susceptibility Scores | | | |
	High (15-19)	Moderate (9-14)	Low (9)	Total
More than monthly	9	1	0	10
Monthly	31	5	0	36
6-11 times	11	3	0	14
1-15 times	19	3	0	22
less than yearly	5	1	0	6
Never	13	10	1	24
Total	88	23	1	112

Table 20.11 Data Modified from Table 20.10 to Meet Criteria for Chi Square Test of Independence

	High (15-19)	Low and Moderate (less than 15)	Total
12 or more times per year	40	6	46
1-11 times per year	30	6	36
less than yearly or never	18	11	30
Total	88	23	112

However, in doing this, we arrive at a decision exactly the opposite that of the authors ($\chi^2(2)=7.24$, $p<0.05$). With $\alpha=0.05$ there is a significant relationship between risk factors and the volunteers practice of BSE. Also, note in the original table that the frequency of the BSE variable did not represent mutually exclusive and exhaustive categories. It is assumed that this was a typographical error and the mid-range values should have been 1-5 times and 6-11 times, but it was presented in the article that the two categories overlapped.

If the sample size is too small or data fails to meet the required criteria, a Fisher's exact test should be utilized. The percent of articles with this type of error is approximately 5% (5% by Kanter and Taylor, 1994; and 6% by Felson, 1984). For example, Cruess (1989) discussed an article reporting a significant relationship between reactivity with parasite isolates based on primary or multiple attacks of malaria in subjects studied and presented the follow results:

	Reactivity		
	Positive	Negative	
Primary Attack	1	2	3
Multiple Attacks	5	0	5
	6	2	8

The authors used a chi square test and reported a significant relationship (p=0.03). However, if the more appropriate Fisher's exact test is performed (since there is one empty cell and all expected values are less than five), the result is no significant relationship exists (p = 0.107). An example of the appropriate use of Fisher's exact test is described in the methodology section of an article in <u>Gastroenterology</u>: "The responses to interferon were compared between the cirrhotic and noncirrhotic patients at various times of treatment and follow up, using χ^2 method or Fisher's exact test when appropriate" (Jouet, 1994).

Another type of problem with the chi square test of independence is the correction for continuity when there is only one degree of freedom. This type of error was identified with a frequency of occurring between 2.8% (McGuigan, 1995) and 4.8% (Gore, 1977). The following is a simple clarification in the methodology section by Parsch et al. (1997), which assists the reader in understanding the statistics involved in the manuscript: "Categorical demographic data and differences in clinical outcome were analyzed by χ^2 with Yates correction factor. ... Statistical significance was established at a p-value of less than 0.05."

Summary

The purpose of this chapter has been to identify the most frequent statistical errors seen in the literature to help you better identify these mistakes in your own readings and assist you in avoiding them as you prepare written reports or publishable manuscripts.

One should always view articles published in the literature with caution. Make sure that the drug design and statistical tests are clearly described in the methodology section of the article. Altman (1991), George (1985) and McGuigan (1995) have indicated methods for improving the peer review process. These include requiring authors to indicate who performed the statistical analysis on submissions. Journals should clearly state minimum requirements for submission, even provide a standardized format regarding the nature of the research, the research design and the statistical analyses used in preparing the manuscript. Lastly, papers should be more extensively reviewed by statisticians and possibly include a statistician among the reviewers for any papers submitted for publication. An incorrect or inappropriate statistical analysis can lead to the wrong conclusions and can eventually lead to a false creditability to naive readers (White, 1979).

Additional information on the type of statistical errors can be found in the classic publication by Huff (1954) or a more recent publication by Jaffee and Spirer (1987), which are listed in the suggested supplemental readings. For specific information on designing and evaluation of clinical trails, the reader is referred to the book by Friedman and colleagues (1985), also listed in the suggested readings.

References

Altman, D.G. (1991). "Statistics in medical journals: developments in the 1980s" Statistics in Medicine 10:1897-1913.

Avram, M.J., Shanks, C.A., Dykes, M.H., Ronai, A.K. and Stiers, W.M. (1985). "Statistical methods in anesthesia articles: an evaluation of two American journals during two six-month periods" Anesth Analg 64:607-611.

Badgley, R.F. (1961). "An assessment of research methods reported in 103 scientific articles in two Canadian medical journals" Canadian Medical Association Journal, 85, 246-250.

Cohn, J.B., Wilcox, C.S. and Goodman, L.I. (1993). "Antidepressant efficacy and cardiac safety of trimipramine in patients with mild heart disease" Clinical Therapeutics 15:114-122.

Cruess, D.F. (1989). "Review of use of statistics in the American Journal of Tropical Medicine and Hygiene for January-December 1988" American Journal of Tropical Medicine and Hygiene 41:619-626.

Felson, D.T. , Cupples, L.A. and Meenan R.F. (1984). "Misuse of statistical methods in Arthritis and Rheumatism 1882 versus 1967-68. Arthritis and Rheumatism 27:1018-1022.

Glantz, S.A. (1980). "Biostatistics: how to detect, correct and prevent errors in the medical literature" Circulation 61:1-7.

Goodman, N.W. and Hughes, A.O. (1992). "Statistical awareness of research workers in British anaesthesia" British Journal of Anaesthesia 68:321-324.

Gore, S.M., Jones, I.G. and Rytter, E.C. (1977). "Misuse of statistical methods: critical assessment of articles in BMJ from January to March 1976" British Medical Journal 1:85-87.

Jouet, P., et al. (1994). "Comparative efficacy of interferon alfa in cirrhotic and noncirrhotic patients with non-A, non-B, C hepatitis" Gastroenterology 106:686-690.

Kanter, M.H. and Taylor, J.R. (1994). "Accuracy of statistical methods in Transfusion: a review of articles from July/August 1992 through June 1993" Transfusion 34:687-701.

McGuigan, S.M. (1995). "The use of statistics in the British Journal of Psychiatry" British Journal of Psychiatry 167:683-688.

Parsch, D.J. and Paladino, J.A. (1997) "Economics of sequential ofloxacin versus switch therapy" Annals of Pharmacotherapy 1997;31:1137-1145

Vrbos, L.A., Lorenz, M.A., Peabody, E.H., et al. (1993). "Clinical methodologies and incidence of appropriate statistic testing in orthopaedic spine literature: are statistics misleading?" Spine 18:1021-1029.

White, S.J. (1979). "Statistical errors in papers in the British Journal of Psychiatry" British Journal of Psychiatry 135: 336-342.

Supplemental Suggested Readings

Friedman, L.M., Furberg, C.D. and DeMets, D.L. (1985). Fundamentals of Clinical Trials, second edition, PSG Publishing Company, Inc., Littleton, MA.

Jaffee, A.J. and Spirer, H.F. (1987). Misused Statistics: Straight Talk for Twisted Numbers, Marcel Dekker, Inc., New York.

Huff, D. (1954). How to Lie with Statistics, W.W. Norton and Company, New York.

Appendix A

Flow Charts for the Selection of Appropriate Tests

On the following page are a series of panels which give direction on selecting the most appropriate statistical test to use based on the type of variables involved in the outcomes measurement.

For any given hypothesis being tested, the researcher must first identify the independent variable(s) and dependent variable(s). This begins the process seen in Panel A. Next the researcher must consider if the data presented by the respective variables involves discrete or continuous data (D/C?). Lastly, at various points in the decision making process the researcher must determine if the sample data comes from populations that are normally distributed and, if more than one level of the discrete independent variable, does there appear to be homogeneity of variance (ND/H?).

Panel A

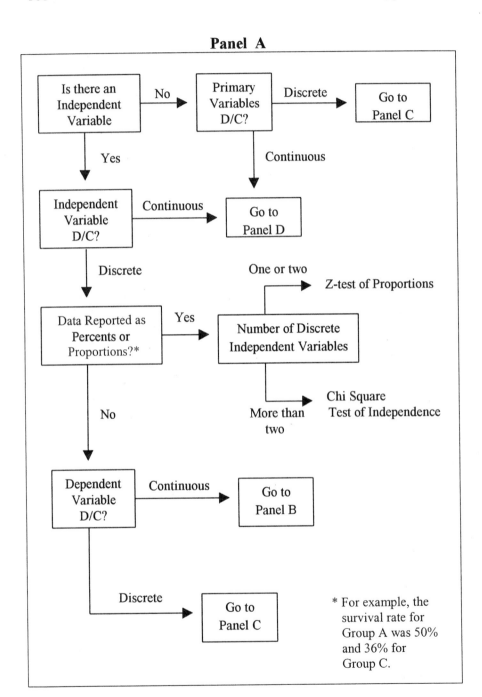

Panel B

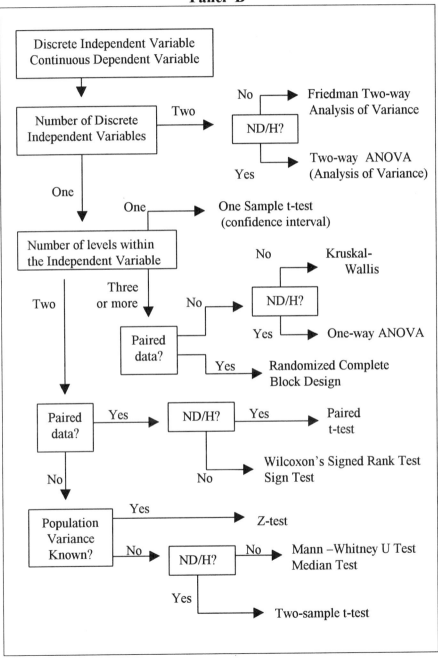

Panel C

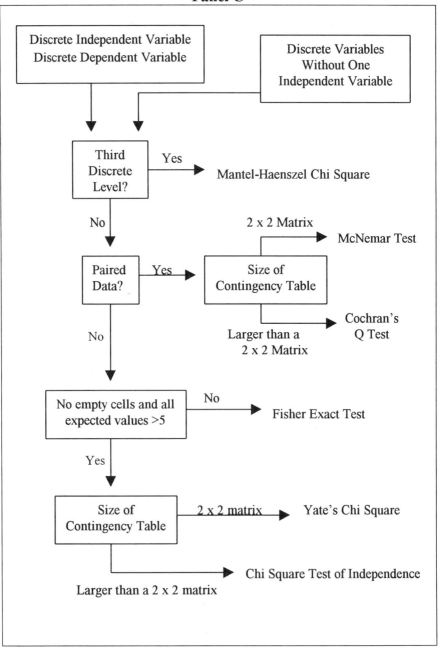

Panel D

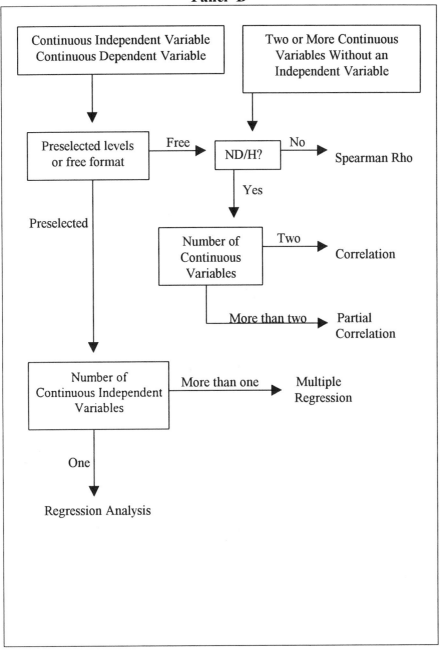

Appendix B

Statistical Tables

Table B1 Random Numbers Table

42505	29928	18850	17263	70236	35432	61247	38337	87214	68897
32654	33712	97303	74982	30341	17824	38448	96101	58318	84892
09241	92732	66397	91735	20477	88736	14252	65579	71724	41661
60481	36875	52880	38061	76675	97108	70738	13808	86470	81613
00548	99401	29620	77382	62582	90279	51053	55882	23689	42138
14935	30864	23867	91238	43732	41176	27818	99720	82276	58577
01517	25915	86821	20550	13767	19657	39114	88111	62768	42600
85448	28625	27677	13522	00733	23616	45170	78646	77552	01582
11004	06949	40228	95804	06583	10471	83884	27164	50516	89635
38507	11952	75182	03552	58010	94680	28292	65340	34292	05896
99452	62431	36306	44997	71725	01887	74115	88038	98193	80710
87961	20548	03520	81159	62323	95340	10516	91057	64979	15326
91695	49105	11072	41328	45844	15199	52172	24889	99580	65735
90335	66089	33914	13927	17168	96354	35817	55119	77894	86274
74775	37096	60407	78405	04361	55394	09344	45095	88789	73620
65141	71286	54481	68757	28095	62329	66628	01479	47433	76801
30755	11466	35367	84313	19280	37714	06161	48322	23077	63845
40192	33948	28043	88427	73014	40780	16652	20279	09418	60695
94528	98786	62495	60668	41998	39213	17701	91582	91659	03018
21917	16043	24943	93160	97513	76195	08674	74415	81408	66525
36632	18689	89137	46685	11119	75330	03907	73296	43519	66437
90668	57765	80858	07179	35167	49098	57371	51101	08015	41710
71063	60441	53750	08240	85269	01440	04898	57359	55221	64656
21036	16589	79605	10277	52852	40111	77130	38429	31212	41578
88085	84496	81220	51929	00903	39425	61281	02201	03726	95044
27162	31340	60963	14372	21057	19015	14858	26932	85648	43430
12046	49063	03168	64138	55123	29232	59462	29850	79201	18349
33052	11252	53477	65078	09199	58814	07790	36148	18962	85602
84187	61668	03267	75095	13486	05438	01962	13994	16834	60262
67887	50033	32275	68259	05930	74797	66309	66181	37093	31528
70457	55716	87554	47943	42819	98810	02729	94043	54642	37974
86336	64926	01880	41598	64455	88602	81755	74262	74591	58802
94323	92053	79740	92794	69032	62871	07447	14192	16290	11747
13869	60770	04022	91154	72841	17275	52936	76317	89963	73241
94585	85528	41527	05795	59929	25458	38851	87484	18897	61470

Table B2 Normal Standardized Distribution

(area under the curve between 0 and z)

z	.00	.01	.02	.03	.04	.05	.06	.07	.08	.09
0.0	.0000	.0040	.0080	.0120	.0160	.0199	.0239	.0279	.0319	.0359
0.1	.0398	.0438	.0478	.0517	.0557	.0596	.0636	.0675	.0714	.0753
0.2	.0793	.0832	.0871	.0910	.0948	.0987	.1026	.1064	.1103	.1141
0.3	.1179	.1217	.1255	.1293	.1331	.1368	.1406	.1443	.1480	.1517
0.4	.1554	.1591	.1628	.1664	.1700	.1736	.1772	.1808	.1844	.1879
0.5	.1915	.1950	.1985	.2019	.2054	.2088	.2123	.2157	.2190	.2224
0.6	.2257	.2291	.2324	.2357	.2389	.2422	.2454	.2486	.2517	.2549
0.7	.2580	.2611	.2642	.2673	.2704	.2734	.2764	.2794	.2823	.2852
0.8	.2881	.2910	.2939	.2967	.2995	.3023	.3051	.3078	.3106	.3133
0.9	.3159	.3186	.3212	.3238	.3264	.3289	.3315	.3340	.3365	.3389
1.0	.3413	.3438	.3461	.3485	.3508	.3531	.3554	.3577	.3599	.3621
1.1	.3643	.3665	.3686	.3708	.3729	.3749	.3770	.3790	.3810	.3830
1.2	.3849	.3869	.3888	.3907	.3925	.3944	.3962	.3980	.3997	.4015
1.3	.4032	.4049	.4066	.4082	.4099	.4115	.4131	.4147	.4162	.4177
1.4	.4192	.4207	.4222	.4236	.4251	.4265	.4279	.4292	.4306	.4319
1.5	.4332	.4345	.4357	.4370	.4382	.4394	.4406	.4418	.4429	.4441
1.6	.4452	.4463	.4474	.4484	.4495	.4505	.4515	.4525	.4535	.4545
1.7	.4554	.4564	.4573	.4582	.4591	.4599	.4608	.4616	.4625	.4633
1.8	.4641	.4649	.4656	.4664	.4671	.4678	.4686	.4693	.4699	.4706
1.9	.4713	.4719	.4726	.4732	.4738	.4744	.4750	.4756	.4761	.4767
2.0	.4772	.4778	.4783	.4788	.4793	.4798	.4803	.4808	.4812	.4817
2.1	.4821	.4826	.4830	.4834	.4838	.4842	.4846	.4850	.4854	.4857
2.2	.4861	.4864	.4868	.4871	.4875	.4878	.4881	.4884	.4887	.4890
2.3	.4893	.4896	.4898	.4901	.4904	.4906	.4909	.4911	.4913	.4916
2.4	.4918	.4920	.4922	.4925	.4927	.4929	.4931	.4932	.4934	.4936
2.5	.4938	.4940	.4941	.4943	.4945	.4946	.4948	.4949	.4951	.4952
2.6	.4953	.4955	.4956	.4957	.4959	.4960	.4961	.4962	.4963	.4964
2.7	.4965	.4966	.4967	.4968	.4969	.4970	.4971	.4972	.4973	.4974
2.8	.4974	.4975	.4976	.4977	.4977	.4978	.4979	.4979	.4980	.4981
2.9	.4981	.4982	.4982	.4983	.4984	.4984	.4985	.4985	.4986	.4986
3.0	.4987	.4987	.4987	.4988	.4988	.4989	.4989	.4989	.4990	.4990

Modified from: Mosteller F., Rourke, R.E.K., Thomas, Jr., G.B. (1970). Probability with Statistical Applications, (Table III), 2nd edition, Addison-Wesley, Reading MA. Reproduced with permission of the publisher.

Table B3   Student t-Distribution (1-α/2)

d.f.	t.90	t.95	t.975	t.99	t.995	t.9975	t.9995
1	3.078	6.314	12.706	31.821	63.657	127.320	636.619
2	1.886	2.920	4.302	6.985	9.924	14.089	31.589
3	1.638	2.353	3.182	4.541	5.840	7.453	12.942
4	1.533	2.131	2.776	3.747	4.604	5.597	8.610
5	1.467	2.015	2.570	3.365	4.032	4.733	6.869
6	1.440	1.943	2.446	3.143	3.707	4.316	5.959
7	1.415	1.894	2.364	2.998	3.499	4.029	5.408
8	1.397	1.859	2.306	2.896	3.355	3.832	5.041
9	1.383	1.833	2.262	2.821	3.249	3.689	4.781
10	1.372	1.812	2.228	2.764	3.169	3.581	4.587
11	1.363	1.795	2.201	2.718	3.105	3.496	4.437
12	1.356	1.782	2.178	2.681	3.054	3.428	4.318
13	1.350	1.770	2.160	2.650	3.012	3.372	4.221
14	1.345	1.761	2.144	2.624	2.977	3.325	4.140
15	1.341	1.753	2.131	2.602	2.947	3.286	4.073
16	1.337	1.746	2.120	2.583	2.921	3.252	4.015
17	1.333	1.740	2.110	2.567	2.898	3.222	3.965
18	1.330	1.734	2.101	2.552	2.878	3.197	3.922
19	1.328	1.729	2.093	2.539	2.861	3.174	3.883
20	1.325	1.724	2.086	2.528	2.845	3.153	3.850
21	1.323	1.721	2.080	2.518	2.831	3.135	3.819
22	1.321	1.717	2.074	2.508	2.819	3.119	3.792
23	1.319	1.714	2.069	2.500	2.807	3.104	3.767
24	1.318	1.711	2.064	2.492	2.797	3.091	3.7.45
25	1.316	1.708	2.059	2.485	2.787	3.078	3.725
30	1.310	1.697	2.042	2.457	2.750	3.029	3.646
40	1.303	1.683	2.021	2.423	2.704	2.971	3.551
50	1.298	1.675	2.008	2.403	2.677	2.937	3.496
60	1.295	1.670	2.000	2.390	2.660	2.914	3.460
70	1.293	1.666	1.994	2.381	2.648	2.898	3.435
80	1.292	1.664	1.990	2.374	2.638	2.887	3.416
90	1.291	1.662	1.986	2.368	2.631	2.877	3.402
100	1.290	1.660	1.984	2.364	2.626	2.870	3.390
120	1.288	1.657	1.979	2.358	2.617	2.859	3.373
160	1.286	1.654	1.974	2.350	2.607	2.846	3.352
200	1.285	1.652	1.971	2.345	2.600	2.838	3.340
∞	1.282	1.645	1.960	2.326	2.576	2.807	3.291

Table B4 Comparison of One-tailed vs. Two-tailed t-Distributions

	95% Confidence		99% Confidence	
df	Two-Tailed ($\alpha/2$)	One-tailed (α)	Two-Tailed ($\alpha/2$)	One-tailed (α)
1	12.706	6.314	63.657	31.821
2	4.302	2.920	9.924	6.985
3	3.182	2.353	5.840	4.541
4	2.776	2.131	4.604	3.747
5	2.570	2.015	4.032	3.365
6	2.446	1.943	3.707	3.143
7	2.364	1.894	3.499	2.998
8	2.306	1.859	3.355	2.896
9	2.262	1.833	3.249	2.821
10	2.228	1.812	3.169	2.764
11	2.201	1.795	3.105	2.718
12	2.178	1.782	3.054	2.681
13	2.160	1.770	3.012	2.650
14	2.144	1.761	2.976	2.624
15	2.131	1.753	2.947	2.602
16	2.120	1.746	2.921	2.583
17	2.110	1.740	2.898	2.567
18	2.101	1.734	2.878	2.552
19	2.093	1.729	2.861	2.539
20	2.086	1.724	2.845	2.528
21	2.080	1.721	2.831	2.518
22	2.074	1.717	2.819	2.508
23	2.069	1.714	2.807	2.500
24	2.064	1.711	2.797	2.492
25	2.059	1.708	2.787	2.485
30	2.042	1.697	2.750	2.457
40	2.021	1.683	2.704	2.423
50	2.008	1.675	2.677	2.403
60	2.000	1.670	2.660	2.390
70	1.994	1.666	2.648	2.381
80	1.990	1.664	2.638	2.374
90	1.986	1.662	2.631	2.368
100	1.984	1.660	2.626	2.364
120	1.979	1.657	2.617	2.358
160	1.974	1.654	2.607	2.350
∞	1.960	1.645	2.576	2.326

Modified from: Pearson, E.S. and Hartley, H.O. (1970). Biometrika Tables for Statisticians, Vol 1 (Table 12), Biometrika Trustees at the University Press, Cambridge, London. Reproduced with permission of the Biometrika Trustees.

Table B5   Analysis of Variance F-Distribution

v_1	v_2	$F_{.90}$	$F_{.95}$	$F_{.975}$	$F_{.99}$	$F_{.995}$	$F_{.999}$	$F_{.9995}$
	1	39.90	161	648	4050	16200	406000	1620000
	2	8.53	18.5	38.5	98.5	198	998	2000
	3	5.54	10.1	17.4	34.1	55.6	167	266
	4	4.54	7.71	12.2	21.2	31.3	74.1	106
	5	4.06	6.61	10.0	16.3	22.8	47.2	63.6
	6	3.78	5.99	8.81	13.7	18.6	35.5	46.1
	8	3.46	5.32	7.57	11.3	14.7	25.4	31.6
1	10	3.28	4.96	6.94	10.0	12.8	21.0	25.5
	12	3.18	4.75	6.55	9.33	11.8	18.6	22.2
	15	3.07	4.54	6.20	8.68	10.8	16.6	19.5
	20	2.97	4.35	5.87	8.10	9.94	14.8	17.2
	24	2.93	4.26	5.72	7.82	9.55	14.0	16.2
	30	2.88	4.17	5.57	7.56	9.18	13.3	15.2
	40	2.84	4.08	5.42	7.31	8.83	12.6	14.4
	60	2.79	4.00	5.29	7.08	8.49	12.0	13.6
	120	2.75	3.92	5.15	6.85	8.18	11.4	12.8
	∞	2.71	3.84	5.02	6.63	7.88	10.8	12.1
	1	49.5 0	200	800	5000	20000	500000	2000000
	2	9.00	19.0	39.0	99.0	199	999	2000
	3	5.46	9.55	16.0	30.8	49.8	149	237
	4	4.32	6.94	10.6	18.0	26.3	61.2	87.4
	5	3.78	5.79	8.43	13.3	18.3	37.1	49.8
	6	3.46	5.14	7.26	10.9	14.5	27.0	34.8
	8	3.11	4.46	6.06	8.65	11.0	18.5	22.8
2	10	2.92	4.10	5.46	7.56	9.43	14.9	17.9
	12	2.81	3.89	5.10	6.93	8.51	13.0	15.3
	15	2.70	3.68	4.76	6.36	7.70	11.3	13.2
	20	2.59	3.49	4.46	5.85	6.99	9.95	11.4
	24	2.54	3.40	4.32	5.61	6.66	9.34	10.6
	30	2.49	3.32	4.18	5.39	6.35	8.77	9.9
	40	2.44	3.23	4.05	5.18	6.07	8.25	9.25
	60	2.39	3.15	3.93	4.98	5.80	7.76	8.65
	120	2.35	3.07	3.80	4.79	5.54	7.32	8.10
	∞	2.30	3.00	3.69	4.61	5.30	6.91	7.60

Table B5   Analysis of Variance F-Distribution (continued)

v_1	v_2	$F_{.90}$	$F_{.95}$	$F_{.975}$	$F_{.99}$	$F_{.995}$	$F_{.999}$	$F_{.9995}$
	1	53.6	216	846	5400	21600	540000	2160000
	2	9.16	19.2	39.2	99.2	199	999	2000
	3	5.39	9.28	15.4	29.5	47.5	141	225
	4	4.19	6.59	9.98	16.7	24.3	56.2	80.1
	5	3.62	5.41	7.76	12.1	16.5	33.2	44.4
	6	3.29	4.76	6.60	9.78	12.9	23.7	30.4
	8	2.92	4.07	5.42	7.59	9.60	15.8	19.4
3	10	2.73	3.71	4.83	6.55	8.08	12.6	15.0
	12	2.61	3.49	4.47	5.95	7.23	10.8	12.7
	15	2.49	3.29	4.15	5.42	6.48	9.34	10.8
	20	2.38	3.10	3.86	4.94	5.82	8.10	9.20
	24	2.33	3.01	3.72	4.72	5.52	7.55	8.52
	30	2.28	2.92	3.59	4.51	5.24	7.05	7.90
	40	2.23	2.84	3.46	4.31	4.98	6.60	7.33
	60	2.18	2.76	3.34	4.13	4.73	6.17	6.81
	120	2.13	2.68	3.23	3.95	4.50	5.79	6.34
	∞	2.08	2.60	3.12	3.78	4.28	5.42	5.91
	1	55.8	225	900	5620	22500	562000	2250000
	2	9.24	19.2	39.2	99.2	199	999	2000
	3	5.34	9.12	15.1	28.7	46.2	137	218
	4	4.11	6.39	9.60	16.0	23.2	53.4	76.1
	5	3.52	5.19	7.39	11.4	15.6	31.1	41.5
	6	3.18	4.53	6.23	9.15	12.0	21.9	28.1
	8	2.81	3.84	5.05	7.01	8.81	14.4	17.6
4	10	2.61	3.48	4.47	5.99	7.34	11.3	13.4
	12	2.48	3.26	4.12	5.41	6.52	9.63	11.2
	15	2.36	3.06	3.80	4.89	5.80	8.25	9.48
	20	2.25	2.87	3.51	4.43	5.17	7.10	8.02
	24	2.19	2.78	3.38	4.22	4.89	6.59	7.39
	30	2.14	2.69	3.25	4.02	4.62	6.12	6.82
	40	2.09	2.61	3.13	3.83	4.37	5.70	6.30
	60	2.04	2.53	3.01	3.65	4.14	5.31	5.82
	120	1.99	2.45	2.89	3.48	3.92	4.95	5.39
	∞	1.94	2.37	2.79	3.32	3.72	4.62	5.00

continued

Table B5 Analysis of Variance F-Distribution (continued)

ν_1	ν_2	$F_{.90}$	$F_{.95}$	$F_{.975}$	$F_{.99}$	$F_{.995}$	$F_{.999}$	$F_{.9995}$
	1	57.2	230	922	5760	23100	576000	2310000
	2	9.29	19.3	39.3	99.3	199	999	2000
	3	5.31	9.01	14.9	28.2	45.4	135	214
	4	4.05	6.26	9.39	15.5	22.5	51.7	73.6
	5	3.45	5.05	7.15	11.0	14.9	29.7	39.7
	6	3.11	4.39	5.99	8.75	11.5	20.8	26.6
	8	2.73	3.69	4.82	6.63	8.30	13.5	16.4
5	10	2.52	3.33	4.24	5.64	6.87	10.5	12.4
	12	2.39	3.11	3.89	5.06	6.07	8.89	10.4
	15	2.27	2.90	3.58	4.56	5.37	7.57	8.66
	20	2.16	2.71	3.29	4.10	4.76	6.46	7.28
	24	2.10	2.62	3.15	3.90	4.49	5.98	6.68
	30	2.05	2.53	3.03	3.70	4.23	5.53	6.14
	40	2.00	2.45	2.90	3.51	3.99	5.13	5.64
	60	1.95	2.37	2.79	3.34	3.76	4.76	5.20
	120	1.90	2.29	2.67	3.17	3.55	4.42	4.79
	∞	1.85	2.21	2.57	3.02	3.35	4.10	4.42
	1	58.2	234	937	5860	23400	586000	2340000
	2	9.33	19.3	39.3	99.3	199	999	2000
	3	5.28	8.94	14.7	27.9	44.8	133	211
	4	4.01	6.16	9.20	15.2	22.0	50.5	71.9
	5	3.45	4.95	6.98	10.7	14.5	28.8	38.5
	6	3.05	4.28	5.82	8.47	11.1	20.0	25.6
	8	2.67	3.58	4.65	6.37	7.95	12.9	15.7
6	10	2.46	3.22	4.07	5.39	6.54	9.92	11.8
	12	2.33	3.00	3.73	4.82	5.76	8.38	9.74
	15	2.21	2.79	3.41	4.32	5.07	7.09	8.10
	20	2.09	2.60	3.13	3.87	4.47	6.02	6.76
	24	2.04	2.51	2.99	3.67	4.20	5.55	6.18
	30	1.98	2.42	2.87	3.47	3.95	5.12	5.66
	40	1.93	2.34	2.74	3.29	3.71	4.73	5.19
	60	1.87	2.25	2.63	3.12	3.49	4.37	4.76
	120	1.82	2.18	2.52	2.96	3.28	4.04	4.37
	∞	1.77	2.10	2.41	2.80	3.09	3.74	4.02

Table B5 Analysis of Variance F-Distribution (continued)

v_1	v_2	$F_{.90}$	$F_{.95}$	$F_{.975}$	$F_{.99}$	$F_{.995}$	$F_{.999}$	$F_{.9995}$
	1	58.9	237	948	5930	23700	593000	2370000
	2	9.35	19.4	39.4	99.4	199	999	2000
	3	5.27	8.89	14.6	27.7	44.4	132	209
	4	3.98	6.09	9.07	15.0	21.6	49.7	70.6
	5	3.37	4.88	6.85	10.5	14.2	28.2	37.6
	6	3.01	4.21	5.70	8.26	10.8	19.5	24.9
	8	2.62	3.50	4.53	6.18	7.69	12.4	15.1
7	10	2.41	3.14	3.95	5.20	6.30	9.52	11.3
	12	2.28	2.91	3.61	4.64	5.52	8.00	9.28
	15	2.16	2.71	3.29	4.14	4.85	6.74	7.68
	20	2.04	2.51	3.01	3.70	4.26	5.69	6.38
	24	1.98	2.42	2.87	3.50	3.99	5.23	5.82
	30	1.93	2.33	2.75	3.30	3.74	4.82	5.31
	40	1.87	2.25	2.62	3.12	3.51	4.44	4.85
	60	1.82	2.17	2.51	2.95	3.29	4.09	4.44
	120	1.77	2.09	2.39	2.79	3.09	3.77	4.07
	∞	1.72	2.01	2.29	2.64	2.90	3.47	3.72
	1	59.4	239	957	5980	23900	598000	2390000
	2	9.37	19.4	39.4	99.4	199	999	2000
	3	5.25	8.85	14.5	27.5	44.1	131	208
	4	3.95	6.04	8.98	14.8	21.4	49.0	69.7
	5	3.34	4.82	6.76	10.3	14.0	27.6	36.9
	6	2.98	4.15	5.60	8.10	10.6	19.0	24.3
	8	2.59	3.44	4.43	6.03	7.50	12.0	14.6
8	10	2.38	3.07	3.85	5.06	6.12	9.20	10.6
	12	2.24	2.85	3.51	4.50	5.35	7.71	8.94
	15	2.12	2.64	3.20	4.00	4.67	6.47	7.36
	20	2.00	2.45	2.91	3.56	4.09	5.44	6.08
	24	1.94	2.36	2.78	3.36	3.83	4.99	5.54
	30	1.88	2.27	2.65	3.17	3.58	4.58	5.04
	40	1.83	2.18	2.53	2.99	3.35	4.21	4.59
	60	1.77	2.10	2.41	2.82	3.13	3.87	4.18
	120	1.72	2.02	2.30	2.66	2.93	3.55	3.82
	∞	1.67	1.94	2.19	2.51	2.74	3.27	3.48

continued

Table B5   Analysis of Variance F-Distribution (continued)

v_1	v_2	$F_{.90}$	$F_{.95}$	$F_{.975}$	$F_{.99}$	$F_{.995}$	$F_{.999}$	$F_{.9995}$
	10	2.35	3.02	3.78	4.94	5.97	8.96	10.6
	15	2.09	2.59	3.12	3.89	4.54	6.26	7.11
	20	1.96	2.39	2.84	3.46	3.96	5.24	5.85
9	30	1.85	2.21	2.57	3.07	3.45	4.39	4.82
	40	1.79	2.12	2.45	2.89	3.22	4.02	4.38
	60	1.74	2.04	2.33	2.72	3.01	3.69	3.98
	120	1.68	1.96	2.22	2.56	2.81	3.38	3.63
	∞	1.63	1.88	2.11	2.41	2.62	3.10	3.30
	10	2.32	2.98	3.72	4.85	5.85	8.75	10.3
	15	2.06	2.54	3.06	3.80	4.42	6.08	6.91
	20	1.94	2.35	2.77	3.37	3.85	5.08	5.66
10	30	1.82	2.16	2.51	2.98	3.34	4.24	4.65
	40	1.76	2.08	2.39	2.80	3.12	3.87	4.21
	60	1.71	1.99	2.27	2.63	2.90	3.54	3.82
	120	1.65	1.91	2.16	2.47	2.71	3.24	3.47
	∞	1.60	1.83	2.05	2.32	2.52	2.96	3.14
	10	2.30	2.94	3.66	4.77	5.75	8.58	10.1
	15	2.04	2.51	3.01	3.73	4.33	5.93	6.75
	20	1.91	2.31	2.72	3.29	3.76	4.94	5.51
11	30	1.79	2.13	2.46	2.91	3.25	4.11	4.51
	40	1.73	2.04	2.33	2.73	3.03	3.75	4.07
	60	1.68	1.95	2.22	2.56	2.82	3.43	3.69
	120	1.62	1.87	2.10	2.40	2.62	3.12	3.34
	∞	1.57	1.79	1.99	2.25	2.43	2.84	3.02
	10	2.28	2.91	3.62	4.71	5.66	8.44	9.93
	15	2.02	2.48	2.96	3.67	4.25	5.81	6.60
	20	1.89	2.28	2.68	3.23	3.68	4.82	5.38
12	30	1.77	2.09	2.41	2.84	3.18	4.00	4.38
	40	1.71	2.00	2.29	2.66	2.95	3.64	3.95
	60	1.66	1.92	2.17	2.50	2.74	3.31	3.57
	120	1.60	1.83	2.05	2.34	2.54	3.02	3.22
	∞	1.55	1.75	1.94	2.18	2.36	2.74	2.90

Table B6 Upper Percentage Points of the F_{max} Statistic

n-1	α	K = number of variances										
		2	3	4	5	6	7	8	9	10	11	12
4	.05	9.60	15.5	20.6	25.2	29.5	33.6	37.5	41.4	44.6	48.0	51.4
	.01	23.2	37	49	59	69	79	89	97	106	113	120
5	.05	7.15	10.8	13.7	16.3	18.7	20.8	22.9	24.7	26.5	28.2	29.9
	.01	14.9	22	28	33	38	42	46	50	54	57	60
6	.05	5.82	8.38	10.4	12.1	13.7	15.0	16.3	17.5	18.6	19.7	20.7
	.01	11.1	15.5	19.1	22	25	27	30	32	34	36	37
7	.05	4.99	6.94	8.44	9.70	10.8	11.8	12.7	13.5	14.3	15.1	15.8
	.01	8.89	12.1	14.5	16.5	18.4	20	22	23	24	26	27
8	.05	4.43	6.00	7.18	8.12	9.03	9.78	10.5	11.1	11.7	12.2	12.7
	.01	7.50	9.9	11.7	13.2	14.5	15.8	16.9	17.9	18.9	19.8	21
9	.05	4.03	5.34	6.31	7.11	7.80	8.41	8.95	9.45	9.91	10.3	10.7
	.01	6.54	8.5	9.9	11.1	12.1	13.1	13.9	14.7	15.3	16.0	16.6
10	.05	3.72	4.85	5.67	6.34	6.92	7.42	7.87	8.28	8.66	9.01	9.34
	.01	5.85	7.4	8.6	9.6	10.4	11.1	11.8	12.4	12.9	13.4	13.9
12	.05	3.28	4.16	4.79	5.30	5.72	6.09	6.42	6.72	7.00	7.25	7.48
	.01	4.91	6.1	6.9	7.6	8.2	8.7	9.1	9.5	9.9	10.2	10.6
15	.05	2.86	3.54	4.01	4.37	4.68	4.95	5.19	5.40	5.59	5.77	5.93
	.01	4.07	4.9	5.5	6.0	6.4	6.7	7.1	7.3	7.5	7.8	8.0
20	.05	2.46	2.95	3.29	3.54	3.76	3.94	4.10	4.24	4.37	4.49	4.59
	.01	3.32	3.8	4.3	4.6	4.9	5.1	5.3	5.5	5.6	5.8	5.9
30	.05	2.07	2.40	2.61	2.78	2.91	3.02	3.12	3.21	3.29	3.36	3.39
	.01	2.63	3.0	3.3	3.4	3.6	3.7	3.8	3.9	4.0	4.1	4.2
60	.05	1.67	1.85	1.96	2.04	2.11	2.17	2.22	2.26	2.30	2.33	2.36
	.01	1.96	2.2	2.3	2.4	2.4	2.5	2.5	2.6	2.6	2.7	2.7
∞	.05	1.00	1.00	1.00	1.00	1.00	1.00	1.00	1.00	1.00	1.00	1.00
	.01	1.00	1.00	1.00	1.00	1.00	1.00	1.00	1.00	1.00	1.00	1.00

Modified from: Pearson, E.S. and Hartley, H.O. (1970). Biometrika Tables for Statisticians, Vol 1 (Table 31), Biometrika Trustees at the University Press, Cambridge, London. Reproduced with permission of the Biometrika Trustees.

Table B7 Upper Percentage Points of the Cochran C Test for Homogeneity of Variance

n-1	α	k = levels of independent variable							
		2	3	4	5	6	7	8	9
1	.05	.9985	.9669	.9065	.8412	.7808	.7271	.6798	.6385
	.01	.9999	.9933	.9676	.9279	.8828	.8376	.7945	.7544
2	.05	.9750	.8709	.7679	.6838	.6161	.5612	.5157	.4775
	.01	.9950	.9423	.8643	.7885	.7218	.6644	.6152	.5727
3	.05	.9392	.7977	.6841	.5981	.5321	.4800	.4377	.4027
	.01	.9794	.8831	.7814	.6957	.6258	.5685	.5209	.4810
4	.05	.9057	.7457	.6287	.5441	.4803	.4307	.3910	.3584
	.01	.9586	.8335	.7212	.6329	.5635	.5080	.4627	.4251
5	.05	.8772	.7071	.5895	.5065	.4447	.3974	.3595	.3286
	.01	.9373	.7933	.6761	.5875	.5195	.4659	.4226	.3870
6	.05	.8534	.6771	.5598	.4783	.4184	.3726	.3362	.3067
	.01	.9172	.7606	.6410	.5531	.4866	.4347	.3932	.3592
7	.05	.8332	.6530	.5365	.4564	.3980	.3535	.3185	.2901
	.01	.8988	.7335	.6129	.5259	.4608	.4105	.3704	.3378
8	.05	.8159	.6333	.5175	.4387	.3817	.3384	.3043	.2768
	.01	.8823	.7107	.5897	.5037	.4401	.3911	.3522	.3207
9	.05	.8010	.6167	.5017	.4241	.3682	.3259	.2926	.2659
	.05	.8674	.6912	.5702	.4854	.4229	.3751	.3373	.3067
16	.05	.7341	.5466	.4366	.3645	.3135	.2756	.2462	.2226
	.01	.7949	.6059	.4884	.4094	.3529	.3105	.2779	.2514
36	.05	.6602	.4748	.3720	.3066	.2612	.2278	.2022	.1820
	.01	.7067	.5153	.4057	.3351	.2858	.2494	.2214	.1992
144	.05	.5813	.4031	.3093	.2513	.2119	.1833	.1616	.1446
	.01	.6062	.4230	.3251	.2644	.2229	.1929	.1700	.1521

Modified from: Eisenhart, C., Hastay, M.W. and Wallis W.A., eds. (1947). Techniques of Statistical Analysis (Tables 15.1 and 15.2), McGraw-Hill Book Company, New York. Reproduced with permission of the publisher.

Table B8 Percentage Points of the Dunn Multiple Comparisons

Number of Comparisons (C)	α	(N-K) degrees of freedom								
		10	15	20	24	30	40	60	120	∞
2	.05	2.64	2.49	2.42	2.39	2.36	2.33	2.30	2.27	2.24
	.01	3.58	3.29	3.16	3.09	3.03	2.97	2.92	2.86	2.81
3	.05	2.87	2.69	2.61	2.58	2.54	2.50	2.47	2.43	2.39
	.01	3.83	3.48	3.33	3.26	3.19	3.12	3.06	2.99	2.94
4	.05	3.04	2.84	2.75	2.70	2.66	2.62	2.58	2.54	2.50
	.01	4.01	3.62	3.46	3.38	3.30	3.23	3.16	3.09	3.02
5	.05	3.17	2.95	2.85	2.80	2.75	2.71	2.66	2.62	2.58
	.01	4.15	3.74	3.55	3.47	3.39	3.31	3.24	3.16	3.09
6	.05	3.28	3.04	2.93	2.88	2.83	2.78	2.73	2.68	2.64
	.01	4.27	3.82	3.63	3.54	3.46	3.38	3.30	3.22	3.15
7	.05	3.37	3.11	3.00	2.94	2.89	2.84	2.79	2.74	2.69
	.01	4.37	3.90	3.70	3.61	3.52	3.43	3.34	3.27	3.19
8	.05	3.45	3.18	3.06	3.00	2.94	2.89	2.84	2.79	2.74
	.01	4.45	3.97	3.76	3.66	3.57	3.48	3.39	3.31	3.23
9	.05	3.52	3.24	3.11	3.05	2.99	2.93	2.88	2.83	2.77
	.01	4.53	4.02	3.80	3.70	3.61	3.51	3.42	3.34	3.26
10	.05	3.58	3.29	3.16	3.09	3.03	2.97	2.92	2.86	2.81
	.01	4.59	4.07	3.85	3.74	3.65	3.55	3.46	3.37	3.29
15	.05	3.83	3.48	3.33	3.26	3.19	3.12	3.06	2.99	2.94
	.01	4.86	4.29	4.03	3.91	3.80	3.70	3.59	3.50	3.40
20	.05	4.01	3.62	3.46	3.38	3.30	3.23	3.16	3.09	3.02
	.01	5.06	4.42	4.15	4.04	3.90	3.79	3.69	3.58	3.48
30	.05	4.27	3.82	3.63	3.54	3.46	3.38	3.30	3.22	3.15
	.01	5.33	4.61	4.33	4.2	4.13	3.93	3.81	3.69	3.59

Modified from: Dunn, O.J. (1961). "Multiple Comparisons Among Means" Journal of the American Statistical Association, 56:62-64. Reproduced with permission of the American Statistical Association.

Table B9 Percentage Point of the Studentized Range

df	α	number of means or number of steps between ordered means								
		2	3	4	5	6	7	8	9	10
10	.05	3.15	3.88	4.33	4.65	4.91	5.12	5.30	5.46	5.60
	.01	4.48	5.27	5.77	6.14	6.43	6.67	6.87	7.05	7.21
12	.05	3.08	3.77	4.20	4.51	4.75	4.95	5.12	5.27	5.39
	.01	4.32	5.05	5.50	5.84	6.10	6.32	6.51	6.67	6.81
14	.05	3.03	3.70	4.11	4.41	4.64	4.83	4.99	5.13	5.25
	.01	4.21	4.89	5.32	5.63	5.88	6.08	6.26	6.41	6.54
16	.05	3.00	3.65	4.05	4.33	4.56	4.74	4.90	5.03	5.15
	.01	4.13	4.79	5.19	5.49	5.72	5.92	6.08	6.22	6.35
18	.05	2.97	3.61	4.00	4.28	4.49	4.67	4.82	4.96	5.07
	.01	4.07	4.70	5.09	5.38	5.60	5.79	5.94	6.08	6.20
20	.05	2.95	3.58	3.96	4.23	4.45	4.62	4.77	4.90	5.01
	.01	4.02	4.64	5.02	5.29	5.51	5.69	5.84	5.97	6.09
24	.05	2.92	3.53	3.90	4.17	4.37	4.54	4.68	4.81	4.92
	.01	3.96	4.55	4.91	5.17	5.37	5.54	5.69	5.81	5.92
30	.05	2.89	3.49	3.85	4.10	4.30	4.46	4.60	4.72	4.82
	.01	3.89	4.45	4.80	5.05	5.24	5.40	5.54	5.65	5.76
40	.05	2.86	3.44	3.79	4.04	4.23	4.39	4.52	4.63	4.73
	.01	3.82	4.37	4.70	4.93	5.11	5.26	5.39	5.50	5.60
60	.05	2.83	3.40	3.74	3.98	4.16	4.31	4.44	4.55	4.65
	.01	3.76	4.28	4.59	4.82	4.99	5.13	5.25	5.36	5.45
120	.05	2.80	3.36	3.68	3.92	4.10	4.24	4.36	4.47	4.56
	.01	3.70	4.20	4.50	4.71	4.87	5.01	5.12	5.21	5.30
∞	.05	2.77	3.31	3.63	3.86	4.03	4.17	4.29	4.39	4.47
	.01	3.64	4.12	4.40	4.60	4.76	4.88	4.99	5.08	5.16

Modified from: Pearson, E.S. and Hartley, H.O. (1970). Biometrika Tables for Statisticians, Vol 1 (Table 29), Biometrika Trustees at the University Press, Cambridge, London. Reproduced with permission of the Biometrika Trustees.

Table B10 Values of r (Correlation Coefficient) at Different Levels of Significance

d.f.	.01	.05	.01	.001
1	.988	.997	.999	1.00
2	.900	.950	.990	.999
3	.805	.878	.959	.991
4	.730	.811	.917	.974
5	.669	.755	.875	.951
6	.622	.707	.834	.925
7	.582	.666	.798	.898
8	.549	.632	.765	.872
9	.521	.602	.735	.847
10	.497	.576	.708	.823
11	.476	.553	.684	.801
12	.458	.532	.661	.780
13	.441	.514	.641	.760
14	.426	.497	.623	.742
15	.412	.482	.606	.725
16	.400	.468	.590	.708
17	.389	.456	.575	.693
18	.378	.444	.561	.679
19	.369	.433	.549	.665
20	.360	.423	.537	.652
25	.323	.381	.487	.597
30	.296	.349	.449	.554
35	.275	.325	.418	.519
40	.257	.304	.393	.490
50	.231	.273	.354	.443
60	.211	.250	.325	.408
80	.183	.217	.283	.357
100	.164	.195	.254	.321
150	.134	.159	.208	.264
200	.116	.138	.181	.230

Table B11 F Distribution $(1-\alpha)$ for One Numerator df and Smaller Denominator df

v_1	v_2	.90	.95	.975	.99	.995	.999	.9995
	2	8.53	18.5	38.5	98.5	198	998	2000
	3	5.54	10.1	17.4	34.1	55.6	167	266
	4	4.54	7.71	12.2	21.2	31.3	74.1	106
	5	4.06	6.61	10.0	16.3	22.8	47.2	63.6
	6	3.78	5.99	8.81	13.7	18.6	35.5	46.1
1	7	3.59	5.59	8.07	12.2	16.2	29.2	37.0
	8	3.46	5.32	7.57	11.3	14.7	25.4	31.6
	9	3.36	5.12	7.21	10.6	13.6	22.9	28.0
	10	3.28	4.96	6.94	10.0	12.8	21.0	25.5
	11	3.23	4.84	6.72	9.65	12.2	19.7	23.6
	12	3.18	4.75	6.55	9.33	11.8	18.6	22.2
	15	3.07	4.54	6.20	8.68	10.8	16.6	19.5

Modified from: Dixon, W.J. and Massey, F.J. (1983). Introduction to Statistical Analysis (Table A-7c), McGraw-Hill Book Company, New York. Reproduced with permission of the publisher.

Table B12 Chi Square Distribution

d.f.	α=.10	.05	.025	.01	.005	.001
1	2.706	3.841	5.024	6.635	7.879	10.828
2	4.605	5.991	7.378	9.210	10.597	13.816
3	6.251	7.815	9.348	11.345	12.838	16.266
4	7.779	9.488	11.143	13.277	14.860	18.467
5	9.236	11.070	12.832	15.086	16.750	20.515
6	10.645	12.592	14.449	16.812	18.548	22.458
7	12.017	14.067	16.013	18.475	20.278	24.322
8	13.362	15.507	17.535	20.090	21.955	26.125
9	14.684	16.919	19.023	21.666	23.589	27.877
10	15.987	18.307	20.483	23.209	25.188	29.588
11	17.275	19.675	21.920	24.725	26.757	31.264
12	18.549	21.026	23.336	26.217	28.300	32.909
13	19.812	22.362	24.736	27.688	29.819	34.528
14	21.064	23.685	26.119	29.141	31.319	36.123
15	22.307	24.996	27.488	30.578	32.801	37.697
16	23.542	26.296	28.845	32.000	34.267	39.252
17	24.769	27.587	30.191	33.409	35.718	40.790
18	25.989	28.869	31.526	34.805	37.156	42.312
19	27.204	30.144	32.852	36.191	38.582	43.820
20	28.412	31.410	34.170	37.566	39.997	45.315
21	29.615	32.671	35.479	38.932	41.401	46.797
22	30.813	33.924	36.781	40.289	42.796	48.268
23	32.007	35.172	38.076	41.638	44.181	49.728
24	33.196	36.415	39.364	42.980	45.558	51.179
25	34.382	37.652	40.646	44.314	46.928	52.620

Modified from: Pearson, E.S. and Hartley, H.O. (1970). Biometrika Tables for Statisticians, Vol 1 (Table 8), Biometrika Trustees at the University Press, Cambridge, London. Reproduced with permission of the Biometrika Trustees.

Table B13   Values for Use in Grubbs' Test for Outlier (α)

n	0.005	0.01	0.05
3	1.155	1.155	1.153
4	1.496	1.492	1.463
5	1.764	1.749	1.672
6	1.973	1.944	1.822
7	2.139	2.097	1.938
8	2.274	2.221	2.032
9	2.387	2.323	2.110
10	2.482	2.410	2.176
15	2.806	2.705	2.409
20	3.001	2.884	2.557
25	3.135	3.009	2.663

Modified from: Grubbs, F.E. and Beck, G. (1972). "Extension of Sample Size and Percentage Points for Significance Tests of Outlying Observations" Technometrics, 14:847-54.   Reproduced with permission of the American Statistical Association.

Table B14 Values for Use in Dixon's Test for Outlier (α)

Statistic	n	0.5%	1%	5%
τ_{10}	3	.994	.988	.941
	4	.926	.889	.765
	5	.821	.780	.642
	6	.740	.698	.560
	7	.680	.637	.507
τ_{11}	8	.725	.683	.554
	9	.677	.635	.512
	10	.639	.597	.477
τ_{21}	11	.713	.679	.576
	12	.675	.642	.546
	13	.649	.615	.521
τ_{22}	14	.674	.641	.546
	15	.647	.616	.525
	16	.624	.595	.507
	17	.605	.577	.490
	18	.589	.561	.475
	19	.575	.547	.462
	20	.562	.535	.450
	21	.551	.524	.440
	22	.541	.514	.430
	23	.532	.505	.421
	24	.524	.497	.413
	25	.516	.489	.406

From: Dixon, W.J. and Massey, F.J. (1983). <u>Introduction to Statistical Analysis</u> (Table A-8e), McGraw-Hill Book Company, New York. Reproduced with permission of the publisher.

Index